FORENSIC PSYCHOLOGY AND PSYCHIATRY

ANNALS OF THE NEW YORK ACADEMY OF SCIENCES

Volume 347

FORENSIC PSYCHOLOGY AND PSYCHIATRY

Edited by Fred Wright, Charles Bahn, and Robert W. Rieber

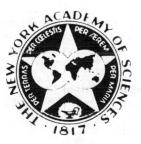

The New York Academy of Sciences
New York, New York
1980

Second printing, June, 1981.

Library of Congress Cataloging in Publication Data

Main entry under title:

Forensic psychology and psychiatry.

(Annals of the New York Academy of Sciences; v. 347)
Papers from a symposium held on September 26–28, 1979 by the New York Academy of Sciences and cosponsored by the United States Dept. of Justice, National Institute of Law Enforcement and Criminal Justice.

1. Psychology, Forensic—Congresses. 2. Forensic psychiatry—Congresses. I. Wright, Fred. II. Bahn, Charles. III. Rieber, Robert W. IV. New York Academy of Sciences. V. National Institute of Law Enforcement and Criminal Justice. VI. Series: New York Academy of Sciences. Annals; v. 347. [DNLM: 1. Forensic psychiatry—Congresses. W1 An626YL v. 347 / W740]
Q11.N5 vol. 347 [RA1148] 500s [614'.1]   80-17982

CCP
Printed in the United States of America
ISBN 0-89766-084-6 (Cloth)
ISBN 0-89766-085-4 (Paper)
ISSN 0077-8923

ANNALS OF THE NEW YORK ACADEMY OF SCIENCES

VOLUME 347

June 20, 1980

FORENSIC PSYCHOLOGY AND PSYCHIATRY*

Editors and Conference Organizers
FRED WRIGHT, *Chair*, CHARLES BAHN, and ROBERT W. RIEBER

CONTENTS

* This volume is the result of a symposium entitled Forensic Psychology and Psychiatry,
held on September 26–28, 1979 by The New York Academy of Sciences and cosponsored by
the United States Department of Justice—National Institute of Law Enforcement and Criminal Justice.

Part VIII. Human Nature, Crime, and Society
Robert W. Rieber, *Chair*

This project was partially supported by Order Number 9-0695-J-LEAA awarded to the
New York Academy of Sciences by the National Institute of Law Enforcement and
Criminal Justice, U.S. Department of Justice, under the Omnibus Crime Control and
Safe Streets Act of 1968, as amended. Points of view or opinions stated in this docu-
ment are those of the authors and do not necessarily represent the official position or
policies of the U.S. Department of Justice.

PREFACE

Fred Wright, Charles Bahn, and Robert W. Rieber

Department of Psychology
John Jay College of Criminal Justice
New York, New York 10019

Recently, in an effort to further understanding and control of crime and the criminal justice process, behavioral scientists have become active on a practical as well as a theoretical level in addressing a number of the problems involved. Substantial contributions have been made in the following areas: competency to stand trial, issues of psychological evidence, crisis intervention and hostage negotiation, violence and the family, treating the offender, and crime and the media.

This symposium has been designed to provide the people working in these areas with an opportunity to present their techniques, research findings, and theoretical advances to the scientific community as well as to the general public. Investigators include those who work in corrections, probation, parole, police departments, and other criminal justice settings as well as those who work in university, hospital, and other non-criminal justice institutions. It is rarely possible for these practitioners and researchers to talk to each other about their respective contributions and thereby influence and enlarge each other's perspective. It is hoped that this symposium will provide this opportunity as well as provide an opportunity for the synthesis and assimilation of this material within a coherent framework. The symposium will also help to establish the field of forensic psychology as one of the areas in which major and important work on the problem of crime is being undertaken.

We, the organizers, would like to take this opportunity to thank the people and institutions that helped make the symposium possible. We would first like to thank our colleagues at the John Jay College of Criminal Justice for working and struggling to keep that institution alive and healthy, thereby helping to keep alive the notion of dealing with crime and justice in an enlightened fashion. This kind of dedication to the task is illustrated by the presence here today of the president of the college, Dr. Gerald Lynch, who has taken the time to chair the symposium's first session. Other colleagues at the college have also shown similar support and dedication to this symposium, and it is most appreciated.

We would also like to thank the New York Academy of Sciences for sponsoring and helping to fund this event. The staff at the Academy functioned in a highly competent and patient fashion, and that too is appreciated. Dr. William Cain, a member of the Academy, was particularly helpful to us as we developed and organized the program.

Further, we would like to thank the National Institute of Law Enforcement and Criminal Justice of the United States Department of Justice for helping to fund this symposium, and to thank Mr. Henry Dogin, director of the Law Enforcement Assistance Administration, for taking the time and effort to be our keynote speaker at the symposium's subscription dinner. Finally, we are indebted to the symposium participants for the time and effort they have given and are continuing to give in preparing themselves and their material for presentation at this event.

COMPETENCY TO STAND TRIAL: OPENING REMARKS

Gerald W. Lynch

John Jay College of Criminal Justice
New York, New York 10019

I would like to congratulate the organizers of this symposium, for bringing together individuals who are concerned with these very pressing questions in forensic psychology. I really can think of no more pressing issues in psychology than those in forensic psychology because of what is at stake. It is not only the liberty, but sometimes the life, of the individual that we are assessing, diagnosing, or evaluating.

I believe that the area of forensic psychology is one in which there will be breakthroughs in the near future. I think they will make a difference to the fields of criminal justice and psychology.

Probably the reason I'm so hopeful is that I think that the present state of our knowledge is so lacking. We have great difficulty agreeing on the diagnosis in any one case. We fall even farther apart in attempting to explain the reason for the diagnosis, and of course we are at our most vulnerable in trying to predict future behavior. And all these three functions—diagnosis, explanation, and prediction—are what the public and the criminal justice system and the legal system expect of us, and we really haven't been able to provide the answers that we wish we could. I think many who are now in the field are saying that we don't know as much as we perhaps thought we did. But now we are working on it, and systematically we are trying to find the answers, and we are making progress. It is for that reason that we at John Jay College of Criminal Justice established a couple of years ago a Master's Degree in Forensic Psychology and just last year an undergraduate major in forensic psychology.

I see this symposium as a further step in making progress in this crucial field. So I am very pleased to join with you in this symposium.

THE INTERFACE OF THE MENTAL HEALTH AND CRIMINAL JUSTICE SYSTEMS: HANDLING THE VIOLENT RELEASED MENTAL PATIENT

Charles Bahn*

Temple University
Philadelphia, Pennsylvania 19122

Both the mental health and the criminal justice systems have developed around a common problem: how to understand and cope with bizarre, harmful, and socially unacceptable behavior. Both systems have had to define exactly what kinds of behavior fall within their respective purviews, and these definitions show considerable overlap.

An obvious case in point is the definition of insanity.

The mental health system needs a clear definition of insanity for many reasons, the principal one being to determine who should be involuntarily detained and treated in mental hospitals. In recent years, this definition has been subject to very close scrutiny and modification since Szasz (1961, 1963, 1965),[40-42] Scheff (1966),[37] and Goffman (1961, 1963)[16,17] have persuasively argued that those classified as insane are subject to legal disabilities that allow for the possibility of considerable misuse by individuals or by the government. Groeth (1977)[21] reported that eight states have recently enacted mental health statutes that, in effect, limit involuntary commitment to persons who are dangerous to themselves or to others. One such state, the State of California, changed its statutory definitions through the Lauterman-Petris-Short Act to limit involuntary detention and treatment to those who are dangerous to self or others in an active sense or, in a passive sense, to those who are gravely disabled. Gravely disabled was defined as being "unable to provide for one's basic needs for food, clothing or shelter." In the earlier law, the definition of mental illness justifying involuntary detention and treatment was that the individual be "so mentally ill as . . . to require immediate care, treatment or restraint," a tautology that left the specific judgment strictly to the professionals to make, without limitation.

The new criteria allow for 72 hours of involuntary detention and, if needed, an additional 14 days of involuntary treatment. For those who have attempted suicide, yet another 14-day extension is provided for. After this —although there is a possible judicial commitment for another 90 days in those cases where evidence of dangerousness has been presented—if the patients are not gravely disabled, they must be released on demand.

In these states and in several others, statutory limitations on involun-

* Present affiliation: Department of Psychology, John Jay College of Criminal Justice, New York, N.Y. 10019.

3

tary commitment have been a key factor in the trend to deinstitutionalize mental patients.

Another powerful impetus has come from the decision of the United States Supreme Court in *O'Connor* v. *Donaldson*, which Curran (1975)[10] describes as holding that when a patient is not dangerous to himself or others, is mentally ill, and is not currently receiving any treatment, he must be released from custody at his own request. The court refused to deal with the full scope of the question that it could have examined: If a patient is mentally ill and is dangerous, can he be held involuntarily in a mental facility, or indeed a prison, without treatment? Further questions that emerge involve the definition of treatment: Do given procedures and methods require specified outcomes in order to be acknowledged as treatment (Miller, 1977)?[26]

All of these issues, decisions, and questions have contributed to the growing deinstitutionalization of mental patients.

The criminal justice system has its own distinctive needs for definitions of insanity, as Goldstein (1967) explained so clearly in *The Insanity Defense*.[18] If, for example, an individual commits a crime as a result of unconscious and irrational forces over which he has no control, do we wish to hold him responsible?

In 1843, Lord Chief Justice Tindal of the British court declared "not guilty, on the grounds of insanity," one M'Naghten who had shot and killed the personal secretary to Sir Robert Peel.

The acquittal stirred such controversy, whipped up by the newspapers and supported by the queen, that the House of Lords convened a commission of 15 distinguished judges to elucidate the law regarding insanity in a criminal proceeding. The rule that was drawn up stated that:

> to establish a defense on the grounds of insanity, it must be clearly proved that, at the time of committing the act, the party accused was laboring under such a defect of reason, from disease of mind, as not to know the nature and quality of the act he was doing. Or, if he did know it, that he did not know he was doing what was wrong.

Eule (1978) analyzed this position as "the presumption of sanity."[13] Goldstein (1968) pointed out that this derived from a time when mental disease was "not yet an extensive concept, when it was widely assumed that only the exceptional offender was sufficiently mentally disordered to warrant dealing differently with him, and when criminal law was not regarded as a treatment device at all."[19]

Smith and Berlin (1974)[39] have concluded that the M'Naghten rule was difficult, and in some cases impossible, to apply in a courtroom situation. Lawyers, judges, and psychiatrists found the terms of the rule both difficult to bring into testimony and not adequate to cover an expanding concept of mental illness. During the past decades, the concept of "irresistible impulse" has been adopted by some states, and others have been tending toward the provisions of the Model Penal Code of the American Law Institute that provides:

> 1. A person is not responsible for criminal conduct if at the time of such conduct as a result of mental disease or defect he lacked substantial capacity to appreciate the

criminality (wrongfulness) of his conduct or to conform to the requirements of the law.
2. As used in this article, the terms mental disease or defect do not include an abnormality manifested only by repeated criminal or otherwise antisocial conduct.

The expanded definitions, while satisfying our current understanding of mental illness, pose serious questions about the place of legal responsibility in a free society. Goldstein (1967)[18] commented that even while we can recognize the forces that contributed to an individual's behavior, the concept of "blame" may be still necessary.

The concept of "blame" and insanity which is its other side, is one of the ways in which culture marks out the extreme beyond which non-conformity may not go.[18]

The point is the most significant one underlying the discussion of the insanity defense. We are back once again to the attempt of society to define insanity so as to delimit the scope of the criminal justice system.

In actual fact, the insanity defense is pleaded in scarcely 2% of all of the criminal cases that are tried annually in the United States (Eule, 1978).[13] Much more significant, in a practical sense, is the definition of insanity as it relates to the determination of competency to stand trial, or even to participate in plea bargaining. This determination—whether the individual is competent to stand trial, to participate in his defense—is not only a very common issue in criminal proceedings, but some states have enacted legislation that a determination of competency be made in all felony cases.

It is an established principle of the American justice system that the defendant have the capacity to participate rationally and effectively in the legal process, but the proportion of cases in which competency determinations are made varies enormously, as do the criteria for establishing competency and those appointed to make this determination. Roesch and Golding[31] reported that in North Carolina, more than half (56%) of judges surveyed reported that they grant a motion for a competency evaluation immediately, without requesting additional facts not included in the motion. In the same study, it was pointed out that competency evaluations were requested on the bases of advice from arresting officers, requests from the defendant's family, prior history of psychiatric treatment, current alcohol/drug abuse, seriousness of charges, suicide threats or attempts, aggressive behavior in jail, and client distress or depression. The fact that prior history of psychiatric treatment is included in the list signifies the likelihood that former patients of mental institutions are likely to be evaluated for competency. The fact is that less than 10% of all referrals in North Carolina are found incompetent (Roesch and Golding, 1977),[34] although here again, the rate varies considerably in other states.

Egon Bittner (1968)[5] has elaborated on the many ways in which the issue of mental abnormality affects the administration of justice outside the courtroom. The most significant area of impact is in the exercise of police discretion. Banton (1964),[2] Bittner (1967),[4] Goldstein (1960),[20] and La Fave (1965)[24] have all demonstrated that the exercise of discretion is especially prominent in the enforcement of the law with regard to common offenses. Bleicher (1967)[6] pointed out that in many jurisdictions, statutory authorization for police intervention in cases of mental illness pertains, and this is defined as being of a civil rather than criminal nature.

The result is that there are significant issues of police discretion in handling cases that could be regarded as either criminal offenses or as mentally unbalanced behavior.

During the past few years, the continuing deinstitutionalization of the mentally ill has spawned extensive research to determine whether released mental patients have arrest rates that exceed those of the general population. Cocozza, Melick, and Steadman (1978) have concluded that

> the public has little to fear from the mentally ill. Few people released from state mental hospitals are involved in violent crime, and very little of the violent crime that occurs results from such persons.[8]

They have explained away repeated studies showing higher arrest rates for released mental patients than for the general population by arguing that among the patient population, there is a subgroup of those with previous criminal histories and that these individuals are indeed more apt to be arrested after release for violent crimes. Their overall conclusion was that "mental illness and violent crime are most often independent and not interactive."[8]

The conclusion seems premature, at very least, because their study and similar research [Abramson (1972);[1] Brill and Maltzburg (1954);[7] Cohen and Freeman (1945);[9] Durbin, Pasewark, and Albers (1977);[12] Giovannoni and Gurer (1967);[15] Guze, Goodwin, and Crane (1969);[22] Paull and Malek (1974);[30] Rappeport and Lassen (1966);[33] Quinsey (1975);[32] Zitrin, Hardesty, Burdock, and Drosaman (1976)[44]] have used arrest rates and sometimes readmission rates as criteria to determine the dangerousness of the released mental patients. One recent comprehensive study of this genre by Fleming was titled "Interface of the Mental Health and Criminal Justice Systems—An Examination of Pennsylvania's Mental Health Procedures Act of 1976."[14] It explored the possibility that a 1976 statute restricting grounds for initiating and continuing involuntary commitment by requiring proof of dangerousness would result in diversion of "less dangerous" mentally ill persons into the criminal justice system. Arrest and commitment trends before and after the enactment of the 1976 law were examined for Philadelphia County, Pennsylvania, and arrest rates from a small sample of persons for whom unsuccessful commitment attempts had resulted from application of the new law's criteria were analyzed. The expected decrease in the number of involuntary commitments did not take place, but the length of time spent in the hospitals by involuntarily committed persons was reduced considerably. Analysis of county-wide arrest rates provided only "tentative support" for the diversion hypothesis: out of 16 public order offenses, only 2 exhibited the hypothesized increase. There was an increase in the frequency of arrests for violent offenses among the mental health system "reject" sample, but the significance of the increase could not be tested. This study, like most preceding studies, found some increase in arrests, but not in every crime category or in large measure.

Arrest rates, even in combination with readmission rates, may well be an inadequate criterion in determining the potential for violent behavior among released mental patients. A sample of 35 New York City police officers attending John Jay College of Criminal Justice responded to a questionnaire that presented four hypothetical situations in which an individual was described as engaged in assaultive behavior (which, though a simple assault, was a felony by definition) while also engaging in bizarre behavior (such as screaming meaningless phrases) that was indicative of mental abnormality. The respondents were asked how they, as police officers, would actually handle and dispose of these incidents. In two of the cases, the assailant was described as a released mental patient; in the other two cases, this specific identification was not made. More than half of the sample (51.4%) indicated that they would bring all four cases to the emergency room of a local hospital with a psychiatric unit. A third of the respondents indicated that they would attempt to calm the individual and then release him. Only three officers identified arrest as the appropriate method of disposition in any of the four cases, and only one officer would have made an arrest in all four cases. Several respondents commented on the questionnaire form that bringing "mentals" to the emergency room was standard procedure, even for the hypothetical case in which the individual attempted to assault the police officers and had to be physically subdued by them. There were no significant differences between the officers' responses to those cases specifically identified as released mental patients and to those not so identified.

If these results are representative (and obviously the small and localized nature of the sample is a limitation of this survey), we may be better able to understand the relatively small differences between the arrest rates of the general population and those of released mental patients. Part of the explanation may lie in the sizeable proportion of elderly people among released mental hospital patients, a group less likely to be engaged in public disorder or violence. The heuristic value of the survey lies in the implication that arrest rates for released mental patients are low because policemen are reluctant to initiate arrests where the possibilities of trial and conviction are minimal. If so, research on comparative arrest rates is of limited relevance, and the appropriate criterion (although more difficult to accumulate and measure) would be total recorded police contacts with released mental patients, particularly including those that result in transient referral to hospital emergency rooms or to psychiatric facilities although not in commitments.

Bauer (1970) has called mental illness and criminality "two sides of the same coin."[3] Their commonality is in the suspicion or judgment of dangerousness in antisocial or eccentric behavior. A strongly held and persistent notion of the American public is that the mentally ill are dangerous (Nunally, 1961;[29] Steadman and Coceozza, 1978[43]).

The prevention of violence—to self and to others—is a common responsibility of the two systems, a responsibility that has been difficult to fulfill (Koerin, 1978).[25] The problem lies in the prediction of violent behavior. While psychiatric and psychological diagnosis can predict

violence at a better than chance ratio, overprediction is still highly prevalent. This means that for every accurate prediction of violence, there will be
many inaccurate predictions of violence, or false positives. Ironically, social
pressure tends toward even less accurate prediction, because society is much
more concerned about the prediction that a given individual will *not* behave
in violent fashion when, in fact, he will (false negatives). Thus, a single instance of a discharged or released patient committing a violent crime invariably raises a hue and cry that release procedures be tightened, that
screening be stricter, that any remote clue suggesting the possibility of
future violence become presumptive evidence that the individual continue to
be detained or, if that is illegal, at least that he be observed and monitored
(Monahan, 1975).[28]

Peszke (1975)[31] contended that the prediction of dangerousness is not,
and should not be, within the competence of medicine, although psychiatrists are competent to judge whether or not the severity of mental illness
impairs a patient's competence to make an informed decision. While agreeing to make some of the required judgments, Peszke is unwilling to make
the judgments that society most desperately requires, arguing that we simply do not have the knowledge at this time. In a recent article by Saleem
Shah (1978) on dangerousness, this point is conceded, in effect, by the conclusion that

> there is abundant evidence to indicate that recidivist offenders account for a dispropor-
> tionate amount of all crimes leading to arrest . . . if a defendant had five or more arrests
> prior to the current arrest, the probability of subsequent arrests began to approach cer-
> tainty . . . defendants that previously committed violent crimes show the highest pro-
> portion of rearrests for violent crime.[38]

Dix (1976)[11] reported similar findings for sexual offenders.

It may well be that the most valid and fair prediction of violence or
dangerousness at this time is simply an empirical prediction based on past
patterns of behavior. Here too, however, all the evidence suggests that we
still will be predicting violence for many individuals who will, in fact, not be
violent.

Abramson (1972)[1] wrote an article on the criminalization of mentally
disordered behavior in which he predicted that the deinstitutionalization of
mental patients would lead to placing the care of the mentally ill ultimately
in the hands of the police. Monahan (1973)[27] responded with an article entitled "The Psychiatrization of Criminal Behavior" in which he identified
the problem as centering on the mentally abnormal offender, who by definition qualifies for entrance into both systems, which leads to each system
asserting priority for controlling and correcting him.

Since these predictions were made, it appears that something else has
taken place. Rather than a struggle for priority in meeting the needs of
society in dealing with mentally abnormal offenders, even those who are
potentially dangerous, the struggle has been to refer or divert these individuals elsewhere. The mental health system has engaged in a massive
deinstitutionalization of hospital populations without building up adequate

community care programs and facilities. The criminal justice system, during the same period, has concentrated on diversion and "community correctional" programs as its court and correctional facilities have become swamped with record numbers of offenders.

This has resulted in informal dispositions made mostly by the police and, sometimes, by prosecutors—referrals that result neither in arrests nor in readmissions. Referrals consist of emergency programs of medication that enable the individual, through sedation, to exert temporary control over his behavior. The contact is a transient one, designed to alleviate the problem briefly; it is a "band-aid" approach. This major interface of the criminal justice and mental health systems is, in fact, one of the sore points of our society. Thus, the estimated 5 to 10% of those apprehended and accused of index crimes (homicide, aggravated assault, rape, and robbery) who are given mental health examinations in order to advise the court about their potential for dangerous behavior really may be only a small proportion of those who actually demonstrate both violent behavior and mental instability (Rubin, 1972).[36]

Obviously, there are other, more positive, interfaces of these two comprehensive service and care systems. The police provide some needed direct mental health services to citizens in their street contacts with them. In many police departments, mental health professionals provide counseling and other mental health services to police officers themselves. Within the juvenile justice system, the treatment model is so prevalent that the principal objective of juvenile courts has been identified as amelioration, if not therapy. Mental health services in corrections, probation, and parole facilities are an intrinsic part of these agencies of criminal justice. Even the most backward states have correctional institutions for the criminally insane—usually those who have committed heinous crimes and show unmistakable evidence of a potential for violence.

A pragmatic overview of the two systems suggests that as the mental health system has been contracting (despite its objective of expanded community care), the criminal justice system has been expanding; this is best demonstrated in growing prison populations. Both systems have been forced by legal challenge to evaluate and monitor the specific formal services rendered to their clientele, particularly when that service is identified as treatment. When these evaluations focus on outcomes in the treatment of mentally abnormal offenders, the conclusion must be that neither system is currently effective in preventing the recurrence of the behavior that brought the individual into the system. We are as far short of "cures" as we are of rehabilitation. Even our definitions and delineations are still inadequate, for in the area of antisocial behavior, we hold widely varying views about what is criminal and what is mental disability. We may agree that some criminals are not insane and that some of the insane are not criminal; but for the great mass of those whose behavior defies simple classification, we have no established way of coping with them or helping them, and are instead shunting them between systems.

REFERENCES

1. ABRAMSON, M. 1972. The criminalization of mentally disordered behavior: possible side effect of a new mental health law. Hosp. Community Psychiatry 23(April): 101–105.
2. BANTON, M. 1964. The Policeman in the Community. Basic Books. New York, N.Y.
3. BAUER, W. 1970. The other side of the coin. Ill. Med. J. 137(February): 158–161.
4. BITTNER, E. 1967. Police discretion of emergency apprehension of mentally ill persons. Social Problems 14: 278–292.
5. BITTNER, E. 1968. The concept of mental abnormality in the administration of justice outside the courtroom. In The Mentally Abnormal Offender. A. de Reuck & R. Porter, Eds.: 201–219. J & A Churchill. London, England.
6. BLEICHER, B. K. 1967. Cleveland-Marshall Law Rev. 16: 93–115.
7. BRILL, H. & B. MALZBERG. 1954. Statistical Report on the Arrest Record of Male ExPatients, Age 16 or Over, Released from New York State Mental Hospitals during the Period 1946–48. American Psychiatric Association–Mental Hospital Service Supplementary Mailing 153, August 1962. New York State Department of Mental Hygiene. Albany, N.Y.
8. COCOZZA, J., M. MELICK & H. J. STEADMAN. 1978. Trends in violent crime among exmental patients. Criminology 16(3): 317–335.
9. COHEN, L. H. & H. FREEMAN. 1945. How dangerous to the community are state hospital patients? Conn. State Med. J. 9(September): 697–700.
10. CURRAN, W. J. 1975. The right to psychiatric treatment: a simple decision in the Supreme Court. N. Eng. J. Med. 293/10: 487–488.
11. DIX, G. E. 1976. Differential processing of abnormal sex offenders: utilization of California's mentally disordered sex offender program. J. Crim. Law Criminol. 67(2): 233–243.
12. DURBIN, J. R., R. A. PASEWARK & D. ALBERS. 1977. Criminality and mental illness: a study of arrest rates in a rural state. Am. J. Psychiatry 134(January): 80–83.
13. EULE, J. M. 1978. The presumption of sanity: bursting the bubble. UCLA Law Rev. 25(4): 637–699.
14. FLEMING, S. 1978. Interface of the Mental Health and Criminal Justice Systems—An Examination of Pennsylvania's Mental Health Procedures Act of 1976. Document No. 78-NI-AX-002. U.S. Department of Justice, LEAA. Washington, D.C.
15. GIOVANNONI, J. M. & L. GURER. 1967. Socially disruptive behavior of ex-mental patients. Arch. Gen. Psychiatry 20(May): 583–591.
16. GOFFMAN, E. 1961. Asylums. Doubleday & Co., Inc. New York, N.Y.
17. GOFFMAN, E. 1963. Stigma. Prentice-Hall, Inc. Englewood Cliffs, N.J.
18. GOLDSTEIN, A. S. 1967. The Insanity Defense. Yale University Press. New York and London.
19. GOLDSTEIN, A. S. 1968. The mentally disordered offender and the criminal law. In The Mentally Abnormal Offender. A. de Reuck & R. Porter, Eds.: 188–201. J & A Churchill. London, England.
20. GOLDSTEIN, J. 1960. Yale Law J. 69: 543–594.
21. GROETH, R. 1977. Overt dangerous behavior as a constitutional requirement for involuntary civil commitment of the mentally ill. Univ. Chicago Law Rev. 44(3): 562–593.
22. GUZE, S. B., D. W. GOODWIN & J. B. CRANE. 1969. Criminal recidivism and psychiatric illness. Arch. Gen. Psychiatry 20(May): 583–591.
23. HALLECK, S. L. 1967. Psychiatry and the Dilemmas of Crime. Harper & Row, Publishers. New York, N.Y.
24. LaFAVE, W. R. 1965. Arrest: The Decision to Take a Suspect into Custody. Little, Brown and Co. Boston, Mass.
25. KOERIN, B. 1978. Violent crime, prevention and control. Crime and Delinquency 24(1): 49–58.
26. MILLER, H. L. 1977. The right to treatment: Can the courts rehabilitate and cure? The Public Interest 46(winter): 96–118.
27. MONAHAN, J. 1973. The psychiatrization of criminal behavior. Hosp. Community Psychiatry 24(February): 105–107.

28. MONAHAN, J. 1975. The prediction of violence. *In* Violence and Criminal Justice. D. Chappel & J. Monahan, Eds. D.C. Heath and Co. Lexington, Mass.
29. NUNALLY, J. D., JR. 1961. Popular Conceptions of Mental Health. Holt, Rinehart & Winston, Inc. New York, N.Y.
30. PAULL, D. & A. A. MALEK. 1974. Psychiatric disorders and criminality. J. Am. Med. Assoc. **228**(June 10): 1369.
31. PESZKE, M. A. 1975. Is dangerousness an issue for physicians in emergency commitment? Am. J. Psychiatry **132/8**: 825–828.
32. QUINSEY, V. C. 1975. Released Oak Ridge patients: a follow-up study of review board discharges. Br. J. Criminol. **45**(3): 264–270.
33. RAPPEPORT, J. R. & G. LASSEN. 1966. The dangerousness of female patients: a comparison of the arrest rate of discharged psychiatric patients and the general population. Am. J. Psychiatry **123**(October): 413–419.
34. ROESCH, R. & S. L. GOLDING. 1977. A Systems Analysis of Competency to Stand Trial Procedures. Department of Psychology. University of Illinois. Urbana, Ill.
35. ROESCH, R. & S. L. GOLDING. 1978. Legal and judicial interpretation of competency to stand trial statutes and procedures. Criminology **16**(3): 420–429.
36. RUBIN, B. 1972. The prediction of dangerousness in mentally ill criminals. Arch. Gen. Psychiatry **77**(September): 397–407.
37. SCHEFF, T. J. 1966. Being Mentally Ill: A Sociological Theory. Aldine. Chicago, Ill.
38. SHAH, S. A. 1978. Dangerousness: a paradigm for exploring some issues in law and psychology. Am. Psychol. **33**(3): 224–239.
39. SMITH, A. B. & L. BERLIN. 1974. Treating the Criminal Offender. Oceana Publications. Dobbs Ferry, N.Y.
40. SZASZ, T. 1961. The Myth of Mental Illness. Harper and Row, Publishers. New York, N.Y.
41. SZASZ, T. 1963. Law, Liberty and Psychiatry. Macmillan Co. New York, N.Y.
42. SZASZ, T. 1965. Psychiatric Justice. Macmillan Co. New York, N.Y.
43. STEADMAN, N. J. & J. J. COCEOZZA. 1978. Selective reporting and the public's misconceptions of the criminally insane. Public Opinion Q. **41**(winter): 523–531.
44. ZITRIN, A., A. S. HARDESTY, E. I. BURDOCK & A. K. DROSAMAN. 1976. Crime and Violence among mental patients. Am. J. Psychiatry **133**(February): 142–149.

PSYCHIATRY ON TRIAL: CLINICAL AND ETHICAL PROBLEMS IN THE PSYCHIATRIC ASSESSMENT OF COMPETENCY TO STAND TRIAL

Henry C. Weinstein

New York University Schools of Medicine and Law
New York, New York 10016

My comments this morning are from a clinical perspective. After a decade of clinical experience, during which I have evaluated thousands of patients as to their competency to stand trial, I find the practice of forensic psychiatry to be a minefield of clinical and ethical problems and conflicts. In my opinion, these clinical and ethical problems and conflicts are so glaring and unacceptable that they cry out for immediate attention and correction. If not, I am afraid that psychiatry will be most harshly judged. This is what I mean by "psychiatry on trial."

The clinical problems are of two sorts. There are the clinical problems that are of general concern in psychiatry—diagnostic reliability and validity, for example. Then there are clinical problems that are specific to the forensic psychiatrist, resulting from the need to apply the findings of the clinical examination to the relevant legal criteria. There are, in addition, special ethical problems, which are ofttimes related to questions of divided professional loyalty or responsibility.

I shall start by making some preliminary remarks about the competency to stand trial process. While competency to stand trial is only one of numerous situations (28 by one count)[1] where a psychiatrist is called to testify in a judicial proceeding in regard to an individual's competency, it is, in my opinion, the most critical interface of psychiatry and the law. This, because it involves the criminal law with its potentially harsh penalties, including the deprivation of liberty, and because it is carried out many times more frequently than the other major criminal law evaluation—that of the insanity defense. As a corollary, many more defendants are involuntarily confined to psychiatric facilities on the basis of questions of incompetency to stand trial than on the basis of having been found not guilty by reason of insanity.

The importance of this issue is highlighted by a consideration of its fundamental rationale. As Stone notes:

> Historically, the legal notion of competency has been thought to serve both ritual and justice. The requirement that the criminal defendant be able to understand the proceedings and aid in his defense flowed from the view that the entering of a plea at trial invoked the judgment of God, sustained the adversarial nature of the court, and aided the discovery of truth.[2]

More specifically, Stone notes that the determination of competency to stand trial serves the following needs of the legal system:

> Guaranteeing the accuracy of the criminal proceedings, especially where competent

accused might provide his counsel with crucial facts known only to the accused . . . .

Guaranteeing the fairness of the trial. There is an ineffable sense in which it has long been felt that an accused has not been fairly convicted, no matter what the extrinsic evidence, unless he is able to understand the nature of the proceedings and the basic defense options and consequences . . . .

Maximizing the efficacy of punishment, both in terms of individual deterrence and attributive catharsis of the rest of society.[2]

Before I turn to specific clinical and ethical problems, I'd like to briefly examine the role of the forensic psychiatrist in the competency to stand trial procedure. In our fellowship training program (in psychiatry and the law) at New York University, we use what we call "the fourfold analysis" of forensic psychiatric questions. This analysis can be utilized to clarify the role of the forensic expert witness in any such situation.

The first part of the analysis is the determination of what is the particular legal issue. The legal issue is a yes-or-no question that is required by the legal situation—a legal question. We are dealing here with the legal issue of competency to stand trial. Is the defendant competent to stand trial or not? The ultimate decision, of course, is made by a judge or jury.

The second step of the forensic psychiatric analysis is the determination of the specific legal criteria that are required to resolve the legal issue. The particular legal criteria are set out in statutes, regulations, or case law. It is important to note that the criteria are *legal* criteria—which in turn are used to resolve the legal issue.

The third aspect of this analysis is the clinical examination of the defendant. This is best done by an expert who is familiar with the legal criteria, because the fourth and final part of the analysis is the application of the findings of the clinical examination to the legal criteria. To put it another way, this fourth step involves a determination of whether the specific legal criteria are or are not met by the clinical findings, i.e., whether there is a *causal relationship* between the findings of the clinical examination and the legal criteria. Obviously, the role of the forensic expert is most importantly related to this last aspect of the evaluation, for it is the forensic expert who—cognizant of the legal issue and the legal criteria—applies the specific clinical findings to those legal criteria.

Turning now to some general problems in the psychiatric assessment of competency to stand trial, let us start with this last-mentioned task of applying the clinical findings to the legal criteria. As is always the case, the criteria are stated in legal terms, not medical, psychiatric, or psychological terms. The legal criteria where competency to stand trial is at issue are generally stated as whether the defendant understands the charges against him and whether he can assist in the defense. This brief statement of the criteria was elaborated somewhat by the U.S. Supreme Court in the *Dusky* case, where the criteria are stated as "whether he [the defendant] has sufficient present ability to consult with his lawyer with a reasonable degree of rational understanding, and whether he has a rational as well as factual understanding of the proceedings against him."[3] However, even this somewhat expanded set of criteria does not significantly assist the forensic expert in the complex task of applying the clinical findings to these criteria. How does one move from a specific set of clinical findings to such concepts as "reasonable degree" of "rational understanding," or "a rational as well as factual understanding of the proceedings"?

As an example, let us start with disorders of mood. At what point does a depression or a mania become so severe that a patient is no longer competent to stand trial? At the forensic psychiatric services of the Bellevue Psychiatric Hospital, many patients are referred following a suicide attempt. That a patient might be depressed in the circumstances during which he is assessed for competency would not be surprising. On the other hand, most would agree that an acutely and severely depressed defendant (so depressed that he is suicidal) would hardly be able to adequately participate in his trial and assist in his defense. But, must the patient be actively and unquestionably suicidal to be incompetent to stand trial? At what point on the depression continuum is this particular line to be drawn? To come to an opinion and present this opinion clearly and understandably to the court is the responsibility of the forensic expert.

Similarly, when a defendant is manic, when is he so manic that he is incompetent to stand trial?[4] As with the depressed patient, it is not the adequacy of the defendant's cognitive functions that is at issue, but the effect of his affective disorganization. These issues of clinical judgment are made even more difficult and complicated by the fact that, in reality (as will be elaborated below), the expert's opinion on competency to stand trial is a prediction of how the defendant will be at a trial.

What of disorders of *thinking*? For example, what of a patient who is delusional? It is difficult enough to determine when a particular belief is a "delusion," but to attempt to decide whether the particular delusion itself (not the mere presence of the delusion) affects the patient's understanding of the charges and his ability to assist in his defense is an almost metaphysical question.

I should note that it was not too long ago that it was generally held that any patient who was actively delusional was, ipso facto, incompetent to stand trial. This was based on the rationale that anyone whose mental functioning was so disordered as to be delusional could not function adequately in the legal process. I believe that forensic experts have become more precise since that time.

I turn now from such general problems of applying clinical data to imprecise and broad legal criteria, to some of the special problems presented to psychiatrists in the competency to stand trial evaluation.

Psychiatrists are often in the position to make "dispositional diagnoses,"[2] i.e., the examiner reaches a particular conclusion and presents to the court a particular opinion in order to achieve a particular result. Most frequently, I have found, this is justified on the basis that it will place the patient into a treatment setting. While some will see this as a subtle misuse of the competency process by psychiatrists, it seems rather to highlight the varied interests served by the psychiatrist in the competency to stand trial procedure.[5] Also note here the interfacing of the criminal justice system with the civil psychiatric hospital system—with the psychiatrist in the role of gatekeeper.

Another special problem presented by the evaluation is the fact that although the competency to stand trial criteria presented (for example by the Supreme Court in the *Dusky* case) are generally related to the defendant's "present ability," it is obvious that—since the clinical examination of the patient usually takes place at a time considerably before the start of the trial—the conclusion arrived at is in reality a prediction of how the defendant will be able to function later—either at his trial or at some other time when he is consulting with his attorney. I need not emphasize to this audience the problems in regard to this type of prediction.

Similarly, the landmark case of *Jackson* v. *Indiana* presents this problem very starkly.[6] This case stands for the proposition that if a defendant cannot, within a reasonable period of time, become competent to stand trial, he must be discharged from the criminal justice system. Thus a prediction must be made.

Still another general clinical problem is that of "fragility." There are defendants who, at the time of the examination, are competent to participate in the judicial process but who cannot, in the opinion of the forensic expert, tolerate the stress and tension of a trial. I would find such a patient not competent to stand trial. Professor Brooks of Rutgers Law School seems to disagree. He states that

> some psychiatrists are prepared to characterize as "incompetent to stand trial" a defendant who is so emotionally disturbed that, in the view of the psychiatrist, if he stands trial, might "decompensate," i.e., become psychotic, or otherwise "breakdown" and become more seriously mentally ill. Is this an accepted grounds for determining the fitness of a defendant to stand trial? If not, should a psychiatrist be permitted to testify to this effect? Many do.[7]

It is somewhat hard for me to understand this position. Surely it is not in the interests of either the defendant or the criminal justice system in general to prematurely return a patient to trial if it means that this will only lead to further delay of his trial. Furthermore, although this is a prediction, psychiatrists are uniquely equipped to evaluate this aspect of competency.

The issue of fragility is closely related to the issue of the foreseeability of improvement in therapy, which is part of the overall issue of the changing clinical picture that a defendant may present. In the first place, the defendant may be undergoing treatment during evaluation, i.e., evaluation in a treatment setting, and may be improving. This in itself is the subject (or at least was until recently) of a serious debate, that is, whether someone could be competent to stand trial at the same time that they were receiving psychotropic medication. A number of years ago, one judge went so far as to label this situation "artificial sanity."

On the other hand, it has been pointed out that many participants in the judicial process use drugs. Hollister, in an article titled "Psychotropic Drugs in Court Competency," noting that "ideally, all parties in criminal litigation should be free of drugs," adds tongue in cheek that

> the world not being ideal, such is seldom the case. The prosecuting attorney may take nicotine during recess by smoking, the defense attorney may take caffeine in a cup. And both of these worthies, as well as the judge, may have been recently exposed to beverages containing ethyl alcohol. A woman juror may have taken a proprietary

medication for relief of her headache that probably contains at least three different painkilling or mood altering drugs. A male juror may have taken a sleeping pill the night before and still have the drug in his circulatory system. If the defendant has been · incarcerated prior to his trial, he may be more free of drugs than any of the other participants, or at least the drug history may be better documented.[8]

Nonetheless, there are serious concerns in regard to drug therapy where the defendant is awaiting trial. At one point, even here in New York City, it was felt to be improper to return a patient to trial who required tranquilizing medication. This is no longer the case, and a majority of jurisdictions (if not all) accept the principle that a patient on medication may be held competent to stand trial. What of the use of ECT—shock treatment—to make a patient competent or to hasten the process? What of the informed consent necessary for such treatment?

As if this were not complex enough, I will interject at this point Dr. Stone's comment that

any defense attorney will recognize that one of the best pieces of evidence for convincing a jury that a person was not responsible for his crime is a defendant who is obviously crazy at the trial. That dramatic impression is blunted by the drugs. The effect of such drugs, when unknown to the jury in its appraisal of the defendant's demeanor, has led to a reversal of a conviction.[2]

I will add an even more serious concern of psychiatrists and lawyers. This is the right of the patient to refuse treatment. I shall not review this complex subject but shall merely ask whether, in light of Stone's comment above, the defendant can refuse treatment—any treatment—or whether, if the patient is not competent to make that decision (notice the accumulating complications), his attorney can act on his behalf and insist on this exercise of this "right." Of course, where it is the patient himself who insists on refusing treatment to protect his "crazy" demeanor before a jury, the question of whether or not he is malingering would be properly raised.

Malingering is another very complicated matter and is a special problem on my unit, where an unusually large proportion of the patients are malingering. The clinical assessment of a patient who is believed to be malingering is itself a highly specialized technique, as is the testimony required to support such an opinion. Malingering often takes the form of a feigned amnesia; a patient says, "I don't remember." It is now established, however, that amnesia in and of itself does not render a patient incompetent to stand trial.[9] It is at this point that some would call for the use of special techniques, such as sodium amytal or hypnosis. Thus, many special ethical problems may be raised for the clinician. For example, how does one satisfy the need for "informed consent" from a patient who is suspected of malingering?

I shall now turn to a series of problems that I have broadly labeled "legal problems." There are those who argue that there is no need for professional assessment of the issue of competency to stand trial, that this can be settled on a common sense basis by the judge or the jury. Others say that the best individual to assess competency to stand trial is the defendant's lawyer.[1] One of the many problems with the latter suggestion is that the lawyer, himself an officer of the court, may have tactical interests in regard to the issue of competency to stand trial. Not only the defendant's lawyer, but the prosecuting attorney and occasionally the judge also may use the competency to stand trial issue for tactical purposes, or for purposes of disposition, plea bargaining, etc., rather than to settle the issue of competency itself.

I also list under "legal problems" the misuse of the psychiatric report. We find ourselves unable to protect the confidentiality of the report, and find the information in our reports on competency being used for various purposes at the trial itself. Our New York State statute specifically prohibits this, but research has shown how these reports are misused in this manner.[10]

A well-known problem is the "battle of the experts," where each side "shops around" for a "well-qualified" professional's opinion that will support its particular perception of the facts. Not only do lawyers shop around, but many judges do also—having formed their own opinion as to competency (but for some reason being unwilling to assert it), they send the patient to various court clinics and inpatient facilities until they receive an opinion consistent with their own.

Another troublesome legal problem is the use of the competency to stand trial question for reasons of preventive detention, where under the guise of an unsettled legal issue (the competency question), a patient is kept in detention because he is felt to be too "dangerous" to be at large in the community.

What of the situation where the findings by "impartial" experts are unsatisfactory to the defendant, and he cannot afford to hire an independent expert? The Legal Aid Society, which represents many of our indigent patients at Bellevue, has very limited funds for these purposes. Corrective legislation is being proposed in many jurisdictions.

I can only briefly mention some of the sociological issues related to the assessment of competency to stand trial, such as the effects of class, racial, or cultural differences between the evaluating doctor and the patient, or for that matter between the judge and the patient, or the lawyer and the patient. Some defendants are very sensitive to the matter of labeling and stigma; some would rather be convicted of a crime than categorized as mentally ill. Indeed, some of these patients attempt to "malinger" mental health: "There's nothing wrong with me. I don't belong here."

What of the misuse of psychiatric evaluation by a government? We castigate the Soviet Union in this regard, since it appears that the misuse of psychiatry in the Soviet Union is quite flagrant. There, dissidents are detained and, for all intents and purposes, silenced by means of various psychiatric procedures and incarcerations. Are there misuses of psychiatry for political purposes in the United States? If so, they rarely involve the competency to stand trial issue. One notorious case was that of Ezra Pound, who, following World War II, was incarcerated in St. Elizabeth's Hospital for many years on the grounds that he was incompetent to stand trial for treason. Thomas Szasz argues very powerfully that this was a "political" misuse of psychiatry.[11]

I will list under political problems the need for self-regulation by the profession to insure adequate training and qualification of experts. For example, I regret to say that I am familiar with a number of "experts" whose work belies their narcissism, egocentricity, grandiosity, and lack of self-control, rather than their clinical skills. As a "political" matter, I wonder how long society will permit the profession to tolerate or ignore such matters.

In the brief time remaining, I shall turn to some ethical issues that concern me in regard to the competency to stand trial procedure. One is the "double agent" conflict,[5] which refers to the fact that in certain situations or settings, there may arise conflict between the psychiatrist's role as an evaluator for the government and his role as a physician for the defendant-patient. This is most serious where the competency to stand trial assessment is made in a "treatment setting."

Similar issues arise in regard to confidentiality. The forensic psychiatrist must take precautions to ensure that the defendant is aware of his, the psychiatrist's, role and responsibilities, i.e., that there is no physician-patient privilege and that the psychiatrist will prepare a report for the court. On the other hand, I believe it is incumbent on the psychiatrist to take every precaution to ensure that the report does not include any material that is not strictly necessary for the purposes of the report and that might be adverse to the interests of the defendant.

Karl Menninger has argued that legal issues such as competency to stand trial involve *moral* questions and judgments in which psychiatrists have no particular expertise and, therefore, that psychiatrists should remove themselves entirely from any participation in the legal process.[12] Still others have suggested that the competency to stand trial procedure is so inherently unfair and unjust that it should be abolished entirely.[7] I cannot agree, for I believe that the law seeks the counsel of the behavioral scientist for good reason in these matters. I believe that with proper precautions, reforms, and changes, many of the clinical and ethical problems that I have cited may be obviated.

There are specific legal reforms that are being attempted. The case of *Jackson* v. *Indiana* and recent legislation in some jurisdictions seek to prevent long criminal incarcerations where a patient is not competent to stand trial. Procedural reforms are being instituted to allow a patient to plead the insanity defense even if he is *not* competent to stand trial.[13]

I believe there are a number of ways in which we psychiatrists who participate in this process can contribute to the resolution of some of these problems. First, as for the clinical problems, the clinician must not only be careful and precise in his application of his clinical data to the legal criteria, but most important of all, must present his reasoning to the court—in his report and his testimony—in a clear and coherent fashion.

Second, we must insure that those who participate in the process of assessment of competency to stand trial are made aware of the clinical, legal, social, ethical, and philosophical issues by means of continuing medical education and in-service education. We have done this on my unit by instituting a weekly seminar for our staff titled "Philosophical and Ethical Issues in the Practice of Forensic Psychiatry." This is led jointly by myself and a Ph.D philosopher. This program recently gained support from the Counsel on the Humanities for a "philosopher in residence" to participate in and to run programs not only for the psychiatric staff, but for the Department of Correction, nursing, and other staffs as well.

Third, it may be necessary to separate the evaluation and the treatment functions of the psychiatrist. I believe this is possible even under the most difficult of circumstances.

Fourth, I think that the judicious use of various instruments that have been developed can be helpful.[13] These instruments cannot replace a good clinical judgment or the skill of the forensic expert, but they certainly can help to organize the clinical evaluation as well as the presentation of the material to the court.

Fifth, we must increase research in these areas. We need larger data bases in regard to these patients. We need further tests of the validity and reliability of our clinical evaluations. We need feedback in regard to the results of our evaluations.

Sixth, we need increased training for experts (both psychiatric and psychological) as to their special roles and responsibilities in the legal process. In this regard, I am glad to see the establishment of boards of certification—both psychiatric and psychological—in regard to forensic matters.

Finally, we need more communication between all of those who participate in this process—communication, for example, between psychiatrists and psychologists. This conference goes a long way in regard to providing such increased communication.

REFERENCES

1. SLOVENKO, R. 1973. Psychiatry and Law: 107, 94. Little Brown & Co. Boston, Mass.
2. STONE, A. A. 1975. Mental Health and Law: A System in Transition: 203–213. National Institute of Mental Health. Bethesda, Md.
3. Dusky v. United States, 362 U.S. 402 (1960).
4. Cf., Faber v. Sweet Style Manufacturing Corp., 40 Misc. 2d 212, 242 N.Y.S. 2d 763 (1963).
5. Hastings Center. 1978. In the Service of the State: The Psychiatrist as Double Agent. Hastings Center Report, Special Supplement. New York, N.Y.
6. Jackson v. Indiana, 406 U.S. 736 (1972).
7. BROOKS, A. 1974. Psychiatry and the Mental Health System: 363, 383. Little, Brown & Co. Boston, Mass.
8. HOLLISTER, L. E. 1972. Psychotropic drugs and court competence. In Law, Psychiatry and the Mentally Disordered Offender. L. M. Irvine & T. B. Brelje, Eds.: 14. Charles C. Thomas. Springfield, Ill.
9. KOSON, D. & A. ROBEY. 1973. Amnesia and competency to stand trial. Am. J. Psychiatry 130: 558.
10. Note: 1976. Protecting the confidentiality of pretrial psychiatric disclosures: a survey of standards. N.Y.U. Law Rev. 51: 409.
11. SZASZ, T. S. 1963. Law, Liberty and Psychiatry. Macmillan Co. New York, N.Y.
12. MENNINGER, K. 1966. The Crime of Punishment: 139. Viking Press, Inc. New York, N.Y.
13. Laboratory of Community Psychiatry, Harvard Medical School. 1973. Competency to Stand Trial and Mental Illness. U.S. Government Printing Office. Washington, D. C.

DIAGNOSIS VERSUS DESCRIPTION IN COMPETENCY ISSUES

John E. Exner, Jr.

Department of Psychology
Long Island University
Brooklyn, New York 11201

Most psychologists and psychiatrists would probably agree that the intent of laws pertaining to the issue of competency seems "clear enough." On the surface, the criteria for competency appear to broach the basic question of cognitive functioning or, more precisely, the extent to which cognitive functioning is "minimally adequate" in the areas of word knowledge, recent and remote memory, perceptual accuracy or reality testing, abstraction, and judgment as it is applied to both the personal and social spheres. These laws, derived from English common law, seem to be designed to insure that a defendant has the capacity to defend himself or herself in the court of law. They hold, in effect, that the subject must possess the ability to cooperate in the formulation of his or her defense, that he or she has an awareness and understanding of the nature and objectives of the legal proceedings, and that the subject has an understanding of the potential consequences of the proceedings.

Translated into the context of psychological functioning, these criteria imply some specific minimal level of intellectual functioning, which becomes the basis from which the contents of a stimulus field are received and processed fairly accurately; and that processing is, in turn, translated in such a way as to make decision actions commensurate with the purpose and nature of the legal procedure. It seems logical, then, to assume that this issue of competency would be most relevant in cases where questions of intellectual disability, or "retardation," occur. Surprisingly, however, the bulk of statutes regarding the issue of competency and a clear majority of cases in which the question has been raised focus on the relevant, but often misleading, issue of "mental illness" as the base from which decisions of competency or incompetency will be derived. The mental illness question typically becomes misleading in that courts, counsels, and expert witnesses are often prone to confuse the issue of competency with the very separate and quite different criteria for criminal responsibility.

Competency involves awareness, participation, and understanding, all of which require some intellectual/cognitive operations. This is not, however, to suggest that evaluations of competency should be reduced to some simplistic measure of intelligence, even if there were such a measure available that was uniformly agreed to by the psychological community and found to be acceptable and legitimate by the legal profession. In other words, the issue of competency cannot be settled by an IQ, yet it would be foolhardy to discard standard intelligence tests from among the various techniques employed in the quest for competency answers. Similarly, it would be foolhardy to discard or disavow the issue of mental illness or psychological disability as relevant to this question. But just as the IQ does not contribute significantly to the solution, neither does the assignment of some psychiatric or psychological label. Such an error is most common among the psychiatric, psychological, and legal communities when the term "schizophrenia" is bandied about. Unfortunately, many people, both lay and professional, tend to equate the diagnosis of schizophrenia with some perpetual state of psychosis that reduces a person's level of functioning to that of legal incompetence. Such a conclusion is, at best, an incompetent fantasy or, worse, a severe distortion of reality. It is quite true that during most "psychotic episodes," the subject of that episode is legally incompetent, just as is the epileptic during or immediately after a seizure, or the alcoholic in a drunken stupor. However, not unlike the epileptic seizure or the alcoholic stupor, the disability created by the psychotic state is usually transient, rarely lasting longer than a few hours or a few days except in those instances of the protracted case that involves organic origins or features. Unfortunately, the professional and lay communities typically devote their attention to the schizophrenic who is psychotic, who requires hospitalization, and who is truly disabled. Little attention has been given to the great majority of schizophrenics who are not psychotic, who are not disabled, and who do not require hospitalization. The fact of the matter is that significant numbers of schizophrenics carry on very productive lives—functioning in most every conceivable occupation, including medicine, psychology, and the law—in spite of the limitations that their condition or "illness" imposes upon them. This is not to suggest that all schizophrenics are legally competent. Some schizophrenics are aware, can participate, and do understand. Others cannot and/or do not.

In the same vein, some subjects with a derived IQ of 65 can and do function quite effectively within specific parameters. It is impossible to work with an intellectually "limited" population without encountering the person who adapts to a regular occupational role, saves money, buys clothes, wends his or her way effectively through the chaos of the mass transit system, recites batting line-ups and home-run records, differentiates "rock" from "disco," a "hook" from a "dunk," and a "safety squeeze" from a "sacrifice." This is not to suggest that all intellectually handicapped people are legally competent; but some are very aware, can participate, and do understand. Others cannot and/or do not.

Obviously, any legitimate evaluation for competency will go well beyond the derivation of some number on an ordinal scale that purports to measure intelligence, or some diagnostic category, often agreed to by consensus, that implies a "simple" yes-or-no answer regarding competency. But the obvious is not always achieved with ease. There are several problems involved in bringing a competency issue to closure. Not the least of these is the vagueness and ambiguity of the law itself. Although it is formulated with the best intent, the term used—competency—is much more legal than psychological. Thus, while seemingly designed to focus on intellectual issues, the actual criteria contained in most statutes clearly open the door to the mental illness issue and, more important, permit dialogue pertaining to "degrees" of competence. The latter are often raised when the magnitude of the purported offense is greater. And this issue cannot be brushed aside by using the parallel of "being a little bit pregnant," for there are indeed degrees of competency, which do vary with circumstances. Consequently, any evaluation for competency must include sufficient data from which questions of psychological disability and degrees of competency may be addressed.

Fortunately, there exists a wide array of assessment techniques that can be drawn upon for the task; and the task remains one of assessing cognitive operations. Under optimal circumstances, the assessment approach will include techniques that will insure that the yield of information is valid. To accomplish this goal, it may well be necessary to generate data from multiple sources that are relevant to the same cognitive issue. For instance, if a subject seems unable to recall a brief sequence of digits (as required in most standardized intelligence tests that are administered individually), it would be vitally important to glean more data from other sources from which the functioning of immediate memory could be viewed more thoroughly. Similarly, where subjects manifest evidence of weak or inadequate judgment in response to standardized test items, such as those contained in the comprehension subtest of the various Wechsler scales, other approaches to the study of the logic of the decision process must be included in the assessment routine. This "call" for cross-validation of data may be overly conservative and more time consuming than is preferred, but it is very important to retain an awareness that *if* a subject is determined to be incompetent, he or she is in jeopardy of being denied due process as guaranteed by the Sixth and Fourteenth Amendments. It may be even more important to recognize that the subject who is found to be incompetent may be placed in a facility that is alien and discomforting for an indeterminate period, after which the subject runs the risk of facing the very legal procedure for which he or she deemed to be incompetent to participate in originally. Thus, it behooves us to proceed carefully toward the goal of providing a thorough and valid description of cognitive functioning in all respects.

The major issues to be addressed in a competency evaluation may overlap with, but are not necessarily identical to, those elements addressed in more routine kinds of psychological assessment oriented toward clinical issues. Again, the focus is on cognitive functioning, and the more important aspects of that functioning will concern higher center operations, such as concept formation, decision processes, abstract and social judgment, reality testing or perceptual accuracy, and the extent to which any or all of these are inhibited or altered by emotional input. Thus, while matters of attention and concentration, immediate and remote memory, and the perception of details may be relevant to any final determination of competency, they are far less important to the three criteria specified in the statutes than are the higher center operations.

The description of the cognitive operations should build from the data much like a "logic tree," that is, proceeding from induction to deduction at each point. Thus, if A is true proceed to B, but if A is not true or, more commonly, if A is questionable, then proceed to descriptive subsections concerning A. Probably the best overall starting point will concern perceptual accuracy, or reality testing. This is relatively easy to assess in that it involves accurate, or reasonably accurate, contour identification. Marked distortions in reality testing typically occur only in instances of severe intellectual limitation, of organic deterioration, or of active psychotic states that may be functional or organic in nature. But even the person who is quite deficient intellectually, or the schizophrenic who is not psychotic, can and does function in reasonably adaptive ways in this area.

Possibly the second most important area in creating the descriptive "logic tree" concerns the clarity of thinking. Unlike the issue of reality testing, this is a much more difficult function to assess, as it is multifaceted. For instance, it is not at all uncommon for the subject of a competency evaluation to claim some form of amnesia for the events in question. Unfortunately, amnesia, or the report of amnesia, can arise from any of a variety of cognitive circumstances. It can occur as a result of severe intellectual deficiency; or it can occur as a result of severe distortions in thinking. Either of those could be produced by organic factors, such as cerebral trauma, senile dementia, acute or chronic toxicity, a Korsakoff syndrome, etc. However, it is also clear that when amnesia is provoked by most organic conditions, some process of confabulation, or memory substitution, occurs. Thus, the ruling out or "ruling in" of the organic possibility becomes an important step in the assessment process as it focuses on the issue of the reported amnesia. Similarly, it is not uncommon for a subject about to be evaluated for competence to present an initial picture of perplexed bewilderment, an impoverishment of ideas, a seeming disturbance of associational processes, and a disorientation for time and place. As with amnesia, such a picture can be produced by toxicity, cerebral trauma, infection, organic decay, or by any of the functional psychoses, or in a situation of very severe intellectual deficiency. It would seem simple to suggest that where such an initial picture is present, the "call" of incompetence is warranted. However, many psychological states can be disruptive to the point of creating this form of detachment and disorientation. Severe anxiety states and marked depressions are especially noted for provoking such behavioral pictures for brief periods. Obviously then, it becomes important to track down the origins of the disorientation and also obtain information concerning the permanence or probable duration of the state. Decisions about competency will probably be quite different if a state of behavioral confusion is provoked by intense anxiety, rather than being an integral part of a chronic illness that produces a major deterioration effect to some of the more important cognitive functions. It is important to note here that, as the clarity or coherence of thinking is evaluated, it is critical to avoid overgeneralizations based on unusual thinking patterns. For example, a subject may produce considerable evidence for a valid conclusion that a well-systematized delusional framework is present. But this does not automatically equate with a decision of incompetence. Some delusional operations do interfere with decision processes to the extent that understanding of charges, cooperation with counsel, and/or understanding of the consequences of proceedings is impossible, while other delusional operations may only interfere with areas of functioning that are not relevant to any of the three criteria of the statutes. It is both impractical and unrealistic to describe inappropriate ideational impulse controls without also specifying those areas of ideation that are particularly vulnerable to the control failure.

This same proposition is applicable to descriptive statements concerning the control and display of emotion. Emotion can and does affect memory, attention, stimulus processing, and decision making. It can have a substantial impact on judgment formulations; but this does not necessarily mean that when the control of emotional impulses is inadequate, the product would be so all pervasive as to routinely affect the areas relevant to the statute criteria. Conversely, poor impulse control could precipitate forms of psychological turmoil that might render the subject unable to be aware, participate, and/or understand.

The last major segment of the description of cognitive functioning should focus on the higher center operations of abstraction, or concept formation. These are important processes in the context of all three criteria of the statutes, as they contribute significantly to the capacity to synthesize information into meaningful patterns from which decision operations can proceed. Unlike the issues of thinking and emotion, these operations are more easily assessed. They are functions less prone to interference by the various functional disorders and consequently can often be used as a kind of baseline from which to study the decay or interference that has occurred to other cognitive activities.

Once the cognitive description is "in place," it can be addressed with the objective of evaluating the various operations as they relate directly to specific features of the legal process. For instance, Lipsett, Lelos, and McGarry[1] have provided a checklist of elements that are critical in the legal procedures and for which various degrees of competency in the subject should be present. This list includes such items as an awareness of available legal defenses, the ability to relate to an attorney, the appraisal of the various roles of judge, jury, and witnesses, appreciation of the charges, the capacity to disclose pertinent facts to one's own attorney, the capacity to testify relevantly, etc. Checklists such as these provide the questions about competency, while the description of cognitive functioning provides the data pool from which answers to most or all of those questions may be derived.

This procedure of extensive assessment from which a valid description of cognitive functioning is derived is cumbersome and not perfect. But it does afford the greatest form of protection to the subject, compared to more simplistic and less time-consuming approaches. This is not to suggest that efforts to establish screening approaches for competency should be avoided or abandoned, because several—such as that developed by the Harvard group under McGarry[2]—hold out considerable potential. But screening for, and final decisions about, are two different matters. Thus, if routine screening suggests incompetency, then a more comprehensive cognitive evaluation is essential. Even if routine screening does not yield suggestions of incompetency, those suggestions may be forthcoming from other data sources, such as a history, prison behavior, etc. In those instances, the comprehensive evaluation continues to be warranted.

Unfortunately, the statutes regarding competency are no more precise or any less ambiguous than statutes pertaining to issues of sanity, irresistible impulse, or diminished capacity. Until the statutes are revised to a more precise definition of competent, professionals responsible for these sorts of evaluations must take into account the full measure of cognitive operations as they are applicable to the legal procedure. An ever increasing tendency of lawyers to call upon the issue of competency as a strategy viable to their respective cases increases the likelihood of a greater number of false positives and false negatives in those instances where the more simplistic procedures of intellectual and/or diagnostic categorization are permitted.

A review of 112 cases from the data pool of Rorschach Workshops in which the issue of competency was broached by the legal community indicates that in only 4 instances were the subjects declared incompetent.. A review of assessment data in those 4 cases—some of which were collected prior to, and some after, the competency hearing—shows that two subjects were severely retarded and obviously the decision in those cases was well founded. In the remaining 2 cases, the decision of incompetency was based mainly on the diagnosis of schizophrenia. However, in the context of the total data bank available concerning those subjects, probably neither was legally incompetent—both could well understand the nature of the charges, both could interact reasonably well with an attorney in the preparation and conduct of their own defense, and both were clearly alert to the outcome.

As an esoteric exercise, we randomly selected 25 cases from the remaining 108 subjects who had been legally deemed competent to stand trial. We employed three clinical psychologists, all diplomates of the American Board of Examiners in Professional Psychology and all with an expertise in assessment procedures. We provided them, independently, with the raw assessment data on each of the 25 subjects, asking them to create a clear professional description of the cognitive functioning for each of the 25 cases and then, using the checklist of Lipsett, Lelos, and McGarry, to identify those areas pertaining to the legal process for which the subject might be deemed incompetent. Our three experts unanimously checked enough of the items positively in 4 cases that there seems to be no question that they were incompetent by legal standards. In 3 other cases, the number of items checked positive was sufficiently large to raise questions about competency at the time of trial. In the remaining 18 cases, there were uniformed negative checks, indicating that the decision of "competent" was appropriate. But the questionable cases comprise more than 20% of a randomly selected sample. The number is frightening! To be sure, the study itself is not a good one because of the lack of controls and in light of the fact that some of the assessment data in each case were collected after the fact, that is, after the hearing had been concluded. But nonetheless, the data are frightening! It is sad to believe that 4, and possibly 7, people were subjected to legal proceedings that they may not have comprehended. It is equally sad to suspect that others may have been denied the right of those proceedings, when they might well have comprehended easily the nature and consequences of those proceedings.

We are often quite critical of our legal colleagues for their adversary approach and, more particularly, for their seemingly distant attitude toward such issues as competency as they may or may not apply to a client. While some of those criticisms are valid, there is no need to reinforce ignorance with our own brand of incompetence. Let us search for the truth and display it in its full splendor. At least if we err, we do so knowing that we offered our best.

REFERENCES

1. LIPSETT, P. D., D. LELOS & A. L. McGARRY. 1971. Competency for trial: a screening instrument. Am. J. Psychiatry **128**: 105–109.
2. McGARRY, A. L., W. J. CURRAN, P. D. LIPSETT et al. 1973. Competency to Stand Trial and Mental Illness. DHEW Publication Number 74–103. National Institute of Mental Health. Bethesda, Md.

PSYCHOLOGICAL ASPECTS OF
COURTROOM TESTIMONY*

Elizabeth F. Loftus

Department of Psychology
University of Washington
Seattle, Washington 98195

In December 1978, the case of *U.S.* v. *Marshall* was tried in Seoul, Korea. The case before the court was rape. The elements in the case were the testimony of the victim and a couple of other witnesses, the testimony of the accused, and the testimony of an expert witness on the reliability of eyewitness accounts. The victim, a young black female soldier, claimed that she had been asleep in the barracks when someone entered her room in the middle of the night, physically assaulted her by striking her in the face with his fists and by choking her, and then raped her. She described her assailant as a black male, but, in part due to heavy drinking, she could not identify the defendant as the person who had raped her.

The defendant, on the other hand, gave a completely different version. He admitted that he had had sex with the victim, but claimed he had been invited. Much to his surprise, the victim then demanded $40. He told her he didn't have the money and would pay her some other time. A witness for the prosecution, a young white woman also living in the barracks, claimed that sometime early that morning she woke up and saw a man standing near her bed. She said, "What are you doing in my room?" to which the man replied something like, "Be cool," and then left. About one month later she identified the defendant as the person who had been in her room, and her version of the events supported the prosecution's contention that the defendant was wandering through the barracks looking for someone to rape, rather than the defendant's version that he had been specifically invited by the victim.

The expert testimony in the case concerned the reliability of eyewitness accounts in general and the specific accounts given in this case. It covered such factors as cross-racial identification and the ability to make an accurate identification after a 32- to 33-day interval of time.

After listening to all the evidence and to instructions from the judge, the jurors retired to deliberate. Shortly thereafter, they acquitted Private Marshall.

As the jurors in a trial (or the judge, if the jury has been waived) listen to testimony, they do more than simply take in the questions and answers. While listening, they construct in their minds an "image" of an incident

* Supported by the National Science Foundation, and by the Andrew Mellon Foundation through its support of the Center for Advanced Study in the Behavioral Sciences where the author held a fellowship during 1978 and 1979.

27

that was, of course, never witnessed by any one of them. If the incident is a crime, their image includes something about the sequence of events, who was involved, and how fleeting or frightening was the crime. If the incident is an accident, their image includes something about what happened, how severe was the accident, and who was at fault. Based on these constructed images, the jurors must then reach a verdict. It is important, then, to understand the factors that influence the construction of an incident in the minds of jurors, as a way of understanding their verdicts.

In every trial, there is a cast of characters, each one of which will impact upon the jury's decision. For each character, it is important to consider both the type of testimony that is presented and the way it is presented.

LANGUAGE AND IMAGE CONSTRUCTION

When a crime or accident occurs, a witness to the event may be asked to recall what happened in as precise detail as possible. Recent research indicates that the language used by the interviewer in questioning a witness can strikingly affect the witness' impression of his or her experience. In one experiment, subject witnesses who had seen a film of an automobile accident were asked about the speed of the vehicles, using one of several question formats. "About how fast were the cars going when they smashed into each other?" led to higher estimates of speed than the same question asked with the verb "hit."[1] Furthermore, witnesses who were queried with the verb "smashed" were later more likely to report that they had seen broken glass, an item that had not existed. The particular words in the question had apparently led the witness to develop a "memory" for the accident that was more severe than the accident actually had been.

Whenever a person experiences an event, some memorial representation is constructed. Postevent information, whether embedded in questions or presented in some other way, can become incorporated into the memory, causing an alteration or distortion in that memory.

If postevent information can so easily alter a person's memory for something that was actually witnessed, it is reasonable to expect that one could alter the construction of an event in the mind of a person who never witnessed that event. Jurors, for example, must construct in their minds a crime or accident that was never witnessed, and must then reach a verdict based upon memorial constructions that are formulated from evidence presented to them. Lawyers have known for some time that the language used in the courtroom can create an impression on the jury. In a 1974 grand jury hearing in which Dr. Kenneth Edelin of Boston, Massachusetts, was charged with manslaughter of a 5- to 7-month-old fetus, the prosecuting attorney used emotionally charged words (e.g., How old was the baby at the time of the abortion? Was the child alive at the time of the abortion?). The defense tended to use less emotional language (e.g., How old was the fetus? Was the fetus viable?). Undoubtedly these versions had very different effects on the construction of the incident in the minds of the jurors.

To study the impact of language in the courtroom, we asked 75 students at the University of Washington to act as jurors, to read some information about a case, and to reach a verdict based on the evidence presented.[2] The incident consisted of a meeting of two men at night at a marina. One man was paying blackmail money to the other. An argument ensued, and the blackmailer ended up in the water and drowned, whereupon the other man was arrested. A witness reported having seen most of the incident. The description of the incident was purposely ambiguous as to whether the blackmailer fell or was pushed in the course of a struggle.

The subject-jurors received one of two versions of the case. One version contained questions with words associated with violence, words intending to evoke emotion, or words that indirectly suggested the blackmailer may have been pushed during a struggle, while the other version contained more neutral language. An example is "How much of the fight did you see?" versus "How much of the incident did you see?"

Jurors who read the emotional version of the case were more likely to return a guilty verdict than those who read the neutral version (41% guilty votes versus 22% guilty votes, respectively). In a follow-up to this study, in which jurors were interviewed individually after returning their verdicts, it was found that those who received the emotional version had a different image of the incident. They tended to think of it as a relatively violent struggle in which the victim pushed the blackmailer over the edge of the pier, resulting in a drowning.

There are many aspects of courtroom language that are worthy of study. For example, the lexical items used by a lawyer can influence the jurors' reactions to evidence. Compare 1 and 2:

1. You testified that the light was red when the car came to the intersection.
2. It was your claim that the light was red when the car came to the intersection.

The language in the first example gives objectivity to the statement that the light was red, whereas the language in the second example gives the impression that the light may or may not have been red. (The statement beginning "It was your contention that . . ." has the same effect.) In a pilot experiment with subjects who played the role of jurors, we found that this simple lexical change influenced how much the jurors believed that the statement was true. Further, in the former case, they were more likely to include a red light in their construction of the accident and to be confident of its existence.

Jurors infer a great deal about lawyers and witnesses from the language they use. For example, during cross-examination, it is common for lawyers to use tag questions of the form: You did X, did you not?, while during direct examination, a more polite form is common: Could you please tell the court what happened on the morning of June 23, 1978? In the courtroom, the tag question is generally very aggressive and leaves the witness little room for formulating an answer. This is often what is desired in cross-examination. Tag questions are not necessarily aggressive and impolite, as when a stranger asks, It's a nice day, isn't it? Juror reactions to aggressive questioning seem to be mixed. Some jurors are impressed by the "strength" exuded by forceful questioning; others are intimidated by the badgering quality of these questions, particularly if the intonation is badgering.

Sociologist Brenda Danet[3] examined the questioning styles of various senators in the Watergate hearings and found that the stance of any particular senator towards the hearing was often given away by the preferred question form. Thus, Senator Sam Ervin relentlessly used tag questions of the form: You did X, didn't you?, while Senator Gurney, the pro-Nixon member of the Watergate committee, frequently used a form like: I am curious to know about X or Could you please tell us about X?, making the hearings sound like a casual conversation between equals, in which one person was inviting the other to fill him in on some details of mere passing interest.

Danet further observed the different tendencies of witnesses to "distance" themselves from some aspect of the situation by using abstract versus concrete terms of reference. Thus, in John Erlichman's testimony before the Ervin committee in the Ellsberg break-in, he referred to the break-in explicitly six different times in a six-minute segment of testimony. But the terms he chose, in sequence, became more and more abstract: (1) "this break-in"; (2) "an activity of this kind"; (3) "an event of this kind"; (4) "this event"; (5) "the thing." Each term is at an increasingly higher level of abstraction, incorporating all previous ones.

There seems to be no doubt that the lexical and syntactic choices that a speaker makes will influence the hearer's ideas, images, and beliefs. John Kennedy recognized this back in 1960 when he was trying to decide whether to run for president. He enlisted the help of Lou Harris and his polls to find out how people felt about politics and religion in general and whether he should openly confront the religious issue in particular. Harris designed some questions specifically to test the depth of religious tension. Example: "Is there a tunnel being dug from Rome so that the Pope can have a secret entrance to the White House if Kennedy wins?" Kennedy was appalled by this question.

"Lou," he asked, "how many people did you poll with this one?"

"About seven or eight hundred people."

"You don't think that's a little dangerous, that you might be planting the idea with some of these people?"

"Well, that's the risk."[4]

In sum, the language that is used in the courtroom and outside of it can reveal a great deal about the speaker. Equally important, it can affect a listener's construction of reality, and thereby influence behavior.

EYEWITNESS TESTIMONY

In a discussion in the House of Lords on March 17, 1973, Lord Gardiner said:

The danger of identification is that anyone in this country may be wrongly convicted on the evidence of a witness who is perfectly sincere, perfectly convinced that the accused in the many they saw, and whose sincerity communicates itself to the members of the jury who therefore accept the evidence.[5]

With these words, Lord Gardiner expressed his recognition of the fact that jurors can be influenced by the testimony communicated by a sincere eyewitness. In fact, many lines of evidence converge to demonstrate the soundness of Lord Gardiner's intuitions.

Because of its enormous impact, eyewitness testimony has been successful in causing juries to convict truly guilty people, but its danger lies in the fact that it occasionally leads to the conviction of the innocent. Honest, but mistaken, identification by prosecution witnesses was the prime cause of two recent miscarriages of justice in England. In view of the serious questions raised by those two cases, a committee was appointed to look into the law and procedures relating to identification. The committee, chaired by Lord Devlin, met for two years—between 1974 and 1976—and during this time, the committee examined all lineups that were held in England and Wales during the year 1973. Their analysis produced the following interesting results: there were 2,116 lineups in all, and the suspect was picked out in 45% of these. After being identified in a lineup, 850 people were prosecuted; but in 347 of these cases, the only evidence against the defendant was the identification by one (169 cases) or more (178 cases) eyewitnesses. Of those 347 prosecutions, 74% resulted in a conviction. This figure of 74% indicates that even when no other evidence is available, the testimony of one or more eyewitnesses can be overwhelmingly influential.

Another way to determine the impact of eyewitness testimony is through a simulated trial experiment in which subjects are asked to play the role of jurors, listen to testimony, and reach a verdict. In one study, subject-jurors were given a description of a grocery store robbery in which the owner and his granddaughter were killed. The subjects also received a summary of the evidence and arguments presented at the defendant's trial, after which each juror arrived at a verdict of guilty or not guilty.

Some of the jurors were told that there had been no eyewitnesses to the crime. Others were told that a store clerk testified that he saw the defendant shoot the two victims, although the defense attorney claimed he was mistaken. Finally, a third group of jurors heard that the store clerk had testified to seeing the shootings, but the defense attorney had discredited him by showing that he had not been wearing his glasses on the day of the robbery and that his vision was too poor to allow him to see the face of the robber from where he stood.

With no eyewitnesses, 18% of the subject-jurors felt the defendant was guilty; this rose to 72% when a single eyewitness account was added to the evidence. Interestingly, of the jurors who heard about the discredited witness, 68% still voted for conviction. The study suggests that jurors give eyewitness testimony a great deal of weight, even when that testimony is suspect.[6]

Finally, in an elaborate two-part study, jurors were asked to indicate their impressions of an eyewitness who testified during a mock trial. The study was conducted in two phases, the crime phase and the trial phase.

During the crime phase, subjects (three in each session) sat for a few minutes, whereupon a "thief" entered, posing as a coparticipant. She soon "discovered" a calculator that had apparently been left by a previous subject. She picked it up and put it in her purse, mumbling something about wanting it, and then she left the experimental room. The entire incident lasted just a few minutes. About a half minute after the "thief" left, the experimenter came into the room, gave each witness a questionnaire requesting a description of the thief, and then asked the witnesses to try to identify the thief from a set of six photographs.

In phase two, the trial phase, a new group of subjects—the jurors—were told about the staged theft and the witnesses' identifications. Then the jurors were asked to watch a cross-examination of one of the witnesses who had made an identification and to decide whether the particular witness was or was not mistaken. Some of the jurors watched the testimony of a correct eyewitness, while others watched the testing of an incorrect eyewitness. Finally, the jurors were asked for their reactions to the eyewitness. The results indicated that jurors tended to believe the eyewitness testimony about 80% of the time. What is striking, however, is that these jurors were just as likely to believe a witness who had made an incorrect identification as one who had made a correct identification.

The confidence of the eyewitness was a crucial determinant of believability. Jurors tended to believe witnesses who were highly confident more than they believed those who were not. As a whole, the data from the experiment lead to the conclusion that eyewitness testimony is likely to be believed by jurors, especially when it is offered with a high level of confidence, even though the accuracy of an eyewitness and the confidence of that witness may not be related to one another at all.[7]

In a follow-up to this work, thefts were staged under conditions designed to yield low, moderate, or high proportions of correct identifications of the thief. Again, jurors listened to the testimony of an accurate or inaccurate eyewitness and indicated how much they believed the eyewitness. Jurors changed their rate of belief of witnesses as a function of the theft conditions, but this change was minimal. Instead they responded largely to the confidence that the eyewitness placed in his or her identification. Overall, jurors were overbelieving of eyewitnesses.[8]

The impact of eyewitness testimony was recently compared experimentally to other types of evidence.[9] Subject jurors were presented with testimony in a hypothetical "bad check" case. The defendant was charged with writing a check for the purchase of a television set, a check that had insufficient funds to cover it. The jurors learned numerous details about the case, including one of four critical details. One quarter of the jurors learned that an eyewitness—a clerk who sold the set—had positively identified the defendant as the person who had passed the check. Another quarter of the jurors learned that a polygraph expert had tested the defendant and found that the defendant was lying when he said he had not written that check. One quarter of the jurors learned that a fingerprint expert had examined a print left on the counter by the person who had passed the check; it matched the prints of the defendant. Finally, one quarter learned of a handwriting expert who claimed that the handwriting on the check matched that of the defendant.

After all the testimony was in, the subject-jurors individually arrived at a verdict. Convictions were highest in the case of the eyewitness (78%) and lowest in the case of the handwriting expert (34%). The testimony of the fingerprint and polygraph experts led to an intermediate number of guilty verdicts (70% and 53%, respectively).

Why does eyewitness testimony carry so much weight? In part, this is due to the fact that people in general, and jurors in particular, lack a full understanding of the workings of memory. Some legal writers have tried to argue that

> jurors daily experience the fragility of their own memories. They know recollection fades with time and is affected by the relative significance of the incident. Probably most have experienced on several occasions their own or another's misidentification in social or business relationships.[10]

I disagree. In most of our life experience, truly precise memory is not demanded of us. Errors in recollection often go undetected because they are not particularly important; thus, people do not "daily experience the fragility of their own memories." Furthermore, a recent survey indicates that jurors are not knowledgeable about the operation of a number of important factors that affect their memories.[11] Because they tend to trust their own memories, they also tend to trust the memories of others. Information provided by an eyewitness, particularly a confident witness, is then accepted by the juror and integrated into the mental construction of the incident about which the witness is testifying. Compared to say a handwriting expert, an eyewitness generally gives a fuller account of the events that had transpired. The account typically consists of a rich description of the events and details of these events, thus providing much material for the mental construction in the minds of the jurors. Other experts provide a mere piece of evidence. Perhaps it is easier for jurors to work with a smooth account, modifying it here and there depending upon subsequent evidence, than to take small fragments and weave them together into a coherent image.

EXPERT TESTIMONY

Rule 702 of the 1975 Federal Rules of Evidence discusses the testimony of experts:

> If scientific, technical, or other specialized knowledge will assist the trier of fact to understand the evidence or to determine a fact in issue, a witness qualified as an expert by knowledge, skill, experience, training, or education, may testify thereto in the form of an opinion or otherwise.[12]

The rule is phrased broadly so that many fields of knowledge may be included. The expert is not viewed in a narrow sense, but as a person qualified in any of a number of ways—by knowledge, skill, and so on. This means that expert testimony is not limited to those with scientific or technical knowledge, such as physicians, psychologists, and economists, but includes those who are occasionally called "skilled" witnesses, such as bankers, or landowners testifying to land values.

The purpose of any evidence, including expert testimony, is to facilitate the acquisition of knowledge by the jury, or trier of fact, thus enabling the jurors to reach a final determination. Because the new federal rules are increasingly liberal in terms of their allowance of expert testimony, it is important to understand what the impact of such testimony is likely to be on the outcome of a trial. A recent study looked at the impact of one type of expert testimony—the testimony of a psychologist about the factors that affect the reliability of eyewitness accounts.[13] Such expert testimony, although relatively new, has already been allowed in numerous states around the country.[14] In this study, experimental jurors were presented with a case modeled after an actual military court-martial that took place during 1977. After reading a summary of the trial, they rendered a verdict. Some of the jurors heard expert psychological testimony, while others did not. The expert testimony described studies that have been conducted, along with experimental results, on people's ability to perceive and recall complex events. Factors that may have influenced the accuracy of the particular identification in the case at bar were related. Individual verdicts were reached. The results indicated that there were fewer convictions when expert testimony was permitted.

In a follow-up experiment, jurors received evidence in a hypothetical crime and then deliberated in "juries" of six to reach a verdict for or against the defendant. Juries who had read about the expert testimony spent much more time discussing the eyewitness account than did juries who had not been presented with expert testimony. Taken together, these studies indicate that one consequence of presenting psychological expert testimony is that it increases the amount of attention that jurors give to eyewitness accounts, perhaps enhancing their scrutinization of those accounts.

It is natural to speculate that other types of experts will similarly affect the amount of attention that jurors give to particular kinds of evidence. Economists undoubtedly increase the attention paid to financial considerations, while physicians enhance the concern for medical injuries. As jurors are constructing mental images of an incident that they hear about, expert testimony can affect the size and shape of the portion that is devoted to a particular aspect of the incident.

Natural shifts in a juror's mental construction will occur throughout the course of a trial as a response to incoming inputs. One particularly powerful phenomenon has been dubbed the "knew-it-all-along" effect.[15] As people come to learn new information, they tend to think that they knew it all along. When a witness is told, either directly or in a more subtle way, that a particular culprit had a mustache or that a given car ran through a red light, it can lead to the belief that this fact was known all along.

Jurors, too, learn information throughout a trial and can come to think that they knew these things all along. This can be worrisome in some trials where it may be necessary to try to restore the jurors to some earlier state of mind. Consider this example. On July 31, 1976, a young man named William Brooks was attending a dental school fraternity picnic at a home on Lake Tapps in the state of Washington. Throughout the day, various students and their companions used different sailboats to sail in the lake. Brooks arrived late at the party, and he and three others took a catamaran sailboat out around 4:00 in the afternoon. While sailing toward the main channel of the lake, the mast of the sailboat came in contact with power lines. The lines carried a current of 12,500 volts, which was transmitted down the mast and through the frame of the boat directly to Brooks. He was electrocuted. A lawsuit was filed by his estate to recover damages for his alleged wrongful death.[16]

The defendants took the position that everyone knows that power lines are dangerous and that death could result if a sailboat makes contact, that Brooks should have known this and should have avoided the power lines, and that the accident was thus his own fault. A critical question then became, Does everyone know that power lines are dangerous . . . ? The jurors who heard this case could not freshly evaluate this question. They were not the same "naive" persons that they had been before the trial began. Rather, they had knowledge that they had not had before; they knew, for example, about this tragic accident. The tendency for people to think that they "knew it all along" undoubtedly caused the jurors to feel that they had known all along a great deal more about sailboats and power lines than they in fact had known. They consequently might have felt that Brooks should have known too.

Can the shifting mental construction be restored to an earlier form? Expert testimony was offered by the plaintiff to try to accomplish this. The testimony took the form of a description and discussion of the "knew-it-all-along" effect. The goal of the testimony was to show how information can change one's state of knowledge, in hopes that the jurors would be less likely to judge the knowledge possessed by William Brooks in terms of the altered knowledge they now possessed.

IMAGE CONSTRUCTION TO VERDICT

In criminal cases in American courts, the burden of proof for determining guilt is the presentation of evidence leading to a belief that is "beyond a reasonable doubt." For civil cases, the standard is a "preponderance of the evidence." These concepts are pivotal. Yet confusion and misunderstanding about the meaning of these terms are widespread. While the courts are haggling the proper meaning of these terms, social scientists are attempting to discover something about the probability judgments that people use in reaching verdicts under these two standards of proof. One study claims that people translate reasonable doubt to mean a probability of guilt higher than 85%;[17] while another claims that under certain conditions, the probability of guilt required by potential jurors is quite low—in some instances as low as 55%—no different from the figure one might expect to find if the jurors were operating under the civil case standard.[18]

The bottom line is, of course, the verdict. Yet to understand how jurors reach verdicts, one must take into account their mental construction of the incidents that they are evaluating. An understanding of these mental constructions will aid in the determination of how much doubt constitutes a "reasonable doubt," or how certain a juror needs to feel that a majority of the evidence favors one party in a lawsuit. The relationship between these images and the final verdicts should become the subject of future research.

SUMMARY

As jurors in a criminal or civil trial listen to testimony, they construct in their minds an "image" of an incident that was never witnessed by them. Many psychological factors influence this mental construction and, consequently, the verdict. Research with experimental jurors has revealed:

1. The images that jurors construct are influenced by the particular words and phrases that are used in the testimony they hear.

2. Jurors tend to be overbelieving of certain types of evidence, such as eyewitness testimony. Jurors are particularly responsive to the confidence with which eyewitnesses relate their testimony, rather than to the likelihood that the testimony is accurate.

3. Expert testimony, particularly on the subject of the reliability of eyewitness accounts, can cause jurors to better scrutinize the evidence they hear.

REFERENCES

1. LOFTUS, E. F. & J. C. PALMER. 1974. Reconstruction of automobile destruction: an example of the interaction between language and memory. J. Verbal Learn. Verbal Behav. **13**: 585–589.
2. KASPRZYK, D., D. E. MONTANO & E. F. LOFTUS. 1975. Effect of leading questions on jurors' verdicts. Jurimetrics J. **16**: 48–51.
3. DANET, B. 1978. Personal communication.
4. HALBERSTAM, D. 1979. The Powers That Be. Alfred A. Knopf, Inc. New York, N.Y.
5. DEVLIN, HONORABLE LORD PATRICK (chair). 1976. Report to the Secretary of State for the Home Department of the Departmental Committee on Evidence of Identification in Criminal Cases. Her Majesty's Stationery Office. London, England.
6. LOFTUS, E. F. 1974. Reconstructing memory: the incredible eyewitness. Psychology Today **8**: 116–119.
7. WELLS, G. L., R. C. L. LINDSAY & T. J. FERGUSON. 1979. Accuracy, confidence, and juror perceptions in eyewitness identification. J. Appl. Psychol. **64**: 440–448.
8. LINDSAY, R. C. L., G. L. WELLS & C. M. RUMPEL. 1979. Juror's Detection of Eyewitness-Identification Accuracy within and across Situations. University of Alberta. Edmonton, Alberta, Canada. (Unpublished manuscript.)
9. LOFTUS, E. F. 1979. Unpublished study. University of Washington. Seattle, Wash.
10. State of Iowa v. James Thomas Galloway, 275 N. W. Rptr. (2nd edit.) 736 (Iowa Supreme Ct. 1975).
11. LOFTUS, E. F. 1979. Eyewitness Testimony. Harvard University Press. Cambridge, Mass.

12. 1975. Federal Rules of Evidence for United States Courts and Magistrates. West Publishing Co. St. Paul, Minn.
13. LOFTUS, E. F. 1980. Impact of expert psychological testimony on the unreliability of eyewitness identification. J. Appl. Psychol. **65:** 9–15.
14. FISHMAN, D. B. & E. F. LOFTUS. 1978. Expert testimony on eyewitness identification. Law Psychol. Rev. **4:** 87–103.
15. FISCHHOFF, B. 1977. Perceived informativeness of facts. J. Exp. Psychol. **3:** 349–358.
16. Brooks v. Puget Sound Power and Light, No. 253270 (Pierce County, Wash., Super. Ct. 1979).
17. SIMON, R. J. & R. J. MAHAN. 1971. Quantifying burdens of proof. Law and Society Rev. **5:** 319–330.
18. NAGEL, S., D. LAMM & M. NEEF. 1978. Decision theory and juror decision-making. Paper presented at the International Society for Political Psychology, New York, N.Y.

COMPETENCY TO STAND TRIAL: DISCUSSION

Discussant: Thomas R. Litwack

Department of Psychology
John Jay College of Criminal Justice
New York, New York 10019

Dr. Bahn's finding that policemen regularly bring assaultive individuals whom they consider to be "mental cases" to hospitals rather than to jails was interesting but not altogether reassuring. Presumably, many such individuals are soon released from the hospitals only to engage again in assaultive behavior. As a citizen, I am not sure that I would not prefer that such individuals be arrested and processed through the criminal justice system, at least initially, even if they were detained—prior to trial, to release on bail, or to some other agreed upon disposition—in a department of corrections hospital rather than jail. At least, then, they would not be released simply to reduce the population of a hospital ward or because they were difficult to manage—as might well be the case now.

However, if such individuals are being brought to hospitals, it should not be surprising to discover—as certain studies referred to by Dr. Bahn suggest—that the patient populations of the psychiatric wards of certain municipal hospitals have higher arrest rates, upon release, than that of the general population. Nevertheless, we have to be careful about how we interpret and present such results. For example, one of the studies cited by Dr. Bahn that found such higher arrest rates for released psychiatric patients was titled "Crime and Violence among Mental Patients."[1] But the patient pool involved was entirely that of Bellevue Hospital patients—hardly a representative sample of "mental patients" generally. Undoubtedly, the title "Crime and Violence among Mental Patients" is likely to stir more interest than the more accurate title: Crime and Violence among Psychiatric Patients Released from Bellevue Hospital. The use of the former title, however, does a great and inexcusable disservice to "mental patients" as a group.

As for the papers of Drs. Exner and Weinstein, I of course agree with Dr. Exner's observation that a particular IQ or psychiatric diagnosis does not render a defendant competent or incompetent—especially since a defendant's competency may depend upon the particular circumstances of the case as well as on his or her state of mind.

In one case that I know of, for example, a defendant charged with murder was found competent to stand trial—and properly so—even though he harbored the delusion that his victims had only *feigned* dying. Since the defendant was willing to allow his attorney to enter a plea of not guilty by reason of insanity, and since the attorney had access to the hospital records necessary to establish that defense, the fact that the defendant was delusional about the events in the indictment would not, and did not, prevent him from receiving a fair trial upon the issue of his insanity.[2] Indeed, his continuing delusions *strengthened* his defense. However, had this same defendant insisted upon going to trial on the sole defense that his alleged victims had not, in fact, died, then he would have been incompetent to stand trial—for then his delusions would have prevented him from rationally and adequately defending himself. (It is also worth noting that, in this case, the defendant's attorney testified on his client's behalf that he, the attorney, needed no further assistance from his client than was forthcoming to adequately defend him on the grounds of insanity. That testimony was crucial—and properly so, I believe—to the ultimate finding of competency. As the court observed, the attorney's testimony regarding the competency of his client was "the most competent source of information on the subject, with the possible exception of the defendant himself.")[2]

Similarly, courts have recognized that a defendant's claimed amnesia for the time period surrounding the crimes with which he or she is charged may or may not render the defendant incompetent to stand trial, depending upon the circumstances. For example, there were reports to the effect that Dan White, who shot and killed the mayor of San Francisco, was claiming amnesia for those events. However, as in that case, when there is no doubt that the defendant had committed the act charged—in other words, when it is clear that no alibi might emerge if the defendant's amnesia should lift (though the defendant's state of mind at the time of the crimes charged might remain in dispute)—then the defendant's amnesia would not interfere with his or her ability to maintain a reasonable defense. Indeed, if such a defendant is claiming some sort of "mental state" defense—either the insanity defense or a defense of diminished responsibility—then his present amnesia is likely to strengthen his claim that, at the time of his criminal acts, he was not "all there."

However, I wish to disagree with Dr. Exner's suggestion that the legal test for competency to stand trial is vague and ambiguous and with Dr. Weinstein's suggestion that the determination of competency or incompetency is often quite difficult. In fact (unlike the various tests for the insanity defense), the criteria for competency (or incompetency) to stand trial are quite clear and precise, and virtually identical from jurisdiction to jurisdiction. Indeed, the criteria for competency are mandated by the Constitution of the United States, since it would be unconstitutional to try a defendant who did not meet certain minimal standards of competency.

In essence, a defendant is competent to stand trial if he is capable of (1) understanding the nature of the charges and the proceedings against him; (2) rationally considering and evaluating the options available to him; (3) cooperating with his attorney in his own defense; and (4) maintaining these functions—and self-control—during a trial. That is *all* that is required for competency, and it is not much. Unless the defendant's mental state would prevent him from receiving a fair trial, the defendant is competent to stand trial—whatever his diagnosis, symptoms, or character defects.

Of course, defendants are often declared incompetent to stand trial when they are in fact competent. But that is because testifying psychiatrists and judges are often ignorant of the criteria for competency; or because—though they know that the defendants at issue are technically competent—mental health professionals and/or judges have decided that certain defendants, for their own good or for the good of society, should be in a hospital rather than in a pretrial detention center or free on bail. In neither case, however, is an erroneous finding of competency made because accurate determinations are difficult to make. In fact, when psychologists are well schooled in the legal criteria for competency, the reliability of their judgments on the subject—even when they are evaluating defendants whose competency is in question—is remarkably high, well over 90%.[3]

Indeed—leaving aside those instances in which defendants may be malingering, i.e., feigning incompetency—it seems to me that the data upon which a defendant's current level of understanding, rationality, and ability to assist his attorney must be judged can always be quickly and simply ascertained. This can be done through questions put to the defendant that directly inquire into the defendant's understanding of his situation,[4] and by questioning the defendant's lawyer as to whether or not the defendant had been able to adequately assist the attorney with the preparation of the defense.

Now this does *not* mean that it will always be easy to ultimately *conclude* whether disturbed defendants are sufficiently informed, rational, and cooperative to be fairly tried. For example, many mentally retarded defendants will have an ability to understand their situation, and to assist their attorney, that is truly on the border line between competency and incompetency. And the determination of whether a defendant has a rational, as well as a factual, understanding of his or her situation may require an equally fine judgment. For example, it may often be difficult to decide whether a defendant who refuses to raise an available defense is acting so irrationally as to be incompetent. But the *data* upon which such difficult judgments must be made will usually be readily obtainable and/or apparent from the facts of the case—the evidence against the defendant and, therefore, the relative likelihood of success of the defenses he is and is not willing to assert—and from the reasons the defendant offers for making his choices.

And whether or not a defendant is sufficiently rational to be tried is *not* an issue for psychiatrists and psychologists to make. Their job is to obtain and describe the data from which the *judge* must determine whether or not the defendant meets the legal criteria for competency. But, of course, mental health professionals can be maximally useful to the court if they present the court with data that are directly relevant to the determination of competency—and *only* with such data.

In fact, it seems to me, traditional psychological tests have no role to play in the determination of competency to stand trial except, perhaps, to aid in the determination of malingering. At least insofar as we are evaluating a defendant's cognitive capacity to stand trial, it would seem that the use of structured interviews that directly assess the defendant's understanding of the legal process and his legal situation would be adequate (assuming, again, that malingering is not in issue). What more information is needed? A broader understanding of the defendant's cognitive capacities—beyond the question of whether or not he understands his legal situation sufficiently well to fairly defend himself—is simply irrelevant.

Thus, I must disagree strongly with the implications of Dr. Exner's finding that, of a sample of cases deemed competent to stand trial, 20% were thought to be incompetent or possibly incompetent by expert clinicians who evaluated the "raw" assessment data—presumably, the results of traditional psychological tests—for each of the 25 cases. Dr. Exner takes those results to mean that numerous defendants who are in fact incompetent to stand trial are, erroneously and unfairly, being declared competent. I take those data only to mean—indeed, to prove—that even expert clinicians cannot validly assess competency to stand trial from "raw" evaluation data— that such data are irrelevant, at best, to competency determinations.

The really difficult problems for mental health professionals (as opposed to judges) in making competency evaluations are (1) determining which defendants are feigning incompetency; and (2) determining which defendants, though presently technically competent, will be unable to proceed to and/or through a trial without suffering an incapacitating breakdown, or worse. More specifically (addressing the second problem first), the fact that a defendant is severely depressed by his predicament does not render him incompetent to stand trial unless he is genuinely too depressed to rationally consider his options or to cooperate with his attorney. But if a depressed patient would be made suicidal by proceeding to trial, then surely he is incompetent to proceed.

Do we have any tools for accurately predicting which disturbed defendants who are presently competent will yet not be able to *remain* competent if forced to undergo the stress of proceeding to trial? I doubt it. So perhaps the only fair way to proceed when a defendant's future competency is in doubt is to give the defendant the benefit of the doubt. That would mean finding defendants incompetent to stand trial when doing otherwise would very possibly cause them grave injury and when they wish such a finding. But it would also mean finding defendants *competent* to stand trial when they are presently competent and wish to proceed, and when the fear that they will not be able to withstand the rigors of a trial is based on less than "clear and convincing evidence."[5] After all, it is usually legally disadvantageous to a defendant who is not incompetent to be found incompetent. Just as no mentally disturbed person's freedom should depend solely upon the demonstrably fallible predictions of psychiatrists,[6] so too a defendant's right to bail, to plea bargain, or to go to trial (perhaps to be found innocent) should not be denied upon mere predictions of incompetence. If it turns out that a defendant cannot, in fact, withstand the pressures of proceeding to or through trial, then of course the judgment of competency can always be reversed.

Moreover, unless a defendant would in fact stand trial—rather than plea bargain—if he or she is found to be competent to proceed, the issue of whether or not the defendant can withstand the stress of a criminal trial, per se, is logically irrelevant to the determination of competency. That is, unless there is good reason to believe that a disturbed defendant's case, if allowed to proceed, will culminate in a trial rather than a negotiated plea, the only legally relevant question becomes whether or not the defendant can rationally understand and participate in the plea-bargaining process.* (Of course, if proceeding to judgment in any manner would engender psychotic or suicidal behavior, then the defendant would be unfit to proceed, regardless of whether a trial or a negotiated plea would otherwise be in the offing.)

As for the issue of malingering, there will no doubt be times when defendants will seek to feign incompetence simply to get transferred from a jail to a hospital; to postpone their trial (when the odds are heavily against them) as long as possible in the hope that witnesses' memories will fade, or the like; or to set the stage for an insanity defense. But at the same time, it should be recognized that the malingering of incompetency will be relatively rare because (with the exceptions just noted) it is rarely in the defendant's interest to successfully feign incompetence. After all, upon a finding of incompetency, the defendant is no longer eligible for bail—since he supposedly needs to be treated in a hospital to be restored to competence—and the prosecutors will lose their incentive to plea bargain. Moreover, unlike the defendant who successfully feigns insanity, the defendant who successfully feigns incompetence is not relieved forever of criminal responsibility for his or her alleged crimes. Once apparent competence returns, the defendant can then be tried. And given how *very disturbed* (or retarded) a defendant must be not to meet the minimal standards required for competency, it is difficult to imagine a defendant feigning for long the overwhelming degree of disturbance that can alone render a person incompetent to stand trial. (The one exception to this would be a feigned claim of amnesia. But, as noted earlier, even true amnesia would not necessarily render a defendant legally incompetent. And the validity of a claim of amnesia can often be determined from a knowledge of the facts surrounding the supposed development of the amnesia and an understanding of the defendant's character structure.) In any case, when the validity of a defendant's apparent incompetency is in doubt, it does little harm to judge the defendant incompetent and to wait and see what develops. The defendant will be hospitalized, and if she or he is malingering, in all likelihood that will soon become apparent.

Finally, I would just like to make one brief comment about Dr. Loftus' paper. If it is true that a witness' recollection of an event is significantly influenced by how she or he is questioned about the event, then the eventual outcome of many trials may well hinge upon who gets to the witness(es) *first,* since people tend to stick to their first account of events. Thus, whether a witness to an automobile accident is first asked (by the plaintiff's attorney) How fast was the other car going when it *smashed* into my client's car? or (by the defendant's insurance company's investigator) How fast was my client's car going when the two cars collided? may well determine how the witness will respond to *either* question in the future.

---

* See Reference 7. Similarly, defendants found incompetent to proceed should not be confined, on the grounds of incompetency per se, for a longer period of time than they would have spent in confinement had they been competent and able to plea bargain.

REFERENCES

1. ZITRIN, A., A. S. HARDESTY, E. I. BURDOCK & A. K. DROSAMAN. 1976. Crime and violence among mental patients. Am. J. Psychiatry **133:** 142–149.
2. People v. Benito Rivera Maldonado, N.Y. St. Supreme Ct. (Preminger, J.)
3. STOCK, H. V. & N. G. Polythress. 1979. Psychologists opinions on competency and insanity: How reliable? Paper presented at the 87th Annual Convention of the American Psychological Association, September 1, 1979.
4. See, e.g., McGARRY, A. L., W. J. CURRAN, P. D. LIPSETT *et al.* 1973. Competency to Stand Trial and Mental Illness. DHEW Publication No. (HSM) 73-9105. National Institute of Mental Health. Bethesda, Md.
5. Cf., Addington v. Texas, 60 L. Ed. 2d 323 (1979).
6. ENNIS, B. & T. R. LITWACK. 1974. Psychiatry and the presumption of expertise: flipping coins in the courtroom. Calif. Law Rev. **62:** 693–752.
7. STEADMAN, H. 1979. Beating a Rap? Defendants Found Incompetent to Stand Trial: 112–114. University of Chicago Press. Chicago, Ill.

COMPETENCY TO STAND TRIAL:
GENERAL DISCUSSION

Moderator: Gerald W. Lynch

John Jay College of Criminal Justice
New York, New York 10019

H. C. WEINSTEIN (*New York University Schools of Medicine and Law, New York, N.Y. 10016*): We should not fail to note that the vast majority of competency-to-stand-trial questions are determined by the lawyer, using common sense. The lawyer discusses the case with his client and decides—usually, no doubt, without thinking much about the matter—that his client is competent to stand trial. If nothing else comes to the attention of the lawyer or the court, the issue is settled. Thus, relatively few cases come to be evaluated by a psychiatrist.

I would like to add my reaction to a number of points made by my colleagues here this morning. Dr. Loftus' discussion of the eyewitness and the jury reminded me of a point relating to the right to refuse treatment as it relates to the competency-to-stand-trial question. In his textbook, Alan Stone points out that "any defense attorney will recognize that one of the best pieces of evidence for convincing a jury that a person was not responsible for his crime is a defendant who is obviously crazy at the trial. That dramatic impression is blunted by the drugs. The effect of such drugs, when unknown to the jury in its appraisal of a defendant's demeanor, has in fact led to the reversal of a conviction."*†

In other words, there is an argument for not treating a patient while he is awaiting trial. The problem here, of course, is that such a patient would be held incompetent to stand trial under ordinary circumstances. On the other hand, however, there is an argument that the best interests of the patient would be served by proceeding with the trial.

Again, I make the same comment about some of Dr. Exner's data; namely, that the judge may have decided (and we sometimes forget it's the judge who decides this, not the psychologist or psychiatrist) that a particular patient is competent, or rather that he should be tried because of certain realities of the matter. For example, the judge may feel that it would be more advantageous to a particular defendant to be tried and get time served and be freed.

So the findings of the psychologists or the psychiatrists, while relevant, may not be the determining factor in a decision by a judge, and yet the data may have shown that the patient was incompetent. These are called dispositional decisions—where the judge, lawyers, and doctors get together and

---

* STONE, A. A. 1975. Mental Health and Law: A System in Transition. National Institute of Mental Health. Bethesda, Md.
† State v. Murphy, 56 Wash. 2d 761, 768, 355 P 2d 323, 327 (1960).

say, in a low-visibility way, This is what we think is best; and Let's call it this way rather than some other way.

Finally, on the issue of malingering, and particularly the case that was cited of a patient who wanted to go to trial—we call that malingering mental health. The patient who is really quite ill and yet says: I want to go to trial. I don't care what you say about me; I want to go to trial. Well, we have to assess that too. Suppose his reason is really a wish to hurt himself, then how do we find that patient? We remember that the classic case in the literature, Hadfield's case in 1800, was of a man who shot at King George III in a theater in the hope that he would be tried and executed; he acted on the basis of a delusion that if he were tried and executed, the world would be saved. Was he competent to stand trial?

VOCAL INDICATORS OF PSYCHOLOGICAL STRESS

Harry Hollien

*Institute for Advanced Study
of the Communication Processes
University of Florida
Gainesville, Florida 32611*

People have been attempting to assess the presence, absence, and/or magnitude of psychological stress from the speech and voice production of other individuals since primitive man added a cognitive overlay to his repertoire of oral signals. Indeed, it is quite probable that crude assessments of this type were attempted even before organized communicative sounds existed among our species. Quite obviously, these analyses were (and are) attempted for a rather substantial number of reasons, some of which are within the scope of forensic psychology. They include assessment of the presence and magnitude of such emotional states as hostility, aggressive intent, fear, and anxiety; behaviors such as deception or divisiveness; even psychopathological states can be included under this rubric.

There is little question but that emotional and/or behavioral conditions of this type exist and their detection is of consequence. For example, it can be important for monitor personnel to be able to determine the levels and types of stress present in individuals who are physically separated from them—i.e., pilots, astronauts, aquanauts, etc.—irrespective of the message content of the spoken interchange. It is desirable also for a worker at a crisis control center to be able to tell if the caller actually is going to commit suicide from the manner in which he or she communicates. Knowledge of the acoustic/temporal speech clues that correlate with psychosis can be important to clinical personnel. In short, many instances can be cited where information about the behavioral intent or emotional states of an individual could be useful.

Law enforcement personnel, also, would find systems or procedures that could reliably identify the emotions felt by the talker, the presence of lying, or the presence/absence of psychosis helpful in their work. Moreover, if such procedures could be carried out rapidly, on-scene decisions sometimes could be made that currently are not possible. In any case, it would appear that the activities of law enforcement, intelligence, and security agencies all would benefit if the various stress states cited above could be instrumentally identified.

Before any attempt is made to discuss the possible vocal correlates of psychological stress, it will be necessary to clarify a number of terms. The concept of stress is, in and of itself, quite difficult to define. For example, sometimes this term is used to refer to the emphasis patterns an individual uses when uttering a spoken message, and, of course, the ways by which such linguistic emphasis is produced have been studied.[11,30,32,33,49,59] However, these speaking characteristics are only of minor importance to the

47

issues considered in this paper. Admittedly, *some* information about an individual possibly could be deduced by careful analysis of the elements that are stressed within the message. Nevertheless, to date, no very good techniques have been developed for this purpose; i.e., we are not able to predict reliably an individual's emotional state by the way he or she emphasizes specific words within an utterance.

Stress, as it is used in this paper, refers to psychological states, and rather specific ones. Moreover, no matter how psychological stress becomes operative, its presence in a person is the result of some sort of threat;[4] or as Lazarus points out,[48] to be stressed, an individual must anticipate confrontation with a harmful condition of some type. He further points out that the strength of the stress response pretty much results from the magnitude of the threat. Unfortunately, however, a particular stressor, or stressful situation, may result in different responses from different individuals. Nevertheless, a threat ordinarily will create some degree of anxiety, fear, or anger in a given individual. These psychological states are often referred to as emotions, but as Arnold points out,[5] it must be remembered that there are many other emotions (for example, love, joy, happiness) that have little or nothing do to with stress. Hence, the Hicks definition of stress will be adopted for this paper: "stress . . . is a psychological state that is a response to a perceived threat and it will be accompanied by specific emotions."[40] The emotions in this case are, of course, anxiety, fear, and anger; they are consistent with the forensic model.

In the forensic milieu, three types of stress-related situations are of interest. First, it may be useful to obtain insight about the stress-related emotions an individual is experiencing at a given moment. As will be seen below, a few studies have been carried out in this area, and some tentative relationships can be established relative to the particular acoustic and temporal voice/speech features that appear to correlate with some of the emotional behaviors investigated. It would be expected that knowledge of those cues that could be used to predict specific emotional states would be of substantial value to law enforcement and related personnel. Unfortunately, however, clear-cut relationships have not yet been found—and for a number of reasons. For example, in some cases the research is carried out in the laboratory, and the "stress" applied is defined only in terms of the stressor; hence, the results of this type of research often are of only minimal use to individuals working in the forensic area. Other research approaches exhibit weaknesses also. To illustrate, when emotions are studied, actors ordinarily are used to portray them, as it is not often possible to study individuals who have talked first while experiencing powerful emotions and then later when the stress-inducing conditions are absent. Indeed, it is rarely possible to carry out controlled research on individuals who are experiencing actual stress, even though a few studies of this type have been reported. In any event, an attempt will be made to synthesize research results of the types cited above and to suggest at least a few voice and speech characteristics that can be thought to accompany stress.

Second, it should be of use to law enforcement (and related) agencies to be able to determine from the vocal signal alone whether a speaker is suffering from some psychosis—particularly a specific (clinical) disorder, such as schizophrenia. Substantial research has been carried out on the speech/voice correlates of such disorders. However, practically all of this research (except some of the earlier subjective work) has used medicated patients as subjects. Nevertheless, some insight can be gained from reviewing this area, and while the vocal correlates of psychosis are not as central to this paper as are the other two issues, relevant research will be summarized briefly. Nor should it be forgotten that information about clinical conditions sometimes can lead to a better understanding of the behavior of individuals not exhibiting pathology.

Finally, it is obvious that law enforcement, security, and intelligence agencies would benefit substantially from having available reliable systems that could detect lying or other forms of spoken deception. Currently, there are electronic systems in existence that are purported to do just that. They are said to be based on the notion that when a person lies, he or she experiences stress (presumably fear or anxiety) and, in doing so, exhibits certain vocal characteristics that can be measured. However, it remains to be seen whether lying and stress correlate to a high degree and whether there are any simple features that will permit the easy and reliable identification of these states. Nevertheless, lie detection by voice analysis appears to be a stress-related issue, and a very important one. Hence, a review of this area constitutes the third topic addressed by this paper.

VOCAL INDICATORS OF STRESS

There are many commonly held notions about the way speech *should* sound when a person is experiencing stress. Some individuals would argue that anger "should" result in loud, harsh speech; fear in a high-pitched, staccato output. Almost any person will venture at least a tentative identification of the voice and speech characteristics they feel accompany some of the more common emotions. But what information about these issues can be found in the relevant research literature? Do the commonly held stereotypes withstand scrutiny when scientific procedures are applied?

Not nearly enough research has been carried out on the voice/speech correlates of emotion and stress. With respect to emotions, a number of authors have indicated that it is possible to perceptually identify some of them (see, among others, Bonner;[12] Costanzo et al.;[18] Davitz and Davitz;[21] Simonov et al.;[78] and Starkweather[81,82]). For example, Fairbanks and Pronovost[28] report correct identification of simulated emotions of up to 88%, and other authors concur; the Lieberman and Michaels[51] listeners correctly identified emotional content 85% of the time. Of course, it should be stressed that much of the research in question has been carried out on emotions simulated by actors. It is possible that actors caricature emotions, or in some manner accentuate a feature (or features) that is easily identifiable; it may not be as easy to identify the emotions of a person who is actually experiencing them. However, there is some suggestion that identifications of this type can be made also.[84] Thus, if it is possible to perceptually recognize emotions from the paralinguistic elements in voice and speech,[77] it likewise should be possible to identify the relevant acoustic and/or temporal features that lead to these identifications.

Frequency

Speaking fundamental frequency (SFF) and patterns of f_0 usage would appear to be one such feature. In 1939, Fairbanks and Pronovost[28] reported SFF data on six actors simulating anger, fear, grief, contempt, and indifference (the message content was held constant). They reported that the highest mean SFF was observed for anger—with fear a close second—and that contempt and especially indifference showed lower mean frequency levels. These authors further indicated that wide frequency ranges were observed for anger and fear (fear exhibited the widest) and narrow ranges for grief and indifference. Finally, they suggested that changes in SFF are rapid for anger and slow for contempt. Thus, it can be seen that some patterns appear to emerge from data even as limited as these. Later, Williams and Stevens[85] carried out a similar study on simulated anger, fear, sorrow (grief?), and a neutral speaking condition. Their results were reasonably similar to those of Fairbanks and Pronovost, except that they found f_0 to be relatively high for anger and only slightly elevated for fear. It should be noted, also, that in an earlier study, Williams and Stevens[84] found that pilots and control tower operators showed an increase in SFF as a function of increased levels of stress—a finding essentially confirmed by Kuroda et al.[47] Since stress probably relates to fear in this case, these results are quite consistent with those cited earlier.

Hicks also has studied SFF as it relates to stress.[40] He defined stress in terms of fear and anxiety, specifically studying the speech of subjects who had stress induced by electric shock and where stress occurred as a result of the subject's making a public speech. He found SFF to be increased somewhat for both stress conditions (especially for the second) but not always significantly so. On the other hand, Markel et al. report that they did not observe any increase in perceived pitch to accompany word-induced hostility or anger but, in some cases, they found lowered pitch to relate to depression.[55] Nor did Almeida et al. find a consistent trend relating f_0 measures to stress (some subjects raised f_0, others lowered it).[1] In a sense, the data reported by Hecker et al.[38] agree with the findings of these authors. Specifically, they required 10 subjects to perform a meter-reading/mathematical task while stress levels were manipulated. These authors report somewhat inconsistent SFF behaviors for their subjects, with some raising f_0 and others lowering it. Finally, the announcer who described the Hindenburg disaster is known to have increased his SFF as a function of emotions he felt during the crash.[84]

In summary, it would appear that—while no definite statements can be made and there is substantial individual variation among subjects—some

TABLE 1

VOICE PARAMETERS THAT APPEAR TO CORRELATE WITH EMOTIONS,
AS CONTRASTED TO NONEMOTIONAL UTTERANCES

Emotion	Feature*		
	Mean SFF Level	Vocal Intensity	Temporal
Anger	+ +	+ +	+
Fear	+	+	+
Grief†	−	−	−
Contempt	−	+	−
Indifference	−	0	+

* + greater than normal; − reduced from normal; 0 not significantly different from normal.
† Sorrow and depression appear to show similar patterns.

patterns emerge relating SFF to stress and/or to certain emotions;* they
may be seen in TABLE 1. Specifically, it would appear that anger and fear
probably are accompanied by raised f_0, and grief, contempt, and indifference by lowered SFF. That is, the presence of either of the two emotions
closely related to stress in the forensic sense (fear/anger) ordinarily can be
expected to result in the individual's raising his or her speaking fundamental
frequency. Of course, it should be remembered that this parameter shifts
with respect to normal usage patterns. Hence, to be helpful to law enforcement agencies, data based on this metric must be compared with baseline
curves for that same individual, obtained from speech produced in a neutral
speaking environment. Currently, comparisons of this type are not easily
made.

Frequency Variability

The data on frequency variability are not very orderly; hence, very little
space will be devoted to this issue. There appears to be some increase in SFF
variability for anger but less of an increase, if any at all, for fear.[28,85] Moreover, if the variability findings are summarized under the general rubric of
stress, the available data permit almost any position at all to be argued, i.e.,
SFF variability related to stress (1) may increase;[28] (2) may decrease;[84,85] (3)
may not change at all;[40] or (4) may vary from speaker to speaker.[38] Thus, a
metric of this type probably would not be of particular use to law enforcement groups, even if it were easily available. A related factor that could
prove helpful, however, is the regularity of speaking fundamental frequency (or lack of it). The authors of the above studies (and others) have noted
that when talking, stressed individuals exhibit behaviors such as voicing

---

* The emotions of grief/sorrow, contempt, and indifference are included to permit better
understanding of the two emotions of primary interest.

irregularities, discontinuities in f_o contours, irregular vocal fold vibration, and even vocal tremor.

Intensity

Vocal intensity as related to stress has been investigated by Hicks.[40] Some of his measurements suggest that intensity is raised as a function of stress; the obtained values increased slightly for his group where fear/anxiety was induced by shock and increased significantly for his "public speakers." Since Hicks was able to measure absolute intensity, it is possible that his data are more powerful than most of the other findings in this area. It must be noted, however, that Markel et al. reported that they did not find significant increases in perceived loudness for anger but that there was a slight trend for loudness reduction associated with depression.[55] On the other hand, in a previous article,[18] Costanzo et al. reported data (a high correlation between perceived loudness and anger) that agree with Hicks—as do Williams and Stevens, who also found some increases in vocal intensity to be associated with anger.[85]

Several other investigators have provided information about vocal intensity–stress relationships. For example, Friedhoff et al. reported that intensity tended to increase when their subjects lied and presumably were experiencing stress.[31] On the other hand, Hecker et al. did not observe consistent intensity differences between their nonstressed and stressed speaking conditions.[38] Of their 10 subjects, 6 showed small and/or inconsistent differences, 1 exhibited increased intensity as a function of stress, and 3 exhibited decreased intensity. Finally, Huttar used semantic differential scales to study emotions and relate them to acoustic measurements.[43] In most cases, his data are consistent with the generalizable findings relating types/levels of stress to vocal intensity. Probably the best evidence, based on a compilation of all the studies reviewed, is that vocal intensity is increased especially for anger, somewhat for fear and perhaps contempt, but is reduced for grief (see again, TABLE 1). However, as with speaking frequency, these data show inconsistencies, and even where the shifts appear stable, it is necessary to compare the obtained values with those related to subjects' control (unstressed) samples.

Time

The temporal analysis of speech and voice—as it relates to stress and emotions—has led to relatively few generalizations. Not many studies have used the same research protocols or, with the exception of rate, similar metrics. However, based on Fairbanks and Hoaglin,[29] Williams and Stevens,[85] Hicks,[40] Bachrach,[6] Ross et al.,[72] and Scherer,[74] at least some relationships can be suggested. It should be noted also that the temporal features column found in TABLE 1 summarizes these findings irrespective of the specific measure. That is, since tendencies only are considered, just the *direction* of the shift—not the type or amount—is indicated. Nevertheless, it can be argued that some intriguing relationships can be found among the time-stress contrasts.

Anger appears to be accompanied by rapid speaking rate and short durations of phonations and pauses;[29] Markel *et al.*[55] agree—at least with respect to rate—as do Williams and Stevens[85] with respect to patterning. According to Fairbanks and Hoaglin,[29] fear is similarly typified, and Bachrach[6] agrees, but Williams and Stevens apparently did not observe parallel relationships (at least they were not systematic). Hicks, also, failed to find that increases in rate correlate with stress (fear/anxiety?). Using another temporal measurement technique, Hicks reported that the number of speech bursts and pauses was significantly reduced as a function of increased stress—a finding consistent with those reported by Fairbanks and Hoaglin, Williams and Stevens, and Hecker *et al.* Specifically, when Hicks carried out a complex analysis of the temporal properties of his subjects' speech (based on the multiple analyses of overall speech patterning), he found significant shifts in his experimental vector accompanying induced stress. Specifically, Hicks' data suggest that when a person is speaking under stress, he or she will exhibit a strong tendency to produce rather long speech bursts—longer, that is, than those to be found in their usual speech rhythms. This particular relationship is one that could be useful to law enforcement personnel in assessing the stress level of a subject. Finally, it is to be noted that nonfluencies may be associated with the speech of individuals who are talking under conditions of stress. For example, Hicks found this to be the case especially for his group where electric shock was the stressor. On the other hand, Silverman and Silverman report that when they threatened to administer electric shock to normal speakers whenever they were nonfluent, their subjects became more fluent.[76] However, these data actually are not in variance with those reported by Hicks as, in this case, the subjects merely demonstrated that they could speak without nonfluencies if they were challenged to do so.

But what of the other emotions? From a synthesis of the findings relative to indifference, it appears that speech rate is somewhat elevated for this emotion. It also appears likely that speech rate and related temporal measures are reduced for contempt and especially for grief (sorrow, depression). In the case of grief, it appears that the reduction in speech rate is due primarily to the prolongation of pauses, particularly between phrases. As stated above, however, these emotions are not as important to law enforcement personnel as are those more closely related to the forensic model. They do provide useful contrasting data, however.

To summarize the acoustic/temporal correlates of stress, the question can be asked, Do the data to be found in TABLE 1 accurately portray the patterns that can be expected in voices reflecting the listed emotions? Unfortunately, only a qualified response can be given to this question. Nevertheless, it is possible to suggest the speech/voice changes that probably would occur when an individual speaks under stressed conditions. Basically, one could expect speaking fundamental frequency to be raised somewhat, vocal intensity to be increased, and, perhaps, the speech rate to be increased slightly. Moreover, there is a very good chance that the stressed individual would exhibit increased nonfluencies and would use relatively long utterances. However, it must be remembered that this description is based on the concept that these features are shifted, or changed, from those exhibited by the same individual in normal or neutral speaking situations. To be of value to more than a very limited forensic model, it will be necessary to specify those acoustic/temporal features that relate directly to stress, since in most instances, a reference profile of a given person's speech probably will not be available. Finally, while some understanding of the speech and voice features that functionally correlate with specific stress and/or emotional conditions is desirable, apparently the parameters identified are not robust enough to be used for the identification of stress and emotions in the field. Indeed, the development of such indicators appears to belong substantially in the future.

Vocal Indicators of Psychosis

There is no question that psychotics experience some form of psychological stress, and there is very good reason to believe that such conditions manifest themselves in the speaking behaviors of these individuals.[15,54] Obviously, then, it is important to identify the vocal correlates of these disorders both for the expected medical reasons and for a reason that is not so clearly recognized, i.e., that information about the relationships of interest possibly can provide useful data concerning the speech characteristics of individuals experiencing short-term stress of a nonclinical type. A secondary purpose for studying the speech of these individuals is one that relates to the forensic milieu: Can a psychotic be recognized as a person who is ill simply by analysis of his or her speech? A brief review of relevant research in this area would appear warranted.†

In order to provide a reasonable structure for this discussion, a system of classifying psychotics has been chosen. It is recognized that there are a number of available and/or acceptable approaches that could be used for this purpose. However, one classification system that would appear defensible divides psychotic states into the following: (1) schizophrenia, with three subcategories according to age: (a) adult, (b) adolescent, and (c) childhood; and (2) affective disorders including: (a) depression (general), (b) involutional depression, and (c) manic-depressive disorders. The present review will use this classification system, in modified form, primarily because most of the reported research uses similar classification categories. The modification will be to reduce these several categories to their two major components: (1) schizophrenia (adult/adolescent) and (2) affective disorders (depression/involutional depression). It is unlikely that organiza-

† For a more thorough review of this area, see Darby and Sherk.[20]

tion of the available data into these two relatively gross categories will do violence to the discussed relationships, since very few of the relevant investigators used subject classifications more rigorous than these.

It must be stressed once again that most of the research to be reported was carried out on patients who had been sedated or who were on a course of psychotropic drugs. For this reason, the observed relationships/data may not reflect the true vocal correlates of any particular psychological disorder. Nevertheless, some insight into the area can be gained from a judicious analysis of the available material. Anyway, if a particular psychotic were found in an unmedicated, acute, and (perhaps) violent state, there probably would be little need to carry out any form of speech analysis in order to discover if that person needed help.

Schizophrenia

One of the earliest of the modern investigators was Moses,[60] who attempted to describe the voice of schizophrenics. He reported that his patients' voices were similar to those of children, that they used very high pitches (in male patients, the phonation apparently was typical of that used by females), and that they exhibited "inappropriate" accents and emphasis as well as "rhythmic repetition of vocal patterns." Moskowitz[61] also was interested in this type of patient. He studied the speech of 40 schizophrenics—roughly matched to 40 controls by means of a rating scale—and observed that his patients exhibited "monotonous and weak speech with a flat colorless tone quality." As may be seen, these comments are somewhat anecdotal in nature; nevertheless, they provide some insight into the speech of schizophrenics and form a base for the more precise research that was carried out subsequently.

Ostwald,[65-67] also a pioneer in this area, was particularly interested in adolescents. For example, in 1964, he reported that he had assessed the speech of an adolescent schizophrenic male; this patient showed patterns of rapid frequency shifts and intermittent sound production.[67] In 1966, he and Skolnikoff published their observations of another male adolescent schizophrenic.[68] They reported his speech to be abnormal primarily as follows: (1) voice quality was nasal; (2) articulation was impaired; and (3) breath control was poor. Moreover, this patient's vocal tract was studied by means of a radiographic technique, and the authors report that sometimes the velum did not seal off the nasopharynx, a condition that presumably resulted in the perceived nasality. Time-frequency-amplitude spectrograms were made of the patient's speech signal, and from them, the authors suggest that (1) certain frictional noises of his consonants were missing; (2) shifts occurred in his vowel formants; (3) articulation of the stop consonant was poor; (4) his intonation patterns were inappropriate; and (5) SFF was abnormally high. These observations appear to be in agreement with those of Moses and Moskowitz, especially with respect to the difficulties in articulation, high SFF, muted voice quality, excessive variability in speech rate/rhythm, and, of course, the apparent lack in this type of patient of a finely tuned, integrated control of the vocal apparatus.

Ostwald[65,66] also is responsible for one of those relatively rare instances where a schizophrenic patient was investigated both before and after treatment. In this regard, he has reported observations of a 16-year-old girl who entered the hospital in an acute state of schizophrenia, characterized by withdrawal and apathy. At that time, he noted that she exhibited "monotonous" voice quality and, hence, carried out an acoustic analysis of her voice. Following five weeks of hospitalization, psychotropic medication, and therapy, Ostwald again evaluated this patient and suggested that several speech changes had taken place: (1) her spectral power curve showed a rise in intensity; (2) her vowel formants showed "appreciable change"; (3) her voice showed less "compactness"; and (4) her oral reading had speeded up by an average of 0.06 seconds per syllable. Stated differently, Ostwald interpreted his observations to mean that his patient's speech improved as a function of therapy and showed improvement in speaking intensity level, SFF and intensity variability, and precision of articulatory gestures.

Spoerri reports that he studied a very large population of schizophrenics ($N = 350$).[80] His listing of the voice/speech correlates of schizophrenia is reminiscent of earlier investigators. He typifies the speech of his patient/subjects as exhibiting (1) strain; (2) harshness; (3) register changes (to falsetto); (4) dysarticulation; (5) volume changes (to loud); (6) speed changes with inappropriate alternations; (7) "gloomy, dull timbre"; and (8) monotonous melody. Moreover, Spoerri related voicing irregularities to schizophrenia, and it will be remembered that this characteristic also was found in the speech of individuals experiencing high levels of stress. Later Chevrie-Muller et al. studied 53 hospitalized adolescent schizophrenics (ages 12–23 years) and an age-matched control group.[17] Their only significant finding was that female schizophrenics tended to show a reduction in frequency variability re normal females; the trend for males was similar but not of statistical significance. They also noted that reading time was longer for the schizophrenics, but not significantly so. Since the Chevrie-Muller et al. findings are somewhat in variance with those of most other investigators, they have attempted to explain their data. Basically, they contend that the (phenothiazine) medications administered to their patients possibly biased their results. Finally, Bannister compared 8 adolescent schizophrenics to 17 hospitalized nonpsychotic patients and to a second control population.[7] In this case, the schizophrenic subjects exhibited significantly reduced f_0 variability when compared to the control groups—these results tend to agree with most other published data.

A classic study was carried out in 1968 by Saxman and Burk.[73] They investigated 37 hospitalized schizophrenic females in relation to speaking fundamental frequency level (SFF), fundamental frequency deviation (FFD), and both mean (overall) and sentence reading rates. They contrasted these data to similar observations of a group of 22 female controls. Perhaps most important, they carried out their research 48 hours after psychotropic medication had been discontinued; hence, they are among the very few investigators to study psychotics who were not medicated. Saxman and Burk report that their schizophrenic population exhibited a higher mean SFF than the controls but that this finding was not of statistical significance. The schizophrenic group, however, did show significant differences (from the normal) relative to oral reading rates (slower) and frequency variability (larger FFD). It should be noted that the Saxman and Burk findings of increased FFD are in contrast to most other studies of schizophrenia. However, since they tested their patients after the discontinuation of medication, it is possible that they were recording an acute schizophrenia process obscured in other studies by the medication effect. Perhaps the single variable of medication is controlling in studies of this type. In any case, this particular investigation suggests that a great deal more research is needed before stable relationships will be found with respect to the vocal correlates of schizophrenia.

Several recent investigations provide additional insights of the speech-schizophrenia interface. Denber investigated the voices of 20 male schizophrenics, 31 controls, and 61 depressed patients.[22] He found that speech power, vocal jitter, and SFF differentiated his schizophrenics from the controls but did not find significant differences between his two psychotic groups. Some of Denber's observations are confirmed by Hollien and Darby,[41] who studied 23 schizophrenics, 15 involutional depressives, and 20 controls. These investigators used perceptual identifications, SFF, FFD, reading time, phonation time, and phonation time ratio (P/T) in an attempt to differentiate among their three populations. They found that their controls were (perceptually) identified as nonpsychotic 88% of the time but that their auditors could not systematically separate the schizophrenics from the depressives. Their findings for SFF were nonsignificant, but the noted trend (lowered SFF for the schizophrenics) was somewhat in variance with the findings of most other investigators—except perhaps Scherer,[74] who observed that for his patients, SFF increased as a function of treatment. It should be noted also that the P/T ratios separated Hollien and Darby's two psychotic populations from the controls; however, the meaning of this relationship is not clear.

Unfortunately, robust voice/speech predictors of schizophrenia do not appear to be available. This lack of strong relationships may be due to a number of factors, such as too general a classification system, the effects of medication, and so on. Of course, it could be due to the fact that there simply are no speech/voice features that systematically correlate with schizophrenia; however, the evidence suggests that there probably are such correlates and that ultimately they will be identified. In the interim, it is possible that the noted tendencies can be used to relate speech parameters to schizophrenia in the following manner: (a) fundamental frequency level (SFF) appears to be somewhat higher for schizophrenics than for normals; (b) fundamental frequency deviation (FFD) tends to be reduced for schizophrenics where patients are medicated but increased where they are not; (c) rate and rhythm phenomena may be important—it appears that the prolongation of pause time, elongation of certain words or phonemes, and increased reading times typify schizophrenics (at least if they are medicated); and (d) it is possible that formant features may be abnormal in schizophrenia and may change with treatment; high-low frequency spectra contrasts may be important also.[74]

Affective Disorders: The Depressed

It should be remembered that there are several classes of depressed patients. The most common (other than mixed or general) are the involutional depressives and the manic-depressives. However, this review will collect all types of affective disorders into a single category—that of depression—primarily because, so far, no voice or speech analyses have been able to differentiate among these groups. Indeed, it has not been conclusively demonstrated that depressives speak differently than do normals. It also should be remembered that, as with schizophrenics, virtually all the research carried out on the communicative attributes of these patients has involved speech samples obtained when the subject/patients have been medicated and the acute effects of the disease may have been obscured by the drugs administered. However, a brief review of the relevant research may provide some information about people who are depressed and how it may be possible (eventually) to identify these conditions from speech and voice analyses.

In 1938, Newman and Mather studied the speech of 40 depressed patients whom they classified into several subgroups.[63] Basically, however, they found that the "classical" depressive patients exhibited voice qualities that were "dead or listless"; had narrow pitch ranges; and exhibited slow speech tempo (with frequent pauses and hesitations) and a lack of emphatic accents. Speaking resonance was described as "pharyngeal" and "nasal," and these patients appeared to have limited syntax and a short length of response. Moses characterized the "depressed" voice as one that exhibits uniformity with a regular repetition of the "same gliding down interval."[60] He indicated that when "tone" was lowered, intensity decreased proportionately and that it is this relationship that is responsible for the monotonous voice quality attributed to depressed states. Eldred and Price appear to agree.[26] They report their impressions of the speech and voice patterns of a single patient whom they studied extensively during a 13-month period of psychoanalysis. They suggest that depressed states are accompanied by decreases in pitch, rate, and/or volume and by narrow pitch ranges. However, it is possible that, since their subject was relatively old, some of the voice/speech characteristics they observed could be due to the physiological changes that accompany aging.

Later, Hargreaves et al. published a study of 32 psychiatrically hospitalized patients classified as depressed.[36] For this research, they correlated mood ratings and power spectra before, during, and after treatment. Predictions of mood ratings from voice spectra correlated significantly for 25 of the 32 patients, and these correlations were largest for those patients who showed the greatest changes in mood; Helfrich and Scherer[39] also discuss a relationship of this type. Subsequently, the 10 patients who showed the greatest change were tested to discover if there was a uniform voice quality for states of depression. Of the 10, 5 were found to exhibit a "depressed" voice, i.e., reduction in loudness and a corollary reduction "in the higher overtones." The authors suggest that this combination resulted in a "dull, lifeless" voice quality, with diminished inflection (see also Rice et al.[71]). Of the remaining 5 patients, 3 exhibited voices that were actually louder and sometimes higher in pitch during depression than otherwise. The authors suggest that depressive symptoms may result in several different clusters of patterns and that each cluster could be associated with some subclass of the disorder.

After a period during which relatively little speech/voice research on depressed patients was carried out, Darby and Hollien report data on six patients before and after electroconvulsive treatment.[19] Prior to treatment, the voices of these patients were perceptually characterized by a speech pathologist as "dull" and lacking in vitality. Following treatment and with moderate clinical improvement, the voices were judged by the same speech pathologist to have regained some of their normal vitality. Further perceptual analysis resulted in the observation that improvement occurred in articulation and pitch inflection (five patients) and in linguistic stress (four patients). Instrumental analysis also was carried out, but significant trends were not detected in speech power spectra, SFF, FFD, or speaking rate. The lack of significant instrumental findings in this study is of interest. Further, the results would appear to be at variance with those from several other investigations (for example, see Helfrich and Scherer[39]) and especially with Ostwald's[66] findings of increased intensity centered around 500 Hz following electroconvulsant therapy. Possible explanations of these differences could relate to the different methods of analyzing the data. First, Darby and Hollien's subjects were not studied individually but rather as a group, since it is safe to generalize only those relationships that are universal (or pretty much so). Thus, in this instance, the pretreatment spectral curves were averaged and then compared to the mean posttreatment curves. Since no statistically significant differences appeared, the frequency bands centering around 500 Hz were not individually compared, nor were other frequency regions within the overall spectra. Another investigator, Denber,[22] who studied 61 male depressives, 31 controls, and 20 schizophrenics, appears to have found some evidence that a related measure—power—is increased as a function of depression. However, he did not section his spectrograms into high and/or low frequency bands either; and, as a matter of fact, his finding that speech power is increased for depressives tends to run counter to the findings of most other investigators. It also is interesting to note that of Denber's 20 other measures, only the 2 parameters of SFF and jitter differentiated the psychotics from the normals, and jitter alone appeared to separate the groups on a three-way basis.

Finally, two studies have been reported recently. As stated, Hollien and Darby used perceptual ratings, SFF, FFD, reading time, phonation time, and P/T ratios in an attempt to differentiate among their three groups of subjects (15 involutional depressives, 23 schizophrenics, and 20 controls).[41]

It will be remembered that they found the controls could be identified as normal 88% of the time, that the psychotics usually were identified as clinical cases, but that the judges could not differentiate systematically between the two clinical groups. These authors do note, however, that the depressive patients exhibited slightly lower SFF than did the controls (nonsignificant), as well as a slower reading time; the P/T ratios also proved useful in identifying the depressives. Scherer used somewhat smaller groups (9 depressives contrasted to 11 schizophrenics) in order to study the vocal correlates of psychosis.[74] He also carried out speech/voice analyses before and after his subjects received treatment. Of his several measures, only frequency differentiated Scherer's groups; he reports a mean decrease of 9.5 Hz in SFF *following* treatment, and these data are in variance with most other authors. On the other hand, Scherer's reported findings on spectral bands appear to agree with Ostwald and others. In this case, he found an increase in low frequency energy (260–440 Hz) following therapy. Finally, Scherer concludes that treatment causes patients' voices to become more resonant and flexible—a change that, he suggests, is the result of increases in muscle tone.

To summarize, a review of the vocal correlates of affective disorders suggests that such patients probably use different speaking patterns than do normals. While there may be no classical pattern of the speech/voice characteristics of depression, an approximation might be as follows: these patients probably exhibit (1) reduced speaking intensity; (2) reduced FFD, or pitch range; (3) slower speech; (4) reduced intonation; and (5) a lack of linguistic stress. It should be noted also that, with the exception of SFF and its perceptual correlate pitch, this description essentially parallels those for the emotions grief and sorrow. Thus, just as (with certain exceptions) anger/fear appear to correlate with schizophrenia, the vocal correlates of depression suggest related emotional states also. While it probably is somewhat dangerous to push these analogies too far, the suggestion remains that such relationships may have merit, and they may be useful as guides to further research. It must be stressed, however, that all of the relationships suggested in TABLE 2 are tenuous; indeed, conflicting data exist in several instances. Hence, it is necessary to be a little cautious when attempting to generalize the speech/voice characteristics of psychotics for any purpose whatsoever.

LIE (STRESS) DETECTION

As has been pointed out in the preceding two sections, there may be voice and speech attributes that correlate with the emotional or psychological conditions experienced by an individual. Admittedly, the current state-of-the-science makes it difficult to predict precisely which of these factors relate to specific psychological states, and even whether those relationships that apparently have been established can be assumed for all individuals. Nevertheless, the commonly held opinion that high levels of stress produce gross changes in speech rate, vocal intensity, voice frequen-

TABLE 2

PRESUMED SPEECH/VOICE DEVIATIONS (FROM THE NORMAL) OF
TWO BROAD CLASSIFICATIONS OF PSYCHOSIS*

Parameter	Schizophrenia[†]	Depression[†]
Speaking Fundamental Frequency	+	0
Fundamental Frequency Deviation	?	−
Speaking Rate	0	−
Speaking Tempo	+	0
Vocal Intensity	0	−

* Only acoustical and perceptual parameters are included.

[†] + greater than normal; 0 not significantly different from normal; − reduced from normal; ? conflicting data.

cy, and possibly vocal quality probably is a defensible one. However, for the present, it may be unrealistic for a phonetician or psychologist to claim that he or she can identify behavioral states—such as types of emotion, level of stress, lying, and/or psychosis—solely from an analysis of an individual's speech and voice characteristics. That is, it appears obvious that the speech features correlating with the specific psychological conditions are not robust enough to permit these states to be accurately identified in the field. As stated, development of such indicators appears to be the responsibility of future investigators.

Nevertheless, a number of commercial firms are now marketing equipment that they claim can be used to detect stress, and ultimately lying, from live or recorded samples of a person's speech.[62,79] Chief among them are the Psychological Stress Evaluator (PSE), manufactured by Dektor Counterintelligence and Security, Inc., the Mark II Voice Analyzer, produced by Law Enforcement Associates, Inc., and the Voice Stress Analyzer (VSA), a product of Decision Control, Inc. Several additional devices include the Psychological Stress Analyzer, or PSA (Burns International Security Services), the Hagoth (see Bennett[9]), the Voice Stress Monitor, or ESM-4000 (Security Specialists Marketing Group), and others. Of course, if devices such as these actually were able to detect when an individual was practicing deception, they would be of substantial worth to law enforcement agencies. Even if they were only able to provide some estimation of the level of stress being experienced by a suspect, they would have considerable value. In any case, a number of these devices are being manufactured and marketed. Questions can be raised relative to the principles upon which they are based and as to their accuracy and effectiveness.

Before considering these questions, however, it should be noted that there has been some notoriety associated with voice analyzers, particularly the PSE. For example, analysis of the speech samples associated with the assassinations of both John and Robert Kennedy has led to much sensationalism (see, for example, Newsweek,[2] Dick,[24] and O'Toole[64])—as has the processing of speech related to the Patty Hearst kidnapping[25] and the so-called Washington scandals (see, for example, Dick[23] and Haines[35]). Moreover, the fact that the manufacturers claim that their devices can be used to analyze speech transmitted over the telephone, or be used in other covert ways, has resulted in the possibility that their use could lead to abuse of civil rights. Accordingly, in 1976, a congressional committee placed a ban on their use by federal agencies.[3] The proponents of these devices apparently are not deterred by such rulings, and a substantial number of them are in use today throughout the United States. Thus, there is a need to understand the basic premises upon which psychological stress evaluators are predicated and the validity of their output.

It is almost impossible to identify the bases upon which the Voice Stress Analyzer and most of the other systems operate. The manufacturer of the Mark II claims that its characteristics are "different" from those of the PSE, but this unit probably operates in a fashion similar to the PSE. On the other hand, the PSE manufacturers have gone to considerable effort to describe how their unit works. Moreover, their device is somewhat more complex than many of the others—it has several modes of operation, and the operator has to carry out a fairly complex analysis of a graphic trace, whereas many of the other devices use colored lights for readout (green for "the truth" and red for "a lie," of course). As would be expected, no details are given about the actual PSE circuitry. However, analysis of the device (including those elements embedded in molded plastic) reveals that its operational modes probably parallel those of a low-pass filter. Hence, it is necessary to look elsewhere for the theoretical constructs or empirical evidence upon which the operation of this device is based. In this regard, the PSE manufacturers claim that they detect and measure the very slight tremblings (often called microtremors) that occur in the muscles of the human body, in order to accomplish their intended task. That is, they contend that they can evaluate stress, and presumably lying, by demodulating the "subsonic frequencies" that are caused by minute oscillations in the muscles of the vocal mechanism. They argue that these microtremors are normal to *any* voluntary muscle activity but that in the stress situation, they are suppressed. The PSE, then, presumably measures the frequency modulation (FM) of the (vocal) utterance, which is present for normal speech but is reduced (or disappears) for stress (see, among others, Kupec[46]).

There is no question that such microtremors do exist—at least in the long muscles—and at rates varying from 8-14 Hz.[16,52] As noted above, the PSE proponents claim that this tremor exists in the *voice* also, presumably created by some interaction between the laryngeal muscles and the airstream. But do these microtremors exist in the small muscles of the larynx as well as in the large muscles of the extremities? Indeed, it is difficult to understand how an action that is so miniscule as to require sophisticated electromyography (EMG) to be recorded can affect the acoustic speech signal to such a degree that it can be detected in the manner described. In any event, a substantial number of questions such as these can be asked, but, at present, there are very few scientific reports on the subject, and the data reported often appear contradictory.

Perhaps it would be useful to examine first the possibility that microtremors may be present in the muscles associated with the vocal tract.

Four studies appear relevant in this regard. First, Shipp and McGlone, who are highly experienced electromyographists, used hook-wire electrodes embedded in both lip and laryngeal muscles to study this issue.[75] They report that these muscles did not show tremor patterns similar to those of the long muscles and thereby were forced to conclude that if voice analyzers work, their operation has to be based on some other set of principles. In discussing these conclusions, plus additional data that demonstrate this same lack of a relationship, McGlone argues that microtremors of the type in question are most readily found in the large muscles, especially those of the extremities.[57] He further indicates that such tremors are usually associated with isometric contractions, which seldom occur in the small, fast-acting muscles of the vocal tract. On the other hand, Inbar *et al.* claim that they were able to observe a laryngeal tremor of the type specified.[44] However, they used surface electrodes coupled to a low-pass filtering system in their research. As is well known, surface electrodes will pick up activity created by any muscles in their vicinity, and there is no way of knowing whether the muscle action potentials analyzed are from a single muscle set, from groups of muscles, or simply, perhaps, from some sort of interaction among the muscles. Indeed, when surface electrodes are placed over a structure as complex as the larynx, it even is possible to speculate that the EMG system is triggered by structural movement rather than by action potentials. An EMG study by Faaborg-Anderson appears to bear on this issue.[27] He studied the discharge frequency of the vocalis muscle single motor units for three subjects and found that these rates rose from 10 to 40 per second at the onset of phonation, maintained a 25-39 firing rate during phonation, and fell off to about 15 firings per second after the cessation of sound. While it must be conceded that Faaborg-Anderson did not measure microtremors directly, it also can be argued that microtremors result from neural control of this type. Hence, it is of interest that the firing rate varied as a function of voicing and did not remain at the specified level of 8-14 Hz during phonation. Finally, a comment by Almeida *et al.* appears germane to this discussion.[1] They indicated that the PSE literature does not restrict microtremor origin to the glottal region. However, they suggest that if such undulations were to originate in the supraglottal tract, "one would have to presuppose a fine synchronization of the discharge frequencies in the different articulator muscles. But since the innervation of different muscles displays continuous phase difference, an acoustic neutralization of [such] possible effects . . . must be expected." Obviously, this relationship also would appear consistent with laryngeal operation and, if true, would negate any potential for a microtremor to occur in the voice. In short, it would appear that the neurological evidence supporting the claims of the PSE proponents is sketchy and contradictory at best; the case they present can hardly be considered as well established.

Studies that have attempted to locate evidence of the microtremor within the acoustic signal itself also have been carried out. McGlone and Hollien[58] report that Dabbs performed fast Fourier transforms on the speech of speakers in stressed and unstressed situations. For the unstressed condition, he found a peak of energy between 10 and 15 Hz, and this peak disappeared in high stress situations; however, peaks also occurred between 0 and 5 Hz in the unstressed speaking condition, and these peaks did not disappear as a function of stress. In an attempt to provide additional data and perhaps clarify these relationships, McGlone and Hollien spectrographically studied the 5–100 Hz frequency band for 30 male subjects producing unstressed speech and compared the obtained results to those from the speech of 10 males stressed by electric shock.[58] They report that there appeared to be no systematic evidence of energy at frequencies below the subjects' speaking fundamental frequency levels for either of their two groups. Almeida *et al.* report that they investigated this issue also but by means of a somewhat different technique.[1] They analyzed the acoustic output of 14 subjects who were placed in a situation where a lie was required. Examination of time-expanded oscillograms showed that most of their subjects had a tendency to maintain constant f_o throughout all tests and retests. These measurements were subjected to statistical analysis, and the hypothesis that deception causes a modification in the average period duration of an answer was rejected. Further inspection of their measurements demonstrated that subjects react variably to induced stress, that is, with regard to their response patterns. For example, measurement of the average fluctuation values (an FM phenomenon) did not show any significant rise or fall among the answers. This issue is further confused by Inbar *et al.,* who claim to have found evidence of a "tremor" occurring in the third formant of vowels.[44] As can be seen, this statement does little to clarify the controversy. Moreover, it contradicts accepted acoustic theory relative to the operation of the vocal tract, i.e., a very low frequency existing within the signal would modulate the entire signal, not just one resonance region within it. Finally, based on studies in this area, Bachrach concludes that "there appears to be no conclusive evidence that . . . a microtremor exists in the vocal apparatus and the transfer from normal physiological tremor to vocal cords appears unwarranted."[6]

To summarize, currently there appears to be a serious question as to whether the tremor that the PSE and other like units are purported to measure actually is present in the voice and speech of talkers and, indeed, whether the voice analyzers really are not measuring some other feature or event. The very fact that the manufacturers of these units indicate that they can be used over the telephone argues against detection of very low frequencies. That is, if the effects of the microtremor are in the frequency region of 8–14 Hz—and the low-pass cutoff of the telephone is 250 Hz at best—the frequency of interest could not be detected; hence, it must be some other feature that is being measured. In any case, it appears from the above review that all of the propositions suggested by Papcun[69] have been violated, viz., (1) that oscillation occurs in the vocal muscles during speech; (2) that this oscillation is manifest in the acoustic speech signal; and (3) that the oscillation is reduced or modified by psychological stress.

Conceivably, it could be immaterial how a system operates if it does indeed perform the tasks required of it. Unfortunately, the available research does not provide a clear-cut answer about the effectiveness of voice analysis in this regard either. There are some indications that the devices in question can be used to detect stress if the level is high enough[58] but that they are ineffective if the stress level is relatively low.[8,56,57] The above studies would appear to provide useful information, because if it holds that high stress can be detected by voice analyzers and high stress is present during lying, then these devices should be able to detect lying also. However, are these relationships/contentions supported by relevant investigations?

Brenner reports that when he required 24 students to recite a poem before 0–22 spectators, his PSE analyses showed stress to increase as a function of audience size.[13] In this case, it would appear that there were identifiable differences in the PSE patterns and that these patterns correlated with levels of stress. The findings of Leith et al. are not so clear-cut.[50] By PSE analysis, he did find an apparent lowering of stress as his subjects serially made telephone calls, i.e., the adaptation effect was identified. However, the PSE did not discriminate between his two groups: the first were stutterers, who were clearly experiencing severe distress at having to make the telephone calls; and his controls were nonstutterers, who apparently experienced no fear or anxiety as a result of this task. The VanderCar et al. results are mixed also.[83] In their first study, these investigators correlated PSE analyses with stress measures of heart rate and scores on a test of anxiety. Their subjects were stressed by fear of electric shock and by requiring that they "speak taboo words." In the first study, all three measures were found to reflect the expected levels of stress and to correlate significantly with each other. However, when the study was replicated under only slightly different conditions, the PSE analyses did not correlate with the level of stress or with the other two measures. Thus, VanderCar et al. were forced to conclude that they could not systematically demonstrate the validity of the PSE.

Other conflicting data are available. For example, Brockway et al. report that their obstetrical patients showed similar levels of stress both on the PSE and on a standardized test of stress (anxiety).[14] On the other hand, the data reported by Hollien et al.[42] do not support the Brockway et al. position. This second set of investigators[42] lists data from several studies, one of which involved stress. In that study, a group of young adults produced speech under a high stress condition (as evidenced by experimenter observation, self reports, and high scores on the anxiety scale of the Multiple Affect Adjective Check List) and then under a speaking condition involving little or no stress; a second group of subjects was recorded while speaking under a very low stress condition. PSE traces were made, and three groups of examiners evaluated them. The first group were young adults who received a short training period specifically based on the instructions found in the PSE manual; the second group received substantially more extensive training. The third group was trained in the same manner as was the first but consisted of five scientists who were experienced in analyzing analog traces. The results of this research may be found in TABLE 3. As can be seen from the table, most scores are roughly at chance level; with only the scores of examiner groups A and C for the second unstressed group of talkers above chance.

In short, it does appear the PSE analysis sometimes can provide an in-

TABLE 3

EVALUATION OF PSE TRACES OF STRESSED AND UNSTRESSED SPEECH BY
THREE GROUPS OF AUDITORS*

| | Speech Sample[†] | | | |
Group	Stress	U/S-1	U/S-2	Mean Response
Group A (N = 19)				
Stressed	44			51
Unstressed		45	64	
Group B (N = 10)				
Stressed	35			40
Unstressed		45	39	
Group C (N = 5)				
Stressed	45			53
Unstressed		51	63	

* All values are in percent.
[†] U/S = unstressed condition.

dication of the presence of stress in speech, that is, if the stress level is *very* high. However, it does not appear to work very well when lower levels of stress are investigated. When these data are considered, perhaps the most important observation that can be made is that PSE analysis apparently does not lead to the correct identification of speech and voice where stress is *not* present or where the stress level is very low. The reason this relationship is so important is that, if nonstress speech is often identified as reflecting stress, a danger exists that unfortunate interpretations of the talker's intent will be made.

Research on stress in voice, perhaps, is somewhat off the point, as the psychological stress evaluator's objective is to detect instances of deception in the utterances of individuals being examined. Since such identification also is the goal of the members of the American Polygraph Association (APA), it is surprising that they have not adopted or endorsed the use of psychological stress evaluators. Quite to the contrary, in 1973, the APA Board of Directors disapproved the use of these devices (specifically the PSE-1) because, in their opinion, (1) they can be used covertly and violate an individual's constitutional rights; (2) their reliability and validity have not been demonstrated; and (3) the training programs and standards for examiners are totally inadequate.[10] The APA further indicated that it would reevaluate its position any time the three cited problems were resolved. It should be noted, however, that the fact that the APA does not support the use of the PSE or similar systems alone does not justify the rejection of these devices. Nevertheless, this group's arguments do lead to the postulation of two very important questions: (1) Does stress accompany lying?; and if so, (2) Will the stress levels associated with deception be high enough to be detected by the voice analyzers? Currently, there appears to be no research that bears directly on the first question; hence, it is impossible to experimentally defend either a positive or negative position in this regard.‡ On the other hand, a stress/lying relationship would be of little importance if the psychological stress evaluators actually measured some voice/speech feature that correlates with lying. Anyway, some research is available on the ability of the voice analyzers to detect lying.

Most of the studies to be reviewed are based on PSE analysis. The performance of this particular device has been the one most often studied, primarily because it is the most visible of the units, its use is most widespread, and its manufacturers are slightly more cooperative than are the individuals who make other devices of this type. As with the experiments on stress, the results of PSE evaluations of individuals who engage in deception or lying are conflicting. For example, Heisse reports having tested the PSE by requiring a group of 12 "trained" evaluators to process 258 "evaluation replies."[37] He claims that his examiners were correct 96.12% of the time. On the other hand, both Barland[8] and Kubis,[45] in independent, scientific studies, have challenged the ability of the PSE to detect lying. In his research, Kubis used 174 subjects in a simulated crime involving a thief, a lookout, and an innocent suspect.[45] In order to determine which of his subjects were lying and which were telling the truth, he utilized the polygraph and two "voice-analyzers" (i.e., the PSE and the VSA), as well as reevaluations of the polygraph records by independent examiners and subjective assessment of the recordings by tape monitoring personnel who were present during the interrogations. The primary accuracy level for the polygraph was found to be 76%; the independent polygraph raters scored 50–60%, and the subjective scores of the monitors were equally as high. On the other hand, the results obtained from the psychological stress evaluation systems (PSE, VSA) were roughly chance, even when the voice-analysis operators were provided with partial information about the subject. In any case, the voice analysis scores were well below those of the polygraph. Kubis argues further that, because his monitors were able to perceptually discriminate among his subjects to a significant degree, it is demonstrated that the task resulted in sufficient emotionality to be valid for its stated purpose. Barland's research was somewhat different than that carried out by Kubis; he studied both low risk and high risk deception.[8] He reports that the PSE analysis was not sufficiently sensitive to detect lies if little jeopardy was involved. In the high risk experiment, the voice analysis technique was compared to the polygraph for a number of criminals who were presumed to be lying (deception was later confirmed in a number of instances). In this case, all 14 polygraph evaluations indicated that the subject was lying; 8 of the 14 PSE evaluations agreed with the polygraph results, and the other 6 were inconclusive. Taken in total, Barland's results were not definitive; however, they do little to support the claims of the psychological stress evaluation proponents.

‡ Many would argue, however, that stress does not uniformly accompany lying—in the case of a sociopath (say), the individual probably would exhibit no stress at all when telling a lie.

We are sensitive to the argument that voice analyzers cannot be adequately tested in the laboratory because only low risk lies can be induced in this milieu and only high risk lies can be detected. However, it is our opinion that this argument is not a valid one. Indeed, we are carrying out a series of studies investigating this issue; one of which recently has been reported by Geison.[34] In this case, 12 individuals (plus 7 controls) with very strong feelings about a controversial social issue were induced to read two statements; one endorsing their position, the other endorsing an opinion completely opposed to theirs. Further, until the experiment was over (and they were informed of its true nature), subjects were led to believe that they would be publicly associated with the lie. Their (high) stress level, associated with the lie, was confirmed by a test of anxiety as well as by direct observation by the experimenter. The obtained tape recordings were processed through the PSE, and three groups of judges evaluated the traces: (1) ten individuals without prior knowledge of the technique, (2) five phoneticians experienced in signal analysis, and (3) three experienced PSE operators; the first two groups received training based on the PSE manual. The correct identifications of the stressed and unstressed samples were found to be roughly at the chance level for all three groups of judges. The PSE operators did score 58.3% correct for the unstressed samples, and the phoneticians 61.7% correct for the stressed; but *overall,* the scores were not significantly different from chance. Thus, it was concluded that "the PSE is not a very good tool for . . . the detection of lies."[34]

To summarize, it would appear that voice analyzers are not very effective in detecting low risk lies;[8,56] for high risk lies, the correct identifications appear to range from chance or a little above[34,42] to very high scores.[37] Kubis,[45] Barland,[8] and Puckett[70] have indicated that these devices constitute not nearly as powerful a tool as does the polygraph—and the limitations of the polygraph are well known. Moreover, no one as yet has tested any of the voice analyzers with speech samples that have been transmitted over a telephone, and research of this type is very much needed.

While it is possible to argue that voice analyzers are both valid and effective as lie detectors, it appears that the much stronger case is to the contrary. Moreover, the negative arguments become more compelling when it is remembered that when claims are made about *any* device, it is incumbent upon the proponents of the system to unequivocally demonstrate the validity of their contentions. Perhaps even more serious are the well-documented fears that these devices will be abused, that civil liberties will be violated by their use (especially over the telephone), and that the right to privacy will be invaded. Finally, even though scientists working in this area are keenly aware of the critical need of law enforcement agencies for a valid tool of this type, the inescapable conclusion is that such an aid does not presently exist.

References

1. ALMEIDA, A., G. FLEISCHMANN, G. HEIKE & E. THORMANN. 1975. Short time statistics of the fundamental tone in verbal utterances under psychic stress. Paper read at the Eighth International Congress of Phonetic Sciences, Leeds, England, August 17-23.

2. Anonymous. 1975. Dallas: new questions and answers. Newsweek (April 28): 36–38.
3. Anonymous. 1976. Washington report: house committee calls for ban on government use of polygraph. APA Monitor **1:** 10.
4. APPLEY, M. H. & R. TRUMBULL. 1967. On the concept of psychological stress. *In* Psychological Stress: Issues in Research. M. H. Appley & R. Trumbull, Eds. Meredith Publishing Co. New York, N.Y.
5. ARNOLD, M. B. 1967. Stress and emotion. *In* Psychological Stress: Issues in Research. M. H. Appley & R. Trumbull, Eds. Meredith Publishing Co. New York, N.Y.
6. BACHRACH, A. J. 1979. Speech and its potential for stress monitoring. *In* Proceedings, Workshop on Monitoring Vital Signs in the Diver. C. E. G. Lundgren, Ed.: 78–93. Undersea Medical Society and Office of Naval Research. Bethesda, Md.
7. BANNISTER, M. L. 1972. An instrumental and judgmental analysis of voice samples from psychiatrically hospitalized and non-hospitalized adolescents. Ph.D. Dissertation. University of Kansas. Lawrence, Kans.
8. BARLAND, G. 1973. Use of voice changes in detection of deception. (abst.). J. Acoust. Soc. Am. **54:** 63.
9. BENNETT, R. H., JR. 1977. Hagoth: Fundamentals of Voice Stress Analysis. Hagoth Corp. Issaquah, Wash.
10. Board of Directors. 1973. Resolution Concerning the Dektor Psychological Stress Evaluator (PSE-1). American Polygraph Association. Miami, Fla.
11. BOLLINGER, D. L. 1958. A theory of pitch accent in English. Word **14:** 109–149.
12. BONNER, R. 1943. Changes in the speech pattern under emotional tension. Am. J. Psychol. **56:** 262–273.
13. BRENNER, M. 1974. Stagefright and Stevens' Law. Paper presented at the Eastern Psychological Association Convention, New York, N.Y., April.
14. BROCKWAY, B. F., O. B. PLUMMER & B. M. LOWE. 1976. The effects of two types of nursing reassurance upon patient vocal stress levels as measured by a new tool, the PSE. Nurs. Res. **25:** 440–446.
15. BROWN, B. L., W. J. STRONG & A. C. RENCHER. 1973. Perceptions of personality from speech: effects of manipulations of acoustic parameters. J. Acoust. Soc. Am. **54:** 29–35.
16. BRUMLIK, J. & C. YAP. 1970. Normal Tremor: A Comparative Study. C. C. Thomas. Springfield, Ill.
17. CHEVRIE-MULLER, C., F. DODART, N. SEQUIER-DERMER & D. SALMON 1971. Étude des parametres acoustiques de la parole au cours de la schizophrenia de l'adolescent. Folia Phoniat. **23:** 401–428.
18. COSTANZO, F. S., N. N. MARKEL & P. R. COSTANZO. 1969. Voice quality profile and perceived emotion. J. Counsel. Psychol. **16:** 267–270.
19. DARBY, J. K. & H. HOLLIEN. 1977. Vocal and speech patterns of depressive patients. Folia Phoniat. **29:** 279–291.
20. DARBY, J. K. & A. SHERK. 1979. Speech studies in psychiatric populations. *In* Current Issues in the Phonetic Sciences. H. & P. Hollien, Eds.: 599–608. J. Benjamin, B.V. Amsterdam, The Netherlands.
21. DAVITZ, J. R. & L. J. DAVITZ. 1959. The communication of feelings through content-free speech. J. Commun. **9:** 6–13.
22. DENBER, M. A. 1978. Sound spectrum analysis of the mentally ill. Master's Thesis. University of Rochester. Rochester, N.Y.
23. DICK, W. 1975. Scientific evidence proves Ted told the truth about Chappaquidick. National Enquirer **49** (July 1).
24. DICK, W. 1975. Sirhan was hypnotized to kill Bobby Kennedy. National Enquirer **50** (October 27).
25. DWORKEN, A. 1975. Patty Hearst not guilty. Voice test proves she was forced to lie. National Enquirer **50** (September 23).
26. ELDRED, S. H. & D. B. PRICE. 1958. A linguistic evaluation of feeling states in psychotherapy. Psychiatry **21:** 115–121.
27. FAABORG-ANDERSON, K. 1957. Electromyographic investigation of intrinsic laryngeal muscles in humans. Acta Physiol. Scand. **41**(Supplement): 140.
28. FAIRBANKS, G. & W. PRONOVOST. 1939. An experimental study of the pitch characteristics of the voice during the expression of emotion. Speech Monogr. **6:** 87–104.

29. FAIRBANKS, G. & L. W. HOAGLIN. 1941. An experimental study of the durational characteristics of the voice during the expression of emotion. Speech Monogr. **8**: 85-90.
30. FONAGY, I. 1966. Electrophysiological and acoustic correlates of stress and stress perception. J. Speech Hear. Res. **9**: 231-244.
31. FRIEDHOFF, A. J., M. ALPERT & R. L. KURTZBERG. 1964. An electro-acoustical analysis of the effects of stress on voice. J. Neuropsychiatry **5**: 265-272.
32. FRY, D. B. 1955. Duration and intensity as physical correlates of linguistic stress. J. Accoust. Soc. Am. **27**: 765-768.
33. FRY, D. B. 1958. Experiments in the perception of stress. Lang. Speech **1**: 126-152.
34. GEISON, L. L. 1979. Evaluation of high stress lying by voice analysis. M.A. Thesis. University of Florida. Gainesville, Fla.
35. HAINES, R. 1976. Elizabeth Ray told the truth about the Washington sex scandal: Congressman Hayes did not. National Enquirer **51** (September).
36. HARGREAVES, W. A., J. A. STARKWEATHER & K. H. BLACKER. 1965. Voice quality in depression. J. Abnorm. Psychol. **70**: 218-220.
37. HEISSE, J. W. 1976. Audio stress analysis—A validation and reliability study of the Psychological Stress Evaluator (PSE). *In* Proceedings, 1976 Carnahan Conference on Crime Countermeasures, University of Kentucky, Lexington, Ky.: 5-18.
38. HECKER, M. H. L., K. N. STEVENS, G. VON BISMARCK & C. E. WILLIAMS. 1968. Manifestations of task-induced stress in the acoustic speech signal. J. Acoust. Soc. Am. **44**: 993-1001.
39. HELFRICH, H. & K. R. SCHERER. 1977. Experimental assessment of antidepressant drug effects using spectral analysis of voice. Paper presented at the fall meetings of the Acoustical Society of America, Miami Beach, Fla., December 13-16.
40. HICKS, J. W., JR. 1979. An acoustical/temporal analysis of emotional stress in speech. Ph.D. Dissertation. University of Florida. Gainesville, Fla.
41. HOLLIEN, H. & J. K. DARBY. 1979. Acoustic comparisons of psychotic and non-psychotic voices. *In* Current Issues in the Phonetic Sciences. H. & P. Hollien, Eds.: 609-614. J. Benjamin, B. V. Amsterdam, The Netherlands.
42. HOLLIEN, H., L. L. GEISON & J. W. HICKS, JR. 1980. Stress/lie studies utilizing the PSE. Paper read at the annual meeting of the American Academy of Forensic Sciences, New Orleans, La., February 20-23.
43. HUTTAR, G. L. 1968. Relations between prosodic variables and emotions in normal American English utterances. J. Speech Hear. Res. **11**: 481-487.
44. INBAR, G. F., G. EDEN & M. A. KAPLAN. 1977. Frequency modulation in the human voice and the source of its mediation. *In* Proceedings, 1977 Carnahan Conference on Crime Countermeasures, University of Kentucky, Lexington, Ky.: 213-319.
45. KUBIS, J. 1973. Comparison of Voice Analysis and Polygraph as Lie Detection Procedures. U.S. Army Land Warfare Laboratory. Aberdeen Proving Ground, Md.
46. KUPEC, E. W. 1977. Truth or the consequences. Law Enforce. Commun. **4**: 12-18/42-45.
47. KURODA, I., O. FUJUVARA, N. OHAMURA & N. UTSUKI. 1976. Method for determining pilot stress through analysis of voice communication. Aviat. Space Environ. Med. **47**: 528-533.
48. LAZARUS, R. S. 1966. Psychological Stress and the Coping Process. McGraw-Hill Book Co., Inc. New York, N.Y.
49. LEHISTE, I. & G. E. PETERSON. 1959. Vowel amplitude and phonetic stress in American speech. J. Acoust. Soc. Am. **31**: 428-435.
50. LEITH, W. R., J. L. TIMMONS & M. D. SUGARMAN. 1977. The use of the Psychological Stress Evaluator with stutterers. Paper read to the Convention of the American Speech and Hearing Association, Chicago, Ill., November 2-5.
51. LIEBERMAN, P. & S. B. MICHAELS. 1962. Some aspects of fundamental frequency and envelope amplitude as related to emotional content of speech. J. Acoust. Soc. Am. **34**: 922-927.
52. LIPPOLD, O. 1971. Physiological tremor. Sci. Am. **224**: 65-73.
53. LYKKEN, D. 1974. Psychology and the lie detector industry. Am. Psychol.: 725-739.
54. MARKEL, N. N. 1969. Relationship between voice-quality profiles and MMPI profiles in psychiatic patients. J. Abnorm. Psychol. **74**: 61-66.

55. MARKEL, N. N., M. F. BEIN & J. A. PHILLIS. 1973. The relationship between words and tone of voice. Lang. Speech 16: 15-21.
56. McGLONE, R. E., C. PETRIE & J. FRYE. 1974. Acoustic analyses of low-risk lies. (abst.) J. Acoust. Soc. Am. 55: S20.
57. McGLONE, R. E. 1975. Tests of the Psychological Stress Evaluator (PSE) as a lie and stress detector. In Proceedings, 1975 Carnahan Conference on Crime Countermeasures, University of Kentucky, Lexington, Ky.: 83-86.
58. McGLONE, R. E. & H. HOLLIEN. 1976. Partial analysis of the acoustic signal of stressed and unstressed speech. In Proceedings, 1976 Carnahan Conference on Crime Countermeasures, University of Kentucky, Lexington, Ky.: 19-21.
59. MOL, H. & E. M. UHLENBECK. 1956. The linguistic relevance of intensity in stress. Lingua. 5: 205-213.
60. MOSES, P. J. 1954. The Voice of Neurosis. Grune and Stratton. New York, N.Y.
61. MOSKOWITZ, E. 1951. Voice quality in the schizophrenic reaction type. Ph.D. Dissertation. New York University. New York, N.Y.
62. NERI, P. A. The Dektor-Psychological Stress Evaluator: an interim report. (Unpublished manuscript.)
63. NEWMAN, S. S. & V. G. MATHER. 1938. Analysis of spoken language of patients with affective disorders. Am. J. Psychiatry 91: 912-942.
64. O'TOOLE, G. 1975. Lee Harvey Oswald was innocent. Penthouse 6(8): 45-46 & 124-132.
65. OSTWALD, P. F. 1961. The sounds of emotional disturbance. Arch. Gen. Psychiatry 5: 587-592.
66. OSTWALD, P. F. 1963. Soundmaking: The Acoustic Communication of Emotion. Charles C. Thomas. Springfield, Ill.
67. OSTWALD, P. F. 1964. Acoustic manifestations of emotional disturbance. In Disorders of Communication. D. Rioch & E. Weinstein, Eds.: 450-465. Williams & Wilkins Co. Baltimore, Md.
68. OSTWALD, P. F. & A. SKOLNIKOFF. 1966. Speech disturbances in a schizophrenic adolescent. Postgraduate Med. 12: 40-49.
69. PAPCUN, G. 1973. The effects of psychological stress on speech. Paper delivered to the fall meeting of the Acoustical Society of America, Los Angeles, Calif., October 30-November 2.
70. PUCKETT, T. 1980. Voice stress analysis procedures vis-a-vis polygraph procedure in real life testing situations. (Unpublished manuscript.)
71. RICE, D. G., G. M. ABRAMS & J. H. SAXMAN. 1969. Speech and physiological correlates of "flat" affect. Arch. Gen. Psychiatry 20: 566-572.
72. ROSS, M., R. J. DUFFY, H. S. COOKER & R. L. SERGEANT. 1973. Contribution of the lower audible frequencies to the recognition of emotions. A.A.D.: 37-42.
73. SAXMAN, J. M. & K. W. BURK. 1968. Speaking fundamental frequency and rate characteristics of adult female schizophrenics. J. Speech Hear. Res. 11: 194-302.
74. SCHERER, K. L. Non-linguistic vocal indicators of emotion and psychopathology. In Emotions and Psychopathology. C. E. Izard, Ed. Plenum Press, New York, N.Y. (In press.)
75. SHIPP, T. & R. E. McGLONE. 1973. Physiologic correlates of acoustic correlates of psychological stress. (abst.). J. Acoust. Soc. Am. 53: S63.
76. SILVERMAN, F. H. & E. M. SILVERMAN. 1975. Effects of threat of shock for being disfluent on fluency of normal speakers. Percep. Motor Skills 41: 353-354.
77. SIMONOV, P. V. & M. V. FROLOV. 1973. Utilization of human voice for estimation of man's emotional stress and state of attention. Aeronaut. Med. 44: 256-258.
78. SIMONOV, P. V., M. V. FROLOV & V. L. TABGKIN. 1975. Use of the invariant method of speech analysis to discern the emotional state of announcers. Aviat. Space Environ. Med. 46: 1014-1016.
79. SMITH, G. A. 1974. The measurement of anxiety: a new method by voice analysis. IRCS (Res. Biomed., Technol., Psychiat. Clin. Psychol.) 2: 1707.
80. SPOERRI, T. H. 1966. Speaking voice of the schizophrenic patient. Arch. Gen. Psychiatry 14: 581-585.
81. STARKWEATHER, J. A. 1961. Vocal communication of personality and human feelings. J. Commun. 11: 63-72.

82. STARKWEATHER, J. A. 1956. Content-free speech as a source of information about the speaker. J. Abnorm. Soc. Psychol. **52:** 394–402.
83. VANDERCAR, D. H., J. GREANER, N. HIBLER, C. D. SPEELBERGER & S. BLOCH. 1980. A description and analysis of the operation and validity of the Psychological Stress Evaluator. J. Forensic Sci. **25:** 174–188.
84. WILLIAMS, C. E. & K. N. STEVENS. 1969. On determining the emotional state of pilots during flight: an exploratory study. Aeronaut. Med. **40:** 1369–1372.
85. WILLIAMS, C. E. & K. N. STEVENS. 1972. Emotions and speech: some acoustical correlates. J. Acoust. Soc. Am. **52:** 1238–1250.

HYPNOSIS AND EVIDENCE: HELP OR HINDRANCE?

Herbert Spiegel*
Department of Psychiatry
College of Physicians and Surgeons
Columbia University
New York, New York 10032

INTRODUCTION

During the past 50 years, there has been a gradual, but definite, emergence of the use of hypnosis in the field of medicine. With this there has been much controversy and, at the same time, an appreciable increase in our knowledge about the phenomenon.[1] More recently, there has been an interest in the uses of hypnosis in the field of forensic medicine. Here the controversies are even more heated, complicated by the intrusion of this controversial subject into legal procedures. Much of the controversy is aggravated and compounded by serious misconceptions about hypnosis itself. In order to minimize the areas of unnecessary friction, it would be well to begin by dealing with the most common misconceptions and clarifying them.

MISCONCEPTIONS

The most common misconception is that hypnosis is sleep. Hypnosis is not only *not* sleep, but is the very opposite of sleep. It is a state of alert, attentive, receptive, integrated concentration characterized by a parallel awareness. That is, the subject in trance can, on the one hand, be aware of a relationship to another person and, at the same time, be intensely involved in another facet of his own life experience. This sensitive capacity to maintain a ribbon of parallel concentration is an indication of extreme alertness, the opposite of sleep. Since the word hypnosis derives from a Greek root meaning sleep, it is an unfortunate term to apply to this phenomenon, but we are historically and traditionally bound to this label.

Another serious misconception is that the hypnotist projects the hypnotic spell onto the subject. This is utter nonsense. The hypnotist projects nothing at all. Instead, he simply taps the natural trance capacity that is inherent in the subject. Trance capacity is a talent that is either genetically determined or learned in an imprint-like manner during early developmental years, or both. The degree of intensity of trance capacity can be measured clinically within 5 to 10 minutes on a 0–5 scale. This measured capability remains stable during adult years except when impaired by some forms of mental illness or by drugs that impair ability to concentrate. A

* Address correspondence to Dr. Spiegel at 19 East 88th Street, New York, N.Y. 10028.

slight reduction of previous capacity can occur with aging, especially by the seventh decade. In everyday life, when a person is highly motivated or highly charged for a specific goal, he is prone to spontaneously shift into his own trance level to facilitate the achievement of a task. What the hypnotist does in formal hypnosis is to simply tap this capacity with the subject's cooperation and compliance.

A third misconception is that only mentally weak or sick people are hypnotizable. This is precisely wrong. It is the mentally healthy population that is usually hypnotizable. For example, psychopaths, persons with character disorders, schizophrenics, the mentally retarded, depressed persons, and persons with neurological deficits that interfere with concentration all have great difficulty concentrating enough in this disciplined way to allow the trance to occur.

Another misunderstanding is that hypnosis occurs only when a hypnotist hypnotizes a subject. We know, of course, that it can occur if the subject cooperates when the hypnotist gives him the signal to go into trance. But more often, hypnosis occurs spontaneously in the person's life, especially under duress or under highly motivating, challenging situations. This fact is especially germane to our topic, which we shall return to later.

A fifth misconception is that hypnosis is dangerous. We now know that hypnosis itself is not dangerous but that the trance state can be used mischievously. One of the features of the trance is that the person goes into such a state of intense concentration that peripheral awareness decreases, customary guardedness decreases, and an assumption of trust—even naive trust—occurs, which makes the subject more vulnerable to deception, exploitation, coercion, or trickery. Such violation of trust by the hypnotist can indeed be dangerous and harmful, but it is not the hypnosis itself that is harmful.

Another misunderstanding about hypnosis is that the hypnotist himself must be some kind of a charismatic, unusual, or weird person in order to evoke a trance state. This is not true. Of course, if the subject perceives the hypnotist as charismatic, that indeed adds to the impact of the interaction; but by and large, any person relating to another person can, if the atmosphere is appropriate, signal a subject to shift into a trance state. Trance induction is simple. It is teachable and learnable; and in a very short time, a novice can be as effective in inducing trance as an experienced hypnotist.

Still another misconception is that women are more hypnotizable than men. Repeatedly, scientific studies have shown that when tested appropriately, there is no difference in distribution of hypnotizability between the adult male and female populations. About 70% of the population is capable of some degree of hypnosis. Roughly, about 15% go into a light trance, which is the peak capacity for that group. Another 15% are capable of very intense trance states, and the remaining are somewhere in the midrange. It is generally observed that whatever capacity a person has can be slightly enhanced by stress or high motivation. With this consideration, it is not an exaggeration to say that well over half of the population is capable of some degree of appreciable trance experience, especially under stress conditions.

Enhanced Memory Recall with Hypnosis

The least controversial use of hypnosis is to enhance memory enough to recall simple, circumscribed data that are subject to further corroboration. For example, a witness sees a car or a truck long enough to scan the license number but, on first effort, is unable to remember the numbers. With the enhanced concentration that occurs in the trance state, it is possible to retrieve the memory of the license plate which at first recall was blurred. In a way, this is simply an extension of an everyday experience where on first effort, thinking about some event in the past is somewhat hazy, but with more effort and determination and collateral associations with the event, a clarifying memory emerges. This often occurs spontaneously, but it can also occur in a more structured way with formal hypnotic trance.

A more dramatic use of hypnosis is the uncovering of amnesic periods. For example, often after a head injury, there is an amnesic phase for the victim. Of course if the trauma leads to unconsciousness, the events that occur during the unconscious phase are called "amnesia"; but in fact, because of the unconsciousness, the events never were perceived by the victim in the first place. After consciousness returns, there is first a patch, then continuous recall of life experience. With head trauma, another kind of amnesia often occurs, that is, a "retrograde" amnesia. This means that even though the patient was conscious up to the point of the impact that led to the unconsciousness, when he recovers his consciousness, he is amnesic for a time frame of seconds to minutes prior to the point of impact. This retrograde amnesia is usually of a psychological nature and is very often recoverable. Here is an example of how hypnosis can facilitate this recovery. A 16-year-old young man was in an automobile accident with his father. The father was driving and was killed by the impact of a truck hitting the car from their right. The young man was also struck with a head injury and became unconscious. He recovered consciousness about an hour later in the hospital. Technically, since the boy's father was dead and the boy himself was amnesic to the entire episode, there was no witness to this accident except the driver of the truck. The driver's account went unchallenged. Some time later, it was discovered that the young man was capable of hypnosis; on a 0–5 scale, he scored a 4. Thus, when instructed to go into trance and regress, he was able to recall certain details of how he and his father had dropped off his aunt and had traveled along a certain road up to a certain point. He could then recall the truck coming down from the right and his father saying he was sure the truck would stop because there was a stop sign at the intersection. It was at this point that everything went blank. He came out of the trance with a sense of disappointment, thinking that he had failed. Actually, what he had done was to uncover the retrograde part of the amnesia. These facts were later confirmed by other testimony, and it now meant that there were technically two witnesses to the accident instead of one. With this new situation, the insurance company agreed to settle the issues rather than go to court.

In another case, a woman in her thirties, divorced, and living with her children in a ground-floor apartment was attacked one night by an intruder who entered her bedroom through the window. He ravaged her with a knife in an apparent attempt to kill her. She was wounded, rushed to the hospital, and almost miraculously recovered. For months she had no memory of what she had seen prior to the knife's coming at her. Police investigations focused upon two suspects but with not enough hard information. To enhance her memory, she asked for help with hypnosis; and it was discovered that she was capable of a midrange trance. While in a trance state and with a great deal of emotion, tears, shouting, and reexperiencing of the event in the present tense, she gave enough descriptive information about the features of the intruder to identify her ex-husband as the person. Although in the trance state she gave specific details that identified him, it was only with great reluctance that she acknowledged that it was, in fact, her ex-husband. When she was brought out of the trance state and asked to review what she had recalled, she expressed dismay at the information and hinted that somehow she had known this but had not wanted to admit it to herself. Perhaps, with time and the practical need to pursue the investigation, she allowed this to surface. But it is also possible that this was a self-serving fantasy. Whether or not the assailant actually was her husband must be verified by other data.

In the *Leyra* case,[2] hypnosis was used along with deception and coercion to elicit a confession. Leyra was apprehended and accused of killing his father and mother. After hours of interrogation at the police station, a doctor was sent to treat Leyra in his cell because he had complained of a headache. Along with other treatment, the doctor hypnotized Leyra and told him that he might as well admit to the murders and that he, the doctor, would see to it that the police would "go easy" with him. Leyra then confessed to the doctor. After this, he was taken to the front of the police station, and in the presence of his business partner, Leyra repeated the confession that he had given to the doctor. He was found guilty and sentenced to the electric chair. The appellate court ordered a new trial on learning that the confession had been coerced. On the basis of that confession alone, they could not sentence Leyra to death. At the second trial, he was again found guilty. This time the prosecution used the second confession, which he had made to his partner shortly after the first one. For the second confession, he had not been in a formal trance state. This case went all the way up to the United States Supreme Court; and on a split decision, a new trial was ordered. The majority opinion, written by Justice Black, held that the confession that was repeated a second time outside of the cell had to be regarded as part of a continuum and, therefore, had the same coerced quality of the first confession. At the third trial, the case against Leyra was built largely around fragmented circumstantial evidence, including some bloody clothes and the testimony of a girlfriend. He again was found guilty. On appeal, the court ruled that the evidence was too circumstantial and fragmented for the court to take Leyra's life, and they reversed the decision. Leyra was subsequently freed of all charges. In this instance, the deception used by the doctor to elicit the confession was perpetrated more easily because the victim was in a trance state, with a reduced level of critical judgment. The state of trust enabled the prisoner to feel freer to expose his inner thoughts and memories. It was this feature of coercion and deception that the court seized upon in reversing the lower court. Further, the Supreme Court recognized that the posthypnotic confession exhibited the same feature of coercion as did the original confession.

In the *Miller* case in Connecticut,[3] the issue of hypnosis became critical because its use was not even mentioned during the first trial. Miller was found guilty of transferring a large amount of heroin from one car to another. He was sentenced to 12 years. The prosecution arguments and the jury decision of guilt were based almost entirely upon the testimony of a French-Canadian named Caron, who at first was vague, then somewhat certain, about identifying Miller. But after he returned from an interrogation in Texas dealing with another aspect of the same case, Caron was positive that Miller was the man he had seen and so testified. After Miller was sentenced, the defense—with the prosecutor's agreement—examined the witness Caron. Caron also agreed to be examined with hypnosis. When he appeared for the examination, Caron revealed that he had already been hypnotized before in Texas by a psychologist working with the prosecuting attorney. It was understood that Caron's own pending sentence as an illegal alien would be influenced by the extent of his cooperation with this prosecutor. It turned out that this prosecutor was innocently exploring some other aspects of the case and wanted to find out if Caron could remember a certain license number. While under hypnosis, the prosecution attorneys kept referring to Miller as the guilty man. Miller was a hairdresser, and they would shift from referring to "the hairdresser" and to Miller—and all during the interrogation, there were repeated inferences that Miller was assumed to be guilty. When Caron returned to Connecticut to participate in the trial there, he suddenly became aware that Miller was the man he had seen and so testified. On testing, it turned out that Caron was capable of a moderate capacity for hypnosis; when the case reached the appellate court, Judge Friendly put his finger on this single issue. He asked the Connecticut prosecutor why he had not mentioned that Caron had been hypnotized in Texas regarding this same case. The prosecuting attorney stated that he had not thought it would be important. Judge Friendly asked the prosecutor if he did not think that the defense could have made quite an issue of this with the jury. The prosecutor allowed that this was a possibility. Largely around that point, the appellate court reversed the decision and ordered a new trial. In the second trial, the issue of possible contamination and fixation of memory with hypnosis was introduced. Miller was acquitted.

What is intriguing is that the district attorney in Texas and the psychologist in Texas were in no way attempting to influence Caron. They only coincidentally referred to Miller as the guilty one; but by so doing, they in effect "brainwashed" an intimidated witness to clear his thinking and to posthypnotically assert in court that he was sure that Miller was the man he had seen, even though at no time prior to the Texas experience had he been so clear and positive about Miller.

THE HONEST LIAR SYNDROME

In 1968, in order to explore further this issue of the reliability of information given under hypnosis and its extension after hypnosis, the following experiment took place: A man in his forties—a successful businessman, not a psychiatric patient—volunteered to be the subject. On a 0–5 scale he scored 5, putting him in the top 15% of the highly hypnotizable population. He agreed to appear at the NBC television studios with Frank McGee and myself. The entire experiment was recorded with a movie camera. While he was in a Grade 5 trance, he was told that the communists were taking over the control of the television networks; that this was the real truth; and that no matter who tried to dissuade him of this belief, he would stick to it. In fact, he would even intensify his conviction if he were to be challenged. He was brought out of the formal trance state locked into this premise, i.e., that the communists were taking over the networks. For quite a period of time, Frank McGee challenged him about this. The more McGee pressed him, the firmer he held to the premise. In fact he went so far as to name names, spelling out details of a meeting that had taken place in a loft above a movie house off Sheridan Square where six people had gathered and talked about this plot. He even gave a specific name and described the physical features of the man who was the leader. After he was given the cutoff signal to come out of this trance bind, he had total amnesia for anything that took place. Five months later, he was shown the movie of this event. He was shocked and astounded at what he had said. He had no knowledge of any such person as he had described and had no memory of any meeting having taken place. He experienced the whole sequence as a blackout. He could not deny that he had said these things, because he saw himself doing so in a sound movie. He was baffled and could not understand where all this information was coming from, because he simply had no knowledge of any such event. What is frightening about this experience is that he was a man whose political orientation is somewhat left of center yet he was talking to Frank McGee as if he, the subject, were an ultraconservative. That is, his allegations and conduct were entirely foreign to his everyday political beliefs. This paradox is critically important to the theme of this paper. During the experiment, in response to the hypnotic signal, the subject created a totally false story to rationalize his compliance. He sincerely believed it to be true. Since he was locked into the hypnotic bind, he suspended his own critical judgment. He lied but did not actually know he was lying. At the time, he was in effect an honest liar.

DISCUSSION

This series of case illustrations was presented to emphasize the Janus-like quality of data obtained through hypnosis. Although it is possible with some people under some circumstances to elicit stunningly accurate information that is otherwise not available, conversely, it is quite possible to so contaminate the memory of the subject that he confuses the hypnotic implantations with his own knowledge. Then, by so fusing them, he cannot tell one from the other. Whether the subject does this for internal reasons of self-defense, because of benign external pressures, or because of blunt coercion to comply, the risk we take in using the hypnotic state to obtain information is that we may wittingly or unwittingly contaminate the memory of the subject in such a way that we cannot be certain of its credibility.

Therefore, the following conclusion is inevitably clear. All data obtained under hypnosis are vulnerable to the counterclaim of memory contamination or coercion (innocent or designed), even though incredibly accurate information can at times emerge. It is thus imperative to document all prehypnosis data as separate and distinct from information obtained during and after hypnotic interrogation. If this is not done, the prehypnosis testimony also risks losing its credibility. The most one can legitimately expect from hypnotic interrogation is further data, which may serve as *leads* for more conventional evidence gathering. Data elicited through hypnosis by itself deserve low or no priority until they are supported by other data. Even confessions of guilt made under hypnosis are vulnerable to counterclaims of coercion and deception, especially in demonstrably highly hypnotizable persons. This certainly does not hold for persons who are not hypnotizable and probably does not apply to those who test low on hypnotizability assessment tests.

However, this is not so simple an issue. It is easy to identify information elicited under *formal* trance interrogation; but it is not so easy to identify posthypnotic influences in testimony after the hypnotic interrogation has occurred and determine to what extent perspectives and facts are contaminated by the interrogation. So far, one could argue that if trance interrogation can be so vulnerable to contamination, why not simply ban all uses of hypnosis in the forensic sphere. That could certainly be done by legislative and judicial fiat but would eliminate only the *formal* use of hypnosis. In no way would it solve the actual dilemma. Such arbitrary orders cannot eliminate the spontaneous trance experience that most persons are prone to, especially under the stress of legal or police interrogation. The Janus-like features described with formal hypnosis can become monstrous perversions of due process when the witness or the accused under duress enters a spontaneous trance state as a desperate way to cope with the intrusion. Fact and fiction can become intertwined and even more confounded when neither the victim nor the interrogator knows that the victim is in trance. Thus, instead of trying to order hypnosis out of existence, it becomes our responsibility to be more knowledgeable about and sensitive to its occurrence.

The best defense against the innocent or calculated abuse of hypnosis is for every person engaged in the interrogation process to become sensitive to the subtle signs of emerging spontaneous trance in the subject being questioned. This requires some training and knowledge; but since trance occurs, is it not the obligation of the professional doing the interrogation to alert himself to it? Of course, the ideal would be for each person to know his own vulnerability to trance under duress and—with this foreknowledge—invoke appropriate safeguards for himself. The details of how this is done are not germane to the discussion here.

DIAGNOSTIC USES OF HYPNOSIS IN THE FORENSIC ARENA

A new and unexpected use of hypnosis has emerged in recent years; that is, using the assessment of hypnotic capacity by means of the Hypnotic Induction Profile (HIP)—a 5- to 10-minute clinical test.[1] The HIP not only determines the hypnotic capacity of the individual, but the configuration of the score also offers a presumptive indication of relative mental health or illness as well as a presumptive indication of personality style. This, in turn, yields information about which pathological syndrome is most likely to occur in that particular person under duress.

Following are actual case illustrations to indicate how this works.

The Reilly Case

Peter Reilly, a Connecticut teenager, was found guilty of murdering his mother.[4-6] The prosecution relied heavily upon a confession that Peter had signed after hours of interrogation and exposure to a lie detector test. Although he had signed a confession, Peter had stated that he still had no memory of killing his mother. The police had explained to him that he had an "amnesia." Peter had accepted this explanation. Friends in the small community who knew him well could not accept the jury's judgment of guilt. Knowing him to be a responsible yet gullible youth, they were perturbed that no medical or psychological testimony had been introduced in the trial. Events snowballed, leading to a hearing for a new trial. Upon examination, the HIP revealed a pattern that indicated that Peter was not the type of person likely to develop amnesia. Careful questioning indicated that he had a clear recall of the entire time span during which the murder had occurred. He had been at a church youth center meeting and had driven home during this time frame. When he had arrived home, he had found his mother dead. He had telephoned for medical help. The HIP pattern was also consistent with a borderline immature personality and poorly developed sense of self with ego diffusion. Peter's extreme modesty and uncertainty about himself along with his long-standing respect for police authority made him vulnerable to charges by the police that he had committed the crime. The polygraph situation was used to make him feel guilty enough to comply with the charges and sign the confession. He accepted the absence of any firsthand knowledge of the murder as due to "amnesia."

The new information about Peter's personality style and immaturity indicated that his having no memory for the event was not due to amnesia but rather was due to the fact that he had not actually been present and had not, in fact, committed the murder. However, he was unable to withstand the accusatory pressure of the police. This along with other points led to a court decision by the same judge who had presided over the original trial that an injustice had been done, and therefore, a new trial was ordered.

Following that decision, it was learned that exculpatory evidence, placing Peter Reilly five miles from the scene at the time the murder was committed, had been withheld by the prosecution during the first trial. Along with other issues, this led to still another court decision by another judge which dropped all charges against Peter; and he was freed.

Because the HIP indicated that Peter was not hypnotizable and not prone to amnesia, and because it further indicated that his confession was due to his immature and uncertain sense of self, the defense had a potent wedge to align with other issues, which led to vindication.

United States v. Thornton

Thornton was a military policeman charged with the kidnapping, rape, and murder of three teenagers as well as the wounding of another.[7] His defense was not guilty by virtue of insanity. This was in essence documented by a videotaped interview, which allegedly demonstrated that under hypnosis, Thornton revealed a dual personality. The "bad" personality committed acts that the "good" personality was not responsible for.

The HIP revealed a pattern of a person barely able to sustain a trance state. It is well established clinically that multiple personalities all have very high capacities for sustained trance experience.

The HIP was also consistent with the category of a sociopathic personality, capable of destructive acting-out, with guile and deceptive ploys to defend itself. Further, a sociopath usually does not qualify as "lacking substantial capacity" under the American Law Institute guidelines. The jury found Thornton guilty as charged. The defense's psychiatrists did not, at any time, assess Thornton's hypnotic capacity and were thus vulnerable to the charge that the accused had simulated a dual personality to deceive his doctors and the jury in his own desperate defense.

The HIP score was thus able to neutralize the drama of the videotaped dual personality thesis and identified Thornton as an ordinary psychopathic personality, responsible for his own acts.

United States v. Leonora Perez and Filipina Narciso

During the summer of 1975, an unusual number of postoperative patients in the Veteran's Administration Hospital in Ann Arbor, Michigan, suffered respiratory arrests.[8] Some died. Those who survived had patchy or hazy memory or no memory at all of what had occurred. Several of the patients had had memory or psychiatric deficits before their surgery. When respiratory arrest with cerebral anoxia episodes were imposed upon this, it was not surprising that accurate and reliable witnesses were difficult to find. It was suspected that a curare-like substance (Pavulon) had been injected into the intravenous tubings to bring about the respiratory arrests. The FBI was authorized to explore for leads with hypnosis. By agreement and design, all testimony of witnesses was put on record and identified as data prior to the hypnotic interviews. It was clearly understood that data obtained with hypnosis were, at best, possible leads for further evidence but were certainly not to be used alone as direct testimony at trial. If they were to be used, they would certainly be vulnerable to charges of contamination. All interviews with hypnosis were recorded on videotape with time and date recorded simultaneously.

The HIP was administered, and several witnesses were eliminated because the test revealed that they were not hypnotizable. About 12 scored well enough to be interrogated further with hypnosis. New information in fact did emerge, which led to indictments of two nurses (Perez and Narciso). At the pretrial hearing, some of the videotaped material was shown. Arguments ensued. The judge ruled that, in principle, information obtained through the use of hypnosis could be presented to the jury. The government case was entirely circumstantial. The data from hypnosis interviews served only to aid the more customary evidence and testimony. The jury voted both nurses guilty.

Later, the judge denied a motion for judgments of acquittal but did grant the defendants' motion for a new trial. The judge concluded that the misconduct of the government did reasonably affect the jury. However, the term "misconduct" did not refer to the manner in which the hypnosis had been used to elicit information. It dealt with other technical issues of conduct unrelated to the hypnosis. Later, with a new district attorney in office, the government decided to drop the case.

In this case, the HIP was used to scan and identify potential witnesses, who were then interviewed with hypnosis with the expectation that the information elicited would aid in discovering other evidence with which to build the case for presentation.

The Torsney Case

Torsney was a white New York City policeman charged with shooting and killing a young black boy. The police had answered an emergency call in a black neighborhood in Brooklyn where an altercation was allegedly occurring. After investigation, as the police had left the apartment, someone had warned them to "be careful since there was a man out there with a gun." As the officers had walked toward their cars, a young boy had moved forward and asked Torsney a question. Torsney had thought he saw a shining object on the boy, so the officer had quickly drawn his unlocked pistol and shot the young boy.[9,10]

Torsney's defense was not guilty by reason of psychosis due to epilepsy. He was tried in a Brooklyn courtroom with an all-white jury. The HIP indicated that he was quite hypnotizable, not psychotic, and prone to respond to stress with hysterical dissociation. In fact, when tested for his hypnotizability in the presence of the defense counsel and the district attorney, Torsney's trance response was so persistent and intense that extra cutoff signals were necessary to get him out of the dissociated trance state. He was obviously not the controlled, vigilant, secure combat officer that one would expect to see at such an assignment. Torsney conveyed a sense of a sad, not too competent man in the wrong job. His general demeanor usually elicited sympathy. During the trial, he sat staring at the table most of the time. Although his defense was largely based on the diagnosis of epilepsy and resulting psychosis, none of the many tests and examinations done by either side revealed any evidence of his ever having had epilepsy. Nor was evidence of psychosis ever elicited in the psychological tests performed by the psychologists for either side. The prosecution's position was that Torsney was simply a frightened, not very competent police officer, who, under stress, had panicked and shown poor judgment by using his gun in a clumsy effort to protect himself against an imagined threat. This is an act that might even be regarded as within normal range in the average person but is certainly not the response of a trained police officer, who has every reason to expect these emergencies in the course of his everyday work. The jury voted to acquit Torsney by reason of insanity.

Torsney was then committed to a state psychiatric facility for treatment and care. Over a year later, the hospital reported that they had at no time found evidence of epilepsy or psychosis and wanted to discharge him. At first, the trial court agreed. Then the appellate court refused, claiming that the hospital had not treated Torsney for the disabilities decided upon by the jury. By a 4–3 decision, the court of appeals reversed the appellate decision and released Torsney. This highlighted the absurdity of making clinical diagnosis for treatment by means of legal tactics in front of a jury. Further, with the jury decision, Torsney now made claim for medical disability from the Police Department.

However, the Police Department was not legally bound to automatically accept the diagnosis without making its own judicial investigation. Accordingly, another hearing was held, and essentially the same arguments were presented by both sides. The presiding officer was obliged to report a summary of the hearings with a recommendation to the police commissioner. Ultimately, the police commissioner ruled that Torsney was not psychotic and not epileptic; because his actions indicated ineptness, Torsney was discharged from the police force without any medical disability.

In many ways, the Torsney case exemplifies the recurrent weaknesses of our adjudicatory process in determining responsibility for an act. The compassionate concept of not punishing authentically mentally ill persons for actions beyond their control was stretched so far in this case that in a perverted way, the state was using a hospital to "punish" a man for committing a crime. Then the state berated the doctors for not playing the punishment game to comply with the jury decision. The doctors balked by discovering, on their own, that Torsney was not psychotic, not epileptic, and did not belong in a hospital. Clever courtroom tactics had convinced the jury, but the state hospital and eventually the Police Department itself viewed the evidence otherwise. The HIP, a 10-minute clinical test, identified the theme of an inept police officer who panicked under stress. This was ultimately concurred with by the hospital and Police Department.

CONCLUSION

Back to the question posed by this paper, Is hypnosis a help or hindrance in coping with the complex issues of evidence? Clearly, the answer is:

1. Used knowledgeably with appreciation of their limits, hypnosis techniques can be helpful.

2. Knowledge about hypnosis enables us to identify its misuse and abuse.

3. Since hypnosis occurs spontaneously with so many people daily, ignorance about the phenomenon obfuscates the judicious discovery and use of evidence. Therefore, I disagree with my medical, psychiatric, and psychology colleagues who would like to preempt this field and deny its use to other professions. Everyday phenomena like spontaneous hypnosis occur regardless of the territorial claims of various guilds or power groups. I strongly advocate that all professionals dealing with interrogation—this includes qualified police officers, prosecuting and defense attorneys—alert themselves, inform themselves, and become even more knowledgeable about this intriguing phenomenon in order to cope with it more expertly.

SUMMARY

Clarifying misconceptions about hypnosis can reduce confusion about the place of hypnosis in forensic medicine. Hypnosis identifies a person's capacity for attentive, receptive concentration with parallel awareness. While in trance concentration, memory recall under interrogation should not only be subject to all the usual investigative safeguards with checks and balances, but even more so because the leverage effect of hypnotically enhanced memory is achieved at the risk of contamination by external and/or internal cues. This Janus-like feature enables incredibly accurate revivification and recall of perceived events but can also evoke false memories, false confessions, and the "honest liar syndrome." The internal and external factors that account for these contradictory possibilities—and the appropriate safeguards—are considered with case illustrations.

In addition, a new use of trance capacity assessment contributes to clarifying diagnosis and the mental defect/disease issue.

Knowledge of the uses and limits of hypnosis by the interrogating professionals enhances the judicious process of eliciting information and evidence.

REFERENCES

1. SPIEGEL, H. & D. SPIEGEL. 1978. Trance and Treatment: Clinical Uses of Hypnosis. Basic Books. New York, N.Y.
2. Leyra v. Denno, 347 U.S. 556 (1954).
3. U.S. v. Miller, 411 F.2d 825 (2d Cir. 1969).
4. Conn. v. Reilly, 5285 (1973).
5. Reilly v. Conn., 0-24981-5 (1976-6).
6. CONNERY, D. S. 1977. Guilty Until Proven Innocent. G.P. Putnam's Sons. New York, N.Y.
7. U.S. v. Thornton (U.S. Dist. Court W.D. Mo. 1977).
8. U.S. v. Narciso and Perez, Crim. No. 7-80149 E.D. Mich., S.D. (1977).
9. N.Y.C. v. Torsney, 3923 (1976).
10. Dept. Hearing, N.Y.C.P.D. Torsney Case, Hon. Nicholas Figueroa (1979).

THE DETERMINATION OF MALINGERING

Israella Y. Bash*

*Psychiatric Associates
Science Park Medical Center
College Park, Maryland 20740*

Murray Alpert†

*Department of Psychology
New York University Medical Center
New York, New York 10016*

INTRODUCTION

The problem of malingering presents a frequent and a difficult challenge in clinical psychology, forensic psychiatry, and many other related areas. Scores of studies have investigated the general problem, but the need for a clearer understanding of what we mean by "malingering" and how to detect it is obvious to anyone who has been confronted with the need to evaluate particular cases. Aside from the general considerations of a philosophical, nosological, or clinical nature, the pragmatic difficulties and consequences relating to the patient's disposition within the criminal justice system make the recognition and accurate detection of malingering an issue of some importance. In the forensic setting (the prison ward), we frequently see patients who present a clinical picture that gives rise to the strong suspicion that they are feigning or exaggerating the symptoms of mental illness in order to escape the probable and undesirable consequences of their criminal behavior, i.e., that they are malingering.

At present, the "state of the art" is such that these suspected malingerers are commonly detected by rather vague clinical intuitions, more or less influenced by observations and interpretations of patient behavior as (perhaps selectively) observed by nursing personnel and by certain exaggerated or incongruous aspects of patient behavior. The present study was designed to test promising objective and reliable techniques to evaluate and diagnose malingering in forensic and/or hospital settings.

There are many who regard malingering as evidence of a mental disease in its own right. Therefore, it becomes significant to ask whether malingerers are distinguishable from nonmalingerers in ways that go beyond the specification in the basic definition—for example, with respect to aspects of their personal, social, and psychological histories, or with respect to other psychological characteristics, and so on. The present study has bearing on these questions insofar as they involve a comparison of

---

* Present affiliation: Godding Division, St. Elizabeth Hospital, Washington, D.C. 20020.
† Please address reprint requests to Dr. Alpert.

psychiatrically diagnosed malingerers (individuals feigning psychoses and claiming auditory hallucinations) and nonmalingering, nonpsychotic individuals, both groups being drawn from a population about which there is generally little question that they have recently committed some serious violation of law. In a similar fashion, one can develop the question of whether malingerers can be distinguished from psychotics, i.e., Is the person who feigns schizophrenia the same kind of a person as the one who is actually schizophrenic? Again, the present study has bearing on this question.

Several limitations have been accepted for the present study: (1) we have accepted the psychiatric diagnosis as a criterion of malingering; (2) the subjects (S) are all temporary residents of a prison ward of Bellevue Hospital in New York City, sent there by the courts after being indicted for a crime; (3) the diagnosed malingerers do not cover the gamut of the forms of malingering (i.e., all feign schizophrenia with auditory hallucinations), and thus the outcome of this study could not support the hypothesis that malingerers in general constitute a distinctive group of persons; and (4) the present study is constricted with respect to the range of variables included—it concentrates on the malingering act as such. Our question is whether the malingerer is acting out lines and gestures that are laid out for him or whether he is basically acting out a character. It is harder to *live* or *become* the enacted character; it imposes a greater demand on the person's personality than does carrying out a routine. Following this line of thought leads to a major premise on which this study, in its theoretical aspect, is based. The more narrowly constructed the malingering act is, the less is the likelihood that the actor's own personality is involved. The more differentiatedly adaptive the malingering is to a variety of situations, the greater is the likelihood that the malingerer's own personality is involved. It so happens that the variables we have selected as most promising with respect to the primary concerns of the present study are derived from instruments that are widely used for the investigation of personality, i.e., the Rorschach, Bender-Gestalt, Structured Clinical Interview (SCI), and Wechsler Adult Intelligence Scale (WAIS). With the use of these instruments, differences, if any, between malingerers and the comparison groups will be explored.

The idea of expecting differentiating responses from suspected malingerers stems from the notion that a malingerer does not know how a psychotic patient (schizophrenic) will behave in certain situations and, consequently, will respond in a different way than a real psychotic patient. To evaluate this notion, several tests—each of which has been reported in the literature to have relevant features—were employed: WAIS, Rorschach, Bender-Gestalt, SCI, and the Betts test.

In addition, since the most common complaint of the suspected malingerer in forensic settings is auditory hallucinations, the present study investigated this phenomenon. For that purpose, the Perceptual Characteristic Questionnaire (PCQ) and the Listening Task (both developed by M. Alpert, 1970, 1972) were used. The PCQ is a structured questionnaire intended to give a detailed history and clarification of the patient's hallucinations. The

Listening Task represents an attempt to develop an objective and quantitative method for determining when someone is hallucinating. By controlling the input and requiring the patient to report what he hears, one is able to determine the mismatch between input and report.

The present study was designed to explore and investigate the interrelations among various measures (including psychiatric diagnosis) that have been mentioned in the literature for the detection and diagnosis of malingerers.

REVIEW OF THE LITERATURE

Only a small portion of the immense literature on the topic of malingering will be reviewed here. For a detailed review of the literature on this topic, see Bash.[1]

The concept of malingering has been known throughout history. The Bible and the histories of Greece, Rome, and the Middle Ages[2] cite many instances in which the simulation of insanity was used to avoid execution.

Up to this day, there has been no final agreement among the various authorities as to whether or not malingering should be considered a form of mental disease. Support can be found for either of these viewpoints. Furthermore, a review of the literature on the subject of malingering shows a number of difficulties involved in its diagnosis, detection, and classification.

Perhaps the most difficult problem in the study of malingering is one of classification. Are malingerers a special kind of people? If so, should they be classified as schizophrenics? Psychopathic? Mentally defective? Or, in more general terms, mentally sick? These are only some of the questions treated in the literature with respect to the nosology of malingering.

According to Garner, malingering is used in order to avoid pain or frustration.[3] He assumed that malingering to avoid military service, to gain a dependent position, or to avoid some unpleasantness would indicate an inadequate, asocial, or immature personality. Szasz's views are that malingering is not a diagnosis and therefore should be eliminated from the psychiatric and medical fields, especially as a diagnosis of a disease, and that there is no rational explanation for malingering as a psychopathological syndrome.[4]

The view that malingering is a form of mental illness came to the fore particularly during the Second World War. It was believed that only a "crazy" or "sick" person would malinger. This view was especially supported by Eissler,[5] O'Neil,[6] Moersch,[7] and Hunt,[8] who emphasized that malingering is always a disease, sometimes more severe than a mere neurotic disorder because it involves an arrest of the patient's development at an early age. Wertham's views[9] contrast with those of Eissler; Wertham does not view malingering as a mental disease.

Bleuler seems to have been the first to suggest that the simulation of insanity, irrespective of how conscious or unconscious the patient's motives, should be regarded as a manifestation of a mental illness.[10]

A different view was expressed by Davidson, who stated that malingering by itself does not prove a mental disorder.[11] A person faced with a serious charge would be very sane in trying to escape punishment by being committed to a hospital instead. Jones and Llewellyn pointed to the tendency of the malingerers to exaggerate the behavior.[2] Ossipov described the extremes that the malingerer may exhibit.[12] Macdonald pointed out that the suspect who feigns insanity may be insane but motivated to feign insanity because of his lack of insight into his true condition.[13]

In other studies of the simulation of mental illness, projective tests were found to be of value in differential diagnosis. Rosenberg and Feldberg,[14] Benton,[15] Hunt,[8] and Feldman and Graley[16] tried to detect simulation, using the Rorschach test. Their findings showed that the simulators had few responses, rejected numerous cards, had a large number of popular responses, and perseveration and repetition of previous responses were many. Bizarre responses were seldom seen.

A most difficult aspect in the study of malingering is its diagnosis and detection. As early as 1917, Sir John Collie believed it impossible to find symptoms or to lay down rules for the diagnosis and detection of a malingerer.[17] Eissler[5] and Henderson and Gillespie[18] stressed the importance of having the patient's complete case history, to look for contradictions in the patient's story, for discrepancies, and at his general behavior. For the controversial issues of the Ganser syndrome and hysteria, see Bash.[1]

METHOD

Subjects

Four groups of 30 S each were employed. All S were male patients, age range from 19–50, from the prison ward of Bellevue Hospital. Each S was diagnosed as nonpsychotic or as a genuine or feigned schizophrenic with or without concomitant auditory hallucinations, by two psychiatrists. S represent consecutive admissions who met the requirements of the design. The groups were quite well matched with respect to the distributions of age, race, economic status, and education. Group I consisted of 30 S considered to be malingerers ("diagnosed malingerers") who reported auditory hallucinations. Group II consisted of 30 S diagnosed as schizophrenic who reported auditory hallucinations. Group III consisted of 30 S diagnosed as schizophrenic nonhallucinatory. Group IV consisted of 30 S who were referred to the ward for observations, but who were diagnosed as nonpsychotic, and who were not known to have ever been patients in a psychiatric hospital or to have ever experienced auditory hallucinations.

Materials

The following tests were used: the WAIS, the Rorschach, the Bender-Gestalt, the Listening Task, the SCI, the Betts test, and the PCQ. All of the scoring was done blindly by a rater who did not know the group designation of the *S*. For each test, a special malingering score was devised.

The WAIS

A malingering score was computed based on approximate answers. For **Arithmetic**, the answer given is one above or one below the correct answer (e.g., 4 + 3 = 8 or 6) and was scored +1 for each instance; for **Block Design**, the answer is correct, except for the placement of one block and this block is 90° or less off and is scored +1 for each instance; for **Digit Span**, digits are reported one digit above or below the correct number and the answer is scored +1; for **Picture Arrangement**, all pictures are correct except for one, and this one is placed as the first one or the last one, or *S* does not change the position of the pictures at all, i.e., he leaves the pictures in the same order as experimenter (*E*) puts them, and is scored +1 for each instance; total score is number of picture arrangements scored +1; for **Information**, "I don't know" (DK) answers to easy items, total score number of DK answers to items 1, 2, 3, 4, 5, 6, 8, 11; for **Picture Completion**, "nothing is missing" answers to more than three consecutive items, total score is number of items so answered.

The total approximate answers score for each subtest was translated into a standard score based on the distribution of all *S*. The final approximate answers score for each individual was the sum of the subtest standard scores.

The Rorschach‡

The following items were scored: (1) number of responses; (2) number of cards rejected; (3) mean reaction time (for all cards); (4) number of popular responses; (5) perseveration; (6) number of aggressive and anger responses; (7) number of animal and inanimate movement responses; (8) number of bizarre responses (F−); (9) W:M (usually in the form of W > 2 M); (10) M:C (usually the C outweighs M by 2:1); (11) W% (high W%); (12) failure to interpret popular easy plates; (13) number of color responses = C%. The scoring followed the Klopfer system[19] and was developed as follows: **For item 1,** a distribution of all 120 *S* was computed. *S* got a +1 if his score was below the 25th percentile of the combined distribution. **For item 2,** a distribution of all 120 *S* was computed. *S* got a +1 if his score was above the 75th percentile of the distribution. **For item 3,** a distribution of all 120 *S* was computed. *S* got a +1 if his reaction time was in the top 25th

---

‡ Following are the definitions of the abbreviations used in this paragraph: W = whole or nearly whole blot is used (whole responses); M = human movement responses; C = color responses; F = form level; FM = animal movement responses; m = inanimate responses; and P = popular responses.

percentile of the distribution. **For item 4,** P% was calculated and the distribution for the 120 S was determined; the S then was scored $+1$ if his P% was above the 75th percentile of the distribution. **For item 5,** S was scored $+1$ if he gave the same response to three or more consecutive cards. A distribution was then done. S got a $+1$ if his score was below the 25th percentile of the distribution. **For item 6,** S was scored $+1$ for each response that involved killing, attacking, arguing, a rocket going off, or an explosion. Then a distribution of all the 120 S was done. S got a $+1$ if his score was above the 75th percentile. **For item 7,** the total number of FM and m responses and the (FM + m)% were determined. Here again, a distribution of all 120 S was computed for (FM + m)%. S got a score of $+1$ if his (FM + m)% fell above the 75th percentile of the distribution. **For item 8,** F − % was computed, and S was given a $+1$ if his score was below the 25th percentile of the combined distribution of all 120 S. **For item 9,** the W:M ratio was calculated for each subject, and S was given a $+1$ if his ratio exceeded the 75th percentile of the combined distribution. **For item 10,** S was given a $+1$ if his ratio was above the 75th percentile of the combined distribution of these ratios. **For item 11,** S was scored $+1$ if his W% fell above the 75th percentile of the combined W% distribution. **For item 12,** the reference here is to the rejection of popular responses when asked if he can see them in the course of the testing of the limits. The S was given a $+1$ for each such popular response that he rejected in the testing of the limits. Then a distribution of all 120 S was done. If S's score was above the 75th percentile, he got a $+1$. **For item 13,** it has been reported that malingerers give many color responses as an expression of their emotional state. For each subject (FC + C + C_n + F/C)% was computed (C_n refers to a color naming response, and F/C to the arbitrary use of color, e.g., a "pink dog"). Again, S was given a $+1$ if the ratio was above the 75th percentile of the combined distribution.

A Rorschach "malingering" score was computed as the sum of the point scores on the preceding 13 items. It was expected that the malingerers would score higher than any of the other groups.

The Bender-Gestalt

The Bender's[20] criteria for malingering were used. They are: (1) the drawings are small and inhibited, since the malingerer—attempting to inhibit his intelligence—succeeds only in inhibiting his impulses; (2) uneven performance—some gestalt functions on high level, others on regressed level; (3) actual pattern properties are exactly indicated, e.g., squares do not become loops, etc., order is maintained although the figures' positions are changed; (4) relationship or direction of parts or details may be altered to the point of apparent disorientation, but actual gestalt function will remain on a high level, e.g., the difficult diamond shape will be reproduced accurately; (5) tendency to simplify symbols, e.g., using a continuous line for a series of dots, but retaining the basic shape of the figure; and (6) more complex drawing elements added. This test had been scored on the above six items plus a seventh item—number of items recalled. This additional item, recall, which was employed here, was not mentioned in the literature but was significant to the present study because of the assumption that the malingerers will say that they can't recall or will recall very few items, since this is the way they perceive that a mentally sick person will respond.

The Listening Task

S's task was to report what he heard and to indicate his confidence. Individual product-moment correlations were calculated between the accuracy and the confidence of the response for each *S*. For a more detailed description of the test, see Bash.[1]

The Structured Clinical Interview (SCI)[21]

All 10 categories were used (e.g., anger-hostility, fear-worry, etc.). Scoring was done as follows: On each category for each item that he answered "yes," *S* got a score of + 1. A "no" answer got a zero. The total score for each category was summed separately. Then these raw scores were transformed into standard scores, which are provided in a table, according to age.[21]

The Betts Test

The Sheehan 1967 form was used. All seven modalities were employed. For each modality, *S* was given five items to imagine. *S* was asked to rate the vividness of each image using the following rating scale: 1 = perfectly clear, 2 = very clear, 3 = moderately clear, 4 = not clear but recognizable, 5 = vague and dim, 6 = very vague and dim, 7 = no image present. Some examples of these items are: For the **visual modality**, *S* was asked to imagine some relative or friend and then to rate the vividness of the following: the person's body image, way of walking, different colors of a familiar costume, etc. For the **auditory modality**, *S* was asked to imagine the sound of a whistle of a locomotive, etc. For the **tactual modality**, *S* was asked to imagine the feel of sand, of linen, of fur, etc. For the **kinesthetic modality**, *S* was asked to imagine running upstairs, etc. For the **gustatory modality**, *S* was asked to imagine the taste of salt, etc. For the **olfactory modality**, *S* was asked to imagine the smell of fresh paint, of cooking cabbage, of new leather, etc. For the **somesthetic-organic modality**, *S* was asked to imagine the sensations of fatigue, of hunger, of a sore throat, etc.

The rationale of what we took to be a malingering score was that it was expected that malingerers would attempt to exaggerate the intensity of their imagery, but would have no special reason for doing so more in the context of one of the imagery modalities than in the context of another. Since Sheehan[22] had reported the modality scores separately for a large number of normal *S*, the presumption was that the malingerers particularly would try to make themselves as different as possible from normals by exaggerating the intensity of their imagery. For this reason, we used the Sheehan findings to generate for each modality a transformation into standard scores with a mean of 50 and a standard deviation of 10 in the corresponding Sheehan distribution. These standard scores were then summed, and the total was taken as a malingering score. The higher the score, the greater was the presumption of malingering. As it turned out, the individual modality means standard scores and the total scores were all very much higher than those obtained in the Sheehan distributions. This difference may be worth pursuing in follow-up studies, but there did not seem to be any reason for not using these scores in the comparisons between the groups of the present investigation.

The Perceptual Characteristic Questionnaire (PCQ)

Scoring was done as follows: (1) duration of hallucination—three years or more; (2) aggressive and hostile messages; (3) visual hallucinations; (4) hallucinations occur many times each day (four or more); (5) nonvocal sounds in addition to voices; (6) source localized outside of patient; (7) more frequent with social isolation; (8) more frequent with emotional arousal (e.g., angry, sad, anxious); (9) more frequent with decreased light; (10) medication did not help in reducing frequency.

Each item was scored *one* if present or *zero* if absent. The total score was the sum of the item scores for the subject. For a more detailed description of this test, see Bash.[1]

PROCEDURE

All *S* were tested individually in two sessions with each of the tests. In session I, the SCI, Betts, Listening Task, and Rorschach were employed respectively. In session II, the WAIS, PCQ, and Bender were used respectively.

The testing took place in a separate room at the Bellevue Hospital prison ward. Specific instructions for each test were given by *E*. After reading the instructions for each test, *E* asked *S* if there were any questions, making sure that *S* understood the instructions clearly.

The total time required for each session was approximately 90 minutes.

The same procedure was used with all four groups.

RESULTS

To test the ability of the tests to discriminate between malingerers and the other groups, a one-way analysis of variance (ANOVA), Planned Comparison t-test, and the Student-Newman-Keuls procedure were used for

TABLE 1

MEAN* "MALINGERING" SCORES OF THE FOUR GROUPS

Test	Group I Malingerers	Group II Schizophrenic Hallucinators	Group III Schizophrenic Nonhallucinators	Group IV Nonpsychotic	Groups II–IV Combined Mean
WAIS	357.486	280.192	278.876	283.418	280.829
Rorschach	5.367	2.133	2.567	3.066	2.589
Bender	39.367	11.667	12.667	12.000	12.111
Listening	1.354	0.634	0.545	1.060	0.746
SCI	923.967	1042.533	891.433	722.200	885.389
Betts (Total)	1888.072	1437.635	1387.793	1583.044	1469.480

* The means reported above for the WAIS and the Betts are sums of several standardized scores, each with a mean of 50 and a sigma of 10. See description of these scores in the METHODS section.

each test separately. Results are presented in TABLES 1 and 2. As can be seen, our hypothesis was supported for each of the tests except the SCI, and Group I is significantly discriminated from the other three groups on all of the tests except the SCI ($P = 0.001$).

The hypothesis that the PCQ will discriminate between schizophrenic hallucinators and the suspected malingerers was supported. The PCQ was administered only to the malingerers and the schizophrenic hallucinators. As can be seen from TABLE 3, the two groups are effectively discriminated from one another, and, as anticipated, the malingerers scored lower than the schizophrenic hallucinators group.

A separate analysis was done to determine how well the Listening Task and the PCQ can discriminate between malingerers and others. As can be seen from TABLE 4, the Listening Task had only misdiagnosed 4 S (i.e., false

TABLE 2

SUMMARY OF ANOVA FOR FOUR-GROUP COMPARISON ON THE BETTS TEST

Modality	General Between-Groups Comparisons (df = 3/116)		Student-Newman-Keuls Procedure
	F	P	Homogeneous Subsets and Groups*
Visual	16.294	< 0.001	III, II/II, IV/I
Auditory	15.921	< 0.001	III, II/II, IV/I
Tactual	20.675	< 0.001	III, II/IV/I
Kinesthetic	21.197	< 0.001	III, II/IV/I
Gustatory	16.477	< 0.001	III, II/II, IV/I
Olfactory	19.540	< 0.001	III, II, IV/I
Somesthetic-Organic	10.422	< 0.001	III, II, IV/I
All Modalities Combined	26.418	< 0.001	III, II/IV/I

* Members of homogeneous subsets separated by commas; discriminated subsets (at 0.05 significance level) separated by slashes; order of discriminated subsets is from low to high means.

TABLE 3

RESULTS FOR PERCEPTUAL CHARACTERISTICS QUESTIONNAIRE (PCQ)

Group	Means	df	F	P
I. Malingerers	900.633	1/58	9.394	< 0.003
II. Schizophrenic Hallucinators	1161.100			

positive). The PCQ did not do as well. However, when *both* tests were used, the results were fantastic—no misdiagnoses at all (or false positives).

Inspecting TABLE 5, we see that when the battery of tests was used (except the SCI and PCQ), a substantial phi coefficient was obtained (0.8872). There was only one misdiagnosed S. This phi obtained with the composite score is substantially higher than the highest phi obtained for any of the tests individually.

The one-way ANOVA was used to test the overall differences between the four groups on each modality and the overall modalities of the Betts test. As can be seen from TABLE 6, all modalities are effective in discriminating the malingerers from the other three groups. Furthermore, the tactual, kinesthetic, and the overall modalities are even better discriminators, since Group I is significantly different from Group IV and significantly different from Groups II and III.

To test for statistically significant differences between the four groups on all tests that refer to personal characteristics, a one-way ANOVA was used for the WAIS and the Bender. (For results of the other tests, Rorschach and SCI, see Bash.)[1] The results of the subscores of the WAIS—this time using the conventional scores and the conventional way of scoring—are presented in TABLE 7. As can be seen, the malingerers constituted the lowest scoring group on every WAIS score. However, they were significantly lower by both the Planned Comparison test and the Student-Newman-Keuls procedure only on the Information, Comprehension, Arithmetic, Picture Completion, Verbal, and Full Scale scores. They are not discriminated by the Student-Newman-Keuls procedure on Digit Span, Vo-

TABLE 4

CROSS TABULATION OF PCQ AND LISTENING TASK TEST DIAGNOSIS VS. PSYCHIATRIC DIAGNOSIS*

		Psychiatric Diagnosis		
Test	Test Diagnosis	Nonma-lingerers	Ma-lingerers	
Listening Task	Malingerers	4	26	ϕ = 0.7333
	Nonmalingerers	26	4	sign. at 0.0001
PCQ	Malingerers	9	22	ϕ = 0.4336
	Nonmalingerers	21	8	sign. at 0.002
Listening Task and PCQ	Malingerers	0	20	ϕ = 0.7071
	Nonmalingerers	30	10	sign. at 0.0001

* Malingerers vs. schizophrenic hallucinators.

TABLE 5

CROSS TABULATION OF TEST DIAGNOSIS*

	Psychiatric Diagnosis		
Test Diagnosis	Nonmalingerers	Malingerers	
Malingerers			
	1	26	ϕ = 0.8872
Nonmalingerers	89	4	sign. at 0.0001

* Based on tests, exclusive of SCI and PCQ vs. psychiatric diagnosis.

cabulary, Digit-Symbol, and Performance scores. They are not significantly different on Similarities, Block Design, Picture Arrangement, and Object Assembly. An explanation for this phenomenon may be that Group I deliberately gave wrong answers in order to appear stupid on the assumption that stupidity characterized schizophrenia. Also, because of their extensive use of approximate answers, Group I's scores are lower.

The Bender test results are also given in TABLE 7, this time using Bender's criteria[20] for diagnosing schizophrenia. As can be seen, the Bender successfully discriminated between the nonschizophrenic groups (I and IV) and the schizophrenic groups (II and III). The Student-Newman-Keuls gave the following divisions: Groups I and IV in one subset and Groups II and III in another. The Bender test is a good discriminator.

DISCUSSION

The basic hypothesis bearing on the ability of the seven tests to detect and, thus, to diagnose malingerers was supported by the findings of the present study. Six of the seven tests successfully discriminated the malingerers

TABLE 6

SUMMARY OF ANOVA FOR FOUR-GROUP COMPARISON OF "MALINGERING" SCORES

Test	General Between-Groups Comparisons (df 3/116)		Planned Comparison Group I vs. Other Three (df 116)		Student-Newman-Keuls Procedure
	F	P	t	P	Homogeneous Subsets & Groups*
WAIS	36.075	< 0.001	10.390	< 0.001	II, III, IV/I
Rorschach	26.770	< 0.001	8.642	< 0.001	II, III, IV/I
Bender	25.061	< 0.001	8.667	< 0.001	II, III, IV/I
Listening	33.604	< 0.001	8.067	< 0.001	II, III/IV/I
SCI	8.815	< 0.001	0.750	N.S.	IV, III/I, II
Betts (Total)	26.812	< 0.001	7.985	< 0.001	II, III/IV/I

* Members of homogeneous subsets separated by commas; discriminated subsets (at 0.05 significance level) separated by slashes; order of discriminated subsets is from low to high means.

TABLE 7

SUMMARY OF ANOVA FOR FOUR-GROUP COMPARISON ON
THE WAIS SUBTESTS AND BENDER-GESTALT

Test	General Between-Groups Comparison (df 3/116)		Planned Comparison Group I vs. Other Three (df 116)		Student-Newman-Keuls Procedure
					Homogeneous Subsets and Groups*
	F	P	t	P	
WAIS					
Information	5.854	0.001	3.968	0.001	I/II, IV, III
Comprehension	6.932	0.001	3.971	0.001	I/II, III, IV
Arithmetic	3.567	0.016	3.050	0.001	I/II, III, IV
Similarities	.868	0.460 (N.S.)	1.568	0.120 (N.S.)	I, II, III, IV
Digit Span	2.122	0.101 (N.S.)	2.362	0.020	I, II, III, IV
Vocabulary	3.544	0.017	3.091	0.001	I, II, III/II, III, IV
Digit Symbol	2.023	0.115 (N.S.)	2.166	0.032	I, II, III, IV
Picture Completion	4.514	0.005	3.129	0.002	I/III, II, IV
Block Design	1.586	0.197 (N.S.)	1.947	0.054 (N.S.)	I, III, IV, II
Picture Arrangement	1.717	0.167 (N.S.)	1.324	0.180 (N.S.)	I, III, II, IV
Object Assembly	1.537	0.209 (N.S.)	1.331	0.180 (N.S.)	I, III, IV, II
Verbal Score	5.113	0.001	3.699	0.001	I/II, III, IV
Performance Score	2.481	0.064 (N.S.)	2.369	0.013	I, II, III, IV
Full Scale	4.284	0.007	3.441	0.001	I/III, II, IV
BENDER-GESTALT	7.350	0.001	2.593	0.001	IV, I/II, III

* Members of homogeneous subsets separated by commas; discriminated subsets (at 0.05 significance level) separated by slashes; order of discriminated subsets is from low to high means.

from the other three groups. Four of the seven tests, taken together, yielded a multiple correlation of 0.839 with the psychiatric diagnosis. Both the Listening Task and the PCQ significantly discriminated Group I from Group II.

An additional question of interest to the present study was tested: If the S are classified as malingerers or nonmalingerers separately on the basis of each of the five successful tests (exclusive of the PCQ and SCI), on how many of these tests must the S be so classified in order to be safely characterized as a malingerer? Results showed that when our S were characterized as malingerers on the basis of their scores on at least three of the tests and as nonmalingerers if they were so classified on less than three tests, the phi correlation with the psychiatric classification was 0.8872. However, we would hesitate to generalize from this finding without additional supporting evidence.

In general, the overall performance of the malingerers was significantly more exaggerated and significantly different from that of the schizophrenic or the nonpsychotic S. Thus, it may be said that the malingerers are special kinds of people and may be put in a separate classification. There are common patterns in their malingering, which are manifested in areas of behavior that range far beyond the simulation of a mental disease. In a sense, given an incentive to malinger, what unifies the reported findings is a kind of inner logic of such simulation. Malingerers are recognizable by their conformity to the requirements of this inner logic.

Even so, establishing that there is such a common denominator among malingerers that makes them discriminable from others is a far cry from establishing that there is a core of common traits that disposes certain individuals to malinger and that is lacking in others who do not attempt to do so. As indicated, the failure to establish the kind of unity we have found would throw into doubt the distinctiveness of malingerers in the broader sense. Our success, however, does not establish that malingerers do constitute a distinctive group in the broader sense, that is, as a psychologically and psychiatrically meaningful diagnostic category. This issue is dealt with in Bash.[1]

Conclusions

In reviewing the foregoing, it appears that there is no reason to affirm that malingerers constitute a special class of people, even though we may conclude that they are discriminable from other groups of people. Their difference apparently inheres in what they are doing rather than in what they are. No differences were found between the malingerers and the other subjects that could not be attributed to the act of malingering per se. The nonpsychotic subjects had the same incentive to malinger as did the malingerers, but it is suggested that the simplest explanation of why some individuals malinger and some do not is that the latter are deterred by anxiety about possible consequences of being caught in the deception and by a lack of confidence in their ability to carry it out.

The tests do provide an objective way of detecting malingering, at least in the setting of the prison ward. Apart from their objectivity, the tests may offer the only tenable means of validly diagnosing malingering. Therefore, it is suggested that they should be used whenever possible, especially in a less developed setup.

Finally, it should be noted that the failure to establish distinctive personal characteristics among malingerers in the extreme case of the simulation of psychosis throws some doubt on the likelihood of finding distinctive personal characteristics in other forms of malingering.

References

1. Bash, I. Y. 1978. Malingering: a study designed to differentiate between schizophrenic offenders and malingerers. Ph.D. Dissertation. Department of Psychology. New York University. New York, N.Y.
2. Jones, A. B. & J. Llewellyn. 1917. Malingering. Heinemann. London, England.
3. Garner, H. H. 1965. Malingering. Ill. Med. J. 128: 318–319.
4. Szasz, T. S. 1961. The Myth of Mental Illness. Harper & Row, Publishers. New York, N.Y.

5. Eissler, K. R. 1951. Malingering. *In* Psychoanalysis and Culture. G. B. Wilbur & W. Muensterbegger, Eds.: 218–253. International Universities Press, Inc. New York, N.Y.

6. O'Neil, W. 1943. Goldbricks. Hygeia **21:** 426–427. (Quoted in Reference 5.)

7. Moersch, F. P. 1944. Malingering: with reference to its neuropsychiatric aspects in civil and in military practice. *In* The Medical Clinics of North America, The Mayo Clinic Number: 928–944. W.B. Saunders. Philadelphia, Penn.

8. Hunt, A. 1946. The detection of malingering. U.S. Nav. Med. Bull. **46:** 249–254.

9. Wertham, F. 1949. The Show of Violence. Doubleday & Company, Inc. New York, N.Y.

10. Bleuler, E. 1944. A Textbook of Psychiatry. (Translated by A. A. Brill, 1924.) Macmillan & Company, Ltd. New York, N.Y.

11. Davidson, H. A. 1965. Forensic Psychiatry. Ronald Press Company. New York, N.Y.

12. Ossipov, V. P. 1944. Malingering: the simulation of psychosis. Bull. Menninger Clin. **8(2):** 39–42.

13. Macdonald, J. M. 1969. Psychiatry and the Criminal. Charles C. Thomas. Springfield, Ill.

14. Rosenberg, S. J. & T. M. Feldberg. 1944. Rorschach characteristics of a group of malingerers. Rorschach Research Exchange **8:** 141–158.

15. Benton, A. L. 1945. Rorschach performance of suspected malingerers. J. Abnorm. Soc. Psychol. **40:** 94–96.

16. Feldman, M. J. & J. Graley. 1954. The effects of an experimental set to simulate abnormality on group Rorschach performance. J. Projective Techniques **18:** 326–334.

17. Collie, J. 1917. Malingering and Feigned Sickness. Edward Arnold. London, England. (Quoted in Reference 5.)

18. Henderson, D. & R. D. Gillespie. 1950. A Textbook of Psychiatry. Oxford University Press. New York, N.Y.

19. Klopfer, B., M. D. Ainsworth, W. G. Klopfer & R. R. Holt. 1954. Developments in Rorschach Technique. 1. Technique and Theory. World Book Company. Yonkers-on-Hudson, N.Y.

20. Bender, L. 1938. A Visual Motor Gestalt Test and Its Clinical Use. Research Monograph No. 3. The American Orthopsychiatric Association. New York, N.Y.

21. Burdock, E. I. & A. S. Hardesty. 1968. Structured Clinical Interview (SCI). Springer Publishing Company, Inc. New York, N.Y.

22. Sheehan, P. W. 1967. A shortened form of Betts' questionnaire upon mental imagery (QMI). J. Clin. Psychol. **23:** 386–389.

ISSUES OF PSYCHOLOGICAL EVIDENCE: DISCUSSION

Discussant: Murray S. Miron

Department of Psychology
Syracuse University
Syracuse, New York 13210

The papers of this session all represent issues of singular importance to the problems of criminal justice. Lie or stress detection, voice printing, and hypnosis have been eagerly adopted by law enforcement agencies as means for the detection and identification of the criminal. From the caution and circumspection of the laboratory, these techniques have been rushed into the service of the practitioner whose needs and enthusiasm may make him less wary than is justified by the research on these techniques. There can be no doubt that if we are to deal with the permutated increases in crime, we shall have to bring as much of the power of the scientist's laboratory to bear as we can. But it seems to me that at the same time, we must counsel the caution and skepticism that is the hallmark of the scientist to those who would use the fruits of his researches. There is a disturbing tendency to wishfully imagine that there is a "golden key" solution to our problems of rising and increasingly sophisticated crime. When coupled with the glamour of new and "scientific" discoveries, wish and reality may become hopelessly confused.

Unfortunately, even the scientist is not immune to the temptations of such wishfulness. The respect afforded the scientist—in large measure because of his objectivity—may act to make him less circumspect when called upon to offer his expert assistance, precisely because those who seek his advice often have unrealistic expectations. The world of the courtroom, for example, is dramatically and very often disconcertingly different from the world of the laboratory. More than one expert witness has been trapped into an advocative certainty unwarranted by the probabilistic nature of his own research findings. The courtroom atmosphere appears to encourage such advocacy on the part of the expert, in conformity to the legal style of such proceedings. But when the expert becomes an advocate, I think it fair to say that he loses the essential quality that makes him valuable to such court procedures. It is the scientist's uncertainty—his questions more than his answers—that warrants our respect.

The papers of this session all demonstrated the constraint and caution that mark the best of our scientists. Dr. Hollien points to the paucity of data that would support a conclusion of identifying voice correlates of stress, much less the use of a microtremor indicator of lying. Dr. Spiegel, despite the more optimistic tone of his paper, properly warns against some of the more obvious dangers of the use of hypnosis in evidence gathering and self-induced trance states. The paper by Drs. Bash and Alpert on the detection of malingering in criminal patients can be interpreted as an attempt to make such determination more objective than the ex cathedra pronouncements sometimes offered by the forensic psychiatrist.

Taken as a whole, the papers of this session did not offer much encouragement to those who may have sought their own "golden keys." Nor, I suspect, were they found to be particularly newsworthy to the members of the press who were sent to report on the conference. There was much more drama in the newest "discovery" of the Rahway lifers' solution to juvenile delinquency. The session on issues in evidence appeared to have the character of quibbling over old news—the sort of curmudgeonly crankiness the public often associates with the academic. But what was said and what was implied were neither cranky nor unnewsworthy. The message rang loud and clear to anyone who would have cared to listen. There is no glamorous, easy solution to our problems of crime. Beneath the ballyhoo of the technology that has been applied in the service of our forensic needs there lies a soft substrate of too few data too soon extended. That is not to say that the laboratory and its expert custodians have no place in evidentiary proceedings. But it *is* to say that we must continue to counsel caution whenever we export our products into the exotic countries of their much needed application.

As a member of the psychological community who also has become a part of the growth industry spawned by crime and terrorism, I have come to learn firsthand of the dangers of which I speak. Periodically, I like to remind myself of the comment made by that most outspoken iconoclast, Thomas Szasz. In a letter to the editor of the New York Times, in comment on the use of mental health professionals as negotiators and experts on terrorist problems, Szasz asked the rhetorical question: "What do psychiatrists know about terrorism?" His proffered answer was that either this was merely the natural outgrowth of the increasing "psychiatrizing" of human affairs, or psychiatrists were themselves terrorists and hence well qualified as experts in such matters. Despite the obvious polemics of such hyperbole, it is difficult to deny the evidence of the misuses of psychiatric diagnosis that have been reported by those who have escaped the asylums of Russia. Is there not the seed of such abuse in the claims of sure identification of lying, speaker identity, hypnotic memory reconstruction, and malingering? Perhaps exaggerated in this way, the scientist's crankiness becomes a duty rather than an affectation.

With this rather long-winded (and even perhaps cranky) preamble in mind, I should like to turn to an examination of some of the specifics of the papers presented at this session. The authors have spoken eloquently for themselves, and there is little point in repeating what they have said far better than I as discussant could offer. Instead, I shall use my role as discussant to make some personal observations on the issues of each of the papers. So as not to abuse that role, my remarks should not be interpreted as either endorsed by, or even consonant with the views of, the speakers.

Stress, Lying, and Psychological Stress Evaluation

Among the new technologies, none has received more attention than the psychological stress evaluator (PSE). The storm of controversy and advocacy that has swirled around this technique still rages. It seems to me that the issues involved in the theory and uses of the PSE* are generalizably instructive and hence warrant close examination. There is a veritable army of trained and untrained practitioners of the "science" of lie detection daily practicing their trade in the service of criminal investigation, preemployment screening, and even mischief-making—as, it seems to me, are such things as the assertion that Lee Harvey Oswald was not lying when he said, "I didn't kill nobody, no sir." From a $5000 device only marketed with an instruction course in its use, the offsprings of the PSE have devolved to gadgets of less than $250, offered to anyone and for anything. In a recent visit to one of this nation's most prestigious physics laboratories, my rather mundane talk was monitored by one of these hand-held devices, unashamedly thrust under my nose. In New York State, an amendment to the Labor and Industrial Relations Act makes it a misdemeanor to employ PSE devices for the purposes of preemployment screening, and yet to my certain knowledge they are being so used daily.

If one reviews the data on PSE, a curious dichotomy emerges. On the one hand, laboratory studies of the technique find chance or little better accuracy of deception identification. On the other hand, field studies of its application in actual criminal investigations find perfect or near perfect identification. Such discrepancy has prompted more than one advocate of the device to argue that laboratory studies are both artificial and useless as tests of the efficacy of what was meant to be a tool in criminal investigations. Thus, the laboratory researcher is dismissed from the arena of this controversy, and his findings declared irrelevant to the "real world." Such preemptive dismissal is not new. It has plagued every scientist. In defense, some have left the laboratory to join the ranks of their real-worlder critics, others have defensively declared themselves aloof from the mundane, and still others have tried to tailor their research designs to better reflect reality. The criticism may have validity, but I fear that what I detect is the very old infrasonic note of the antiscience antiintellectualism that would make magic and fraud respectable. Fraud and belief in magic are so far removed from the concern of the scientist that he often is sadly naive to their widespread acceptance. There is nothing more pathetic than the hoodwinked scientist, victim of the charlatan.

Routinely, as a part of my university lectures on the statistics of probability and chance, I demonstrate a series of mental effects that I have either purchased from practicing mentalists or have developed on my own. I can, without failure, appear to read any mind in the classroom, make a perfect run through an ESP deck, and relate facts and circumstances of the

---

* It is merely curious rather than significant that PSE is a palindromic permutation of ESP. My use of the acronym PSE is generic rather than specific to any proprietary device.

students' lives. Before and after each demonstration, I carefully point out that the things I am doing are all tricks that my audience can also purchase from such places as Tannens in New York City. I announce that I am a fraud and that I can no more read minds than the least adept among them. What is startling is that these nascent scientists, these members of the future intelligentsia, invariably ask me if I was born with my talent. Despite my protestations, they respond with awe and even fear of what they presume to be my ability to plumb their minds. That is scary. The unquestioned acceptance of PSE is similarly scary.

Out of an admitted bias, born of my psycholinguistics training, I have always considered truth and deception to be linguistic questions. Only propositions have truth value. The merely physical cannot be true or false. Viewed from this lofty linguistic perspective, the notion that there is a physical basis for deception is just plain silly. Consider the following utterances:

1. This administration has been falsely accused of an attempt to cover up certain facts.
2. No aspirin is more effective than Bayer® Aspirin.
3. No heat costs less than oil heat.

All three statements are tautologically true under translation. In the first, the optional deletion of agent specification permitted by the passive voice serves to conceal the source of the assertion. The existence of any false accuser makes the statement true. In the second, the statement merely proclaims that Bayer Aspirin is aspirin. In fact, the commercial goes on to establish that the Bayer product is nothing but aspirin and hence could not hope to be better or worse than any aspirin. In the third, it is clear that no heat costs nothing and that any other heat or anything else for that matter necessarily costs more. As might be expected, such trickery is not either abnormal or unusual in language. It is, in part, the reason that the subject of the polygraph examination is instructed to restrict his answers to yes-or-no, preprepared questions.

As Professor Hollien's paper observes, there are physical voice correlates of stress, even if fewer than we might hope. It is, however, the inductive leap that would functionally relate stress and deception that transcends these physical correlates. Worse, even the logic of this inductive presumption bears scrutiny. Stated baldly, If deception is presumed to cause stress, why is it not equally plausible to assert that stress causes deception? The circumstances of a lie detection test make such speculation not without merit.

By contrast to the carefully evolved procedures of the polygraph examination, the PSE lends itself to significant carelessness. Where the polygraphist uses both control and irrelevant questions in order to establish experimental-like control conditions, the PSE's attraction is that it can be employed clandestinely and hence potentially without proper controls in both senses of that word.

But such argument presumes what is not entirely certain, namely, that there exists anything at all to measure or even abuse. In a publication of my own, which Professor Hollien had not seen, I tentatively concluded that there was some evidence for a microtremor component in the vocal fold tone of speech. That conclusion was based upon two forms of evidence. First, there are a number of studies of sufficient procedural care that indicate that something claimed to represent the 8–12 Hz microtremor component can reliably be identified. Second, the generally accepted account of the demonstrated microtremor in peripheral musculature as having reflex level origins suggests that the condition should be found in at least all larger, striate musculature. Professor Hollien correctly observes in his paper that the very small, fast-acting musculature controlling the action of the vocal folds is sufficiently different in character from the muscles in which the tremor has been found to warrant suspicion as to generalization. I do not disagree; but at the same time, it should be noted that the entire laryngeal mechanism is supported by a network of large and slow-acting muscles, which could—if subject to such microtremor—superimpose their effect upon the vocal fold tone. Thus, those studies of which I am aware that attempt and fail to record the microtremor from electrodes planted in the smaller musculature need not rule out its presence in other muscles associated with the laryngeal mechanism. Until better evidence is available, prudence dictates that any conclusion regarding the PSE and its use in lie detection should be guarded.

Hypnosis and Memory Enhancement

Professor Spiegel's paper reports a number of cases in which he or others have successfully used hypnosis for the purpose of reconstructing past events significant for criminal investigation. It is of interest that Professor Loftus, in a paper delivered just prior to this session, reported on some aspects of witness testimony that are clearly important to the use of hypnotically induced recall. Professor Loftus found that the content of the questions used to elicit recall of an eyewitness significantly influenced the character of the memory. If one asks a witness whether he saw broken glass at the scene of an accident in which the vehicle had "smashed" into another vehicle, the report is more often positive than if the vehicles had only "collided." Such findings well fit the generalized model of conceptual, rather than sensory, memory storage. It is a model in which the human is viewed as an active processor of stimuli rather than as a passive filterer. Such active processing is a sort of analysis by synthesis. That is to say, the processor actively models—hypothesizes—his inputs in a conceptual framework that predicts and extends the incomplete and unorganized inputs given to his senses. The character of the model used for this sensory organization is dependent upon both the past and future experiences of the organism. Previously formed hypotheses about inputs dictate the meaning of present inputs, and later inputs change and modify the stored models to form new hypotheses for current processing. Such a conception readily accounts for the frequent errors in perception and indeed makes such errors normal, rather than abnormal, aspects of both memory and perception. Memory recall in such a model presupposes that the recaller *reconstructs* the sensory events as deductions from the *hypotheses* that were employed in their perception. Such a view significantly differs from one in which sensory inputs are written on a sort of tabula rasa.

It seems to me that hypnotically induced recall assumes something more like the tabula rasa view of memory. It is significant that the probes for such recall under hypnosis often take the form of suggesting that the subject view the past scene like a movie film that may be slowed and even stopped on particular frames. The clear implication is that memory is a sort of blank film, storing latent images that are merely awaiting development. Such a view is not consonant with the well-documented distortions that characterize memory. The practitioner of hypnosis has typically countered such objection with the assertion that the trance state taps processes that are different from those characterizing the normal waking state—processes that are somehow more elemental and basic than those subject to the effects of preconception, bias, and modeling. This is a strong assertion. In my opinion, it fails to be credible from what we know about the hypnotic state. Hypnotic trance has been described as a heightened state of suggestibility. Professor Spiegel, himself, describes it as a heightened state of awareness and concentrated attention normal to the organism—so ordinary, in fact, that Dr. Spiegel warns that self-induced hypnosis may influence any suspect interview. If the state is so pervasive, then one should expect that its processes should be operative in normal memory research, which favors the analysis by synthesis model. Further, if the hypnotic trance heightens suggestibility, is it not the case that one should expect more, rather than less, susceptibility to the effects of bias in memory? Such questions, at the least, suggest that we should view hypnotically elicited memory with some caution.

Professor Spiegel chose to warn us of another danger. He suggests that the results of a suspect interview may be the contaminated fruit of inadvertent or auto-trance induction. Such warning, in my opinion, goes far too far. If one suspects that one can fall into and out of the trance state without will and with the frequency suggested by Professor Spiegel, then we must be talking about a different process than the one that I would reserve for the term hypnotic trance. I am not suggesting that hypnotic trance is necessarily a qualitatively different state from that which characterizes the normal state; but instead, that the term should be reserved for those quantitative enhancements of concentration and suggestibility that differ from those of nontrance states. Rapport, trust, and openness to cooperation cannot, in my view, be used to define the trance state. Although such effects are observed in trance, they are not definitionally discriminating. If they are erected as the criteria of trance, the term becomes empty of meaning.

Insanity, Irresponsibility, and Malingering

The defense of incompetence by reason of insanity is enjoying one of those fashionable cycles in human affairs reminiscent of the hula hoop craze. The disorder of multiple personality has been used far more often as an account of ordinary criminality than its tenuous psychiatric status would predict to be real. The knowledgeable malingerer, however, knows that schizophrenia is far more frequently the diagnosis of choice when the symptomology is vague and variable. That the unknowledgeable confuse multiple personality with schizophrenia is testimony to the pernicious influence of the mass media on our understanding of mental disorders. Nor would I exclude the self-conscious attempts at manipulating public opinion on the part of the mental health professionals. With the certain knowledge that what I am about to say will raise a hue and cry, I am nonetheless moved to observe that the current public emphasis on mental disorder as disease has done as much harm as good in the shaping of public attitudes. My correspondence files literally bulge with letters from critics who protest that they are proud to be self-confessed psychotics. They claim that, like the cancer victim, they *are* victims who must patiently await their cure and, while suffering, require that we absolve them of any and all responsibility for their state or their recovery. Under such conditions, it is not surprising that psychosis should be feigned as defense against criminal responsibility. In all regards, such malingering in the current climate is adaptive and, under such interpretation, the antithesis of insanity.

Thus, the work of Drs. Bash and Alpert in attempting to detect malingering takes on enormous social significance. Their empirical approach to the problem is refreshing, particularly when it is contrasted with the veritable circus of the expert judgments that has recently characterized some of the more notorious criminal prosecutions. The problem of distinguishing malingering from "true" psychosis, however, is not simple. The problem lies in the slipperiness of either label. Bash and Alpert defined the terms by operational invocation of the judgments made by psychiatric professionals. But such definition assumes both that those judgments are independent of the tests employed by the authors and that they are at least reliable, if not valid. With respect to the first point, Drs. Bash and Alpert observe that the psychiatric judgments were not based upon the explicit use of the tests they themselves subsequently employed. Still, one wonders whether the psychiatric judgments could possibly have been entirely free of the content of these tests, which—if they have any validity at all—must capture diagnostic criteria defining the disorders being diagnosed. Thus, there may remain the question of definitional circularity.

With respect to the assumed reliability and validity of such diagnostic judgments, it is difficult not to resurrect the embarrassment of the Rosenhan study.[1] The central finding of the study of the "sane in insane places" is easily dismissed. One surely would hope that any advanced civilization would admit those who sought mental care to the institutions designed for such care. It is the incidental findings of that study that are disconcerting.

The first is that the bona fide residents of these institutions readily detected the pseudopatients, and the second is what transpired after the study was completed. Challenged by his critics, who argued that such failure to detect malingering could not occur in their hospital, Rosenhan suggested that they endeavor to detect the pseudopatients he might send their way. During the following three-month period, of 193 admissions, 41 patients were judged with high confidence to be pseudopatients by at least one member of the staff. Rosenhan reports that in actuality he sent no one.

Malingerers like Garrett Brock Trapnell, with whom I have had some personal dealings, boastfully attest to the ease with which they are able to deceive those who are vested with the responsibility of detecting their subterfuges. In the ghosted book *The Fox Is Crazy Too*, Trapnell records a lifetime of escape from prosecution by claiming insanity.[2]

None of this is meant to imply pessimism or criticism of the speakers of this session. On the contrary, it is precisely the cautions voiced by each of the speakers that are the firm basis for optimism that we can provide contributions to the issues of psychological evidence.

REFERENCES

1. ROSENHAN, D. L. 1973. On being sane in insane places. Science **179**: 250–258.
2. ASINOF, E. 1976. The Fox Is Crazy Too. William Morrow and Co., Inc. New York, N.Y.

FORENSIC PSYCHOLOGY AND HOSTAGE NEGOTIATION: INTRODUCTORY REMARKS

Dorothy Heid Bracey

Criminal Justice Center
John Jay College of Criminal Justice
New York, New York 10019

Hostage taking is an ancient device for strengthening a bargaining position. Military antagonists as well as criminals and political opponents have often used the means of threatening the life and safety of a third party as a way of increasing their leverage in negotiation. The success of the technique has traditionally depended upon the value placed upon the well-being of the hostage or upon the ability to free the hostage by force. Thus, the outcome of a hostage-taking situation depended on a balance of moral, military, or political power.

That analysis of hostage taking changed irrevocably in 1972. Although the growth of international terrorism had made many individuals in government and law enforcement more conscious of the possibility of hostage situations and the need to deal with them, 1972—the year of the attack upon Lod airport and the massacre at the Munich Olympics—marks the period when hostage negotiation came to be deliberately and systematically developed as a technique for countering hostage takers. Since that time, an ever-increasing amount of data has been gathered and exchanged—not only among agencies, but also among nations—and negotiating practices have been rehearsed and refined on a regular basis. It is common to find hostage negotiation units in medium-to-large-size police departments, while even small forces commonly make use of training in negotiation skills. And if terrorist kidnappings have inspired a new approach to hostage negotiation, those dealing with the phenomenon have found the resulting techniques to be applicable also to hostage situations caused by criminals, spontaneous rioters, and the mentally disturbed.[1]

A successful negotiation is one in which the hostage is released, the hostage taker captured, and no deaths occur among hostages, hostage takers, negotiaters, or bystanders. In order to bring about this situation, a large number of factors must be considered and controlled. Among the things to be faced by any agency faced with a hostage situation are (1) agency policy and priorities concerning negotiable items and the well-being of participants; (2) the existence and extent of interagency cooperation and the joint understanding of jurisdictional boundaries; (3) an agreed-upon chain of command; (4) a mutually supportive relationship with the news media, based upon trust and a common concern for the protection of human life; (5) knowledge of and ability to use whatever support services are available—included here are assault teams and precision firearms capability; (6) familiarity with available equipment, such as ambulances, tear gas, and communications devices; and (7) an intelligence-gathering capability that collects accurate and usable information. Deficiencies in any of these areas can defeat a negotiation attempt before it begins or can cause it to break down anywhere in its duration.

Although the absence of any of these factors can destroy a negotiation, their presence does not ensure its success. Success, it has come to be recognized, depends on the ability to understand and respond to the intra- and interpersonal dynamics taking place during the situation.

It was recognized early in the creation of negotiation techniques that the emotional state of the hostage taker was one of the most crucial variables in deciding the outcome of the situation. Included here is the motivation—the criminal who wishes only to escape must be dealt with differently from the ideological terrorist who is willing to die for a cause. The prison inmates with a concise and well-articulated set of demands call for a style of negotiation different from that to be used with an emotionally disturbed individual who calls for a diffuse and unelaborated "justice." The now-common use of psychologists and psychiatrists in the training of negotiators, and their use as consultants in negotiation situations, testifies to the importance attributed to the understanding of the mind of the hostage taker.

The papers presented here, however, are evidence of a much more sophisticated understanding of the role of the mental health sciences in hostage negotiation. One aspect of this is the realization that the emotional situation is a dynamic one and that the negotiation process itself is a factor in changing it. The technique of negotiation as it exists today is not merely bargaining; instead, it is an attempt to change the emotional relationship between the hostage taker and his surroundings so that he becomes willing to release the hostage unharmed. Bargaining—giving the hostage taker something he wants in return for something he will give up—may be part of this process, but it is not the entirety.

Recognition of negotiation as a technique for changing emotional states and relationships gave rise to the realization that the mental and emotional condition of the hostage taker is not the only factor of concern to forensic psychologists and psychiatrists. The corresponding conditions of the negotiators, other law enforcement agents, and hostages themselves must also be understood if the negotiation is to lead to a successful outcome. At some levels, this statement is self-evident; days of work by a patient, trained negotiator can be quickly undone by an aggressive, undisciplined sharpshooter. Other implications were not immediately obvious but have become accepted as the result of study and experience. For example, close relatives of a hostage taker were often brought to the scene to plead and reason; it is now perceived that the emotional relationship between the hostage taker and members of his family may have been among the factors precipitating or underlying the incident. In such cases, the presence of these individuals may exacerbate the situation rather than improve it. And it is only gradually that we are beginning to get some insights into the dynamics of the relationship between the hostage taker and the victim and that we are able to consider the implications of these dynamics for the negotiating process. This is important because changes in one set of psychological relationships may affect the emotional content of other sets. For instance, the negotiator who is ignorant of the "Stockholm syndrome" may be confused, disturbed, and finally angered by evidence of the victim's affection and concern for the hostage taker. Such a negotiator may come to doubt the legitimacy of an effort to save a victim who is perceived as acting less like a victim than like an accomplice and thereby may seriously undermine the success of the negotiating procedure. The ability to understand and predict such reactions on the part of the victims will enable the negotiator to treat them dispassionately and even to make positive use of them.

Unfortunately, it is the very success of psychological and psychiatric research in dealing with hostage takers that forces upon both researchers and practitioners considerations of confidentiality. It is a familiar paradox that the very dissemination of information that enables researchers and practitioners to benefit from each other's findings and experiences also makes that information available to potential hostage takers. In this area, terrorists pose a greater threat than do criminals or the emotionally disturbed. The high levels of intelligence, education, and discipline frequently found in terrorist groups indicate that terrorists are aware of and capable of utilizing the information to be found in scholarly and professional publications and capable of deducing therefrom the strategies and techniques that will be used by law enforcement. At least since the founding of the *Bulletin of the Atomic Scientists,* researchers have been troubled by the use that may be made of their work. The fact that these questions are not new does not make them any the less perplexing. The free circulation of information is not only one of the ethical underpinnings of science, it is also a practical necessity, for only by such circulation are progress and application possible. To confine psychological research concerning hostage negotiation to scientists and laboratories with high security ratings is unthinkable. At the same time, researchers and practitioners in this area must acknowledge their responsibility. There are no easy answers, although writers and speakers might bear the problem in mind as they consider such things as level of specificity and detail, especially in reporting application and policy. Researchers, such as those represented here, face the difficult task of balancing freedom and safety. May their work continue to be used in the interests of understanding and compassion rather than exploitation and abuse.

REFERENCES

1. MAHER, G. F. 1977. Hostage: A Police Approach to a Contemporary Crisis. Charles C. Thomas, Publishers. Springfield, Ill.

VALUES AND ORGANIZATION IN
HOSTAGE AND CRISIS NEGOTIATION TEAMS

Harvey Schlossberg

Department of Psychology
John Jay College of Criminal Justice
New York, New York 10019

The use of police officers to defuse crisis situations originated in the late fifties with the introduction of family crisis teams. These were regular patrol officers who were selected for special training in the use of some simple psychological tactics for dealing with people in crisis. Sometimes officers were selected because they had attended college and received at least some introductory psychology. It soon became apparent that much of what is considered routine police work really falls into what could be described as crisis situations. One need only consider almost any contact with the public to see that police are called upon when situations get out of hand. Whether it's a simple fender-bender accident, a broken water main, or a person who has become the victim of a crime, the police are called upon to bring order out of overwhelming chaos. Therefore, the intervention tactics should be simple and general enough to apply to a wide range of situations and to be useful to almost every policeman.

Shortly after the 1972 Olympics massacre in Munich, the nations of the world were confronted with the realization that the terrorism that began in the Middle East shortly after the 1967 Arab-Israeli War no longer had geographical limits. In New York City, the author helped develop a program that ultimately was to serve as a model for much of the world. The Hostage Recovery Program was developed to meet the demands that could be put upon the police as the result of an incident of the proportions of the Munich massacre. It soon proved useful to apply the same principles to domestic situations. The success rate and the resulting positive public reaction, coupled with the simplicity of the tactics, spurred many police departments to reach out for and invest in training in crisis tactics.

Domestic and international hostage taking are very similar and lend themselves to the use of the same tactics. There are two basic premises that underlie the Hostage Recovery Program. First is that the hostage, in and of himself, has no value to the holder. This means that the person who takes the hostage is simply using the hostage as a tool or a device to attract an audience and gain attention. Using a hostage, one can go from total obscurity to international fame in a matter of minutes. For this reason, hostage taking must involve some form of announcement so that an audience will respond. Without an audience, the hostage taking is meaningless. The site selected by the criminal is very carefully chosen for its audience potential. For this reason, any event that will draw press coverage or crowds tends to be a fertile ground for the hostage taker. In many ways, the concept "theater of terror" is quite accurate: that is, the criminal is the star, the hostage is the supporting cast, and the police and public are the audience.

113

An important step is for the police to realize that the hostage taker is using the hostage only in order to attract an audience. The importance of this realization for the police is that they can recognize that any threat or actual physical violence inflicted upon the victim is not done to gain victim compliance, since the victim is usually already fully compliant. Just looking at a hostage situation, we can readily see that the hostage is totally and completely under the criminal's control. Being held hostage is about as close as one can come to being an infant, completely and totally dependent on another. In fact, the relationship between the victim and the criminal sometimes can be described as a parent-child relationship, with the hostage taker becoming the surrogate parent. This phenomenon has been described under a variety of headings, such as "Stockholm syndrome," identification with the aggressor, survival identification syndrome, and transference. These concepts have been devised to explain the strong dependence and cooperation that hostages have demonstrated in almost every situation that has occurred. The reaction extends many months and sometimes years after the hostage situation itself has been resolved. Police must recognize, then, that what is done to the hostage is done in order to gain *police compliance*.

The second basic premise underlying the Hostage Recovery Program is that it is just as much in the criminal's interest as it is in the police' interest not to let a situation become violent. The reason for this is based on simple logic—in any situation that becomes violent, the established authorities must be the victor. Outside of an all-out war, the establishment has the manpower and equipment to effect a victory. The simple truth of hostage taking is that for the criminal, a violent interaction can only result in loss; if he is to profit and enjoy the fruits of his labor, then a negotiated solution is the only alternative. The killing of innocent people cannot go unanswered. In fact, a working hypothesis for the police is that most hostage situations are carefully designed by the criminals in such a way as to avoid the taking of life; if in fact the design were to take life, then probably very little could be done to prevent this from occurring. On the other hand, the police themselves can only be governed by one guideline, that is, that human life is the only important consideration. Unless the protection of life is recognized as a fixed and irreversible boundary, the police tactic would consist of escalating force, which could only result in total disaster.

Bearing in mind the two basic principles already stated, hostage taking can be viewed in an entirely different light. The hostage taker is seen as somebody who has reached a point in life where he is totally frustrated and unable to obtain what he desires; the taking of hostages becomes nothing more than his attempt at problem solving.

In training police how to handle hostage situations, the greatest emphasis is placed on recognizing the problem solving without making judgmental values about the goals that the hostage taker is trying to reach. Rather, hostage taking should be recognized as creative, desperate, and intelligent problem solving. When the police arrive at the scene—and the criminal is ranting and raving, threatening violence, or giving deadlines—it is important that the police remember that they are walking in on this individual's problem solving. With this concept as a frame of reference, hostage taking becomes similar to the problem solving one sees people engaged in during a family dispute. In other words, the same dynamics are at work in a family dispute, a threatened suicide, or hostage taking. Once this assumption is made, crisis intervention techniques become appropriate.

The negotiator is the term generally used in law enforcement for the person who will be intervening in the crisis. We would be just as accurate to call him the therapist, since it is the same role. The goal of the negotiator is to establish himself as a significant "other." He will set an atmosphere similar to what one might find at a therapy session. The therapist will not offer any solutions or advice, but rather will set an atmosphere that is conducive to the patient's working through his own solutions. The same holds true for the negotiator: he will not advise the criminal to surrender nor will he offer possible solutions, since they might trigger a negative outcome or establish a direction that the criminal never thought of. In essence, this is clearly a passive therapy, designed to permit the criminal an opportunity to ventilate and explore various alternatives without the fear of total annihilation. Obviously, the negotiator—like the therapist—will be experiencing stress feelings similar to those that the criminal experiences. In essence, as in therapy, there is a mirror relationship between the feelings experienced by the criminal and by the negotiator. As a result, the negotiator is under great stress—not only because of the mirror effect, but also because he has much at stake in terms of outcome. He has a personal investment in terms of his success as a negotiator, and also in terms of his conscience should anyone be killed while he is negotiating. The criminal in many ways has it easier, since he has the negotiator to help him handle the crisis. Recognizing this, we have introduced a concept of negotiating teams.

While the number of members on a team cannot be clearly delineated—and several combinations are possible, as we will explore shortly—the basic number on a team, regardless of departmental size, should be no less than two individuals. The first man, or primary negotiator, deals as a therapist directly with the criminal. The second negotiator is sometimes called the coach, backup, or secondary negotiator. His role varies depending on how many men are on the team. If he is the only other member, he will help gather and screen intelligence information and select those aspects that may be important to the primary negotiator. He will run interference with supervisors by explaining what is happening so that the primary negotiator need not be disturbed or interfered with. In the event the primary negotiator must leave, the backup will replace him, but only after proper introduction to the criminal by the primary. The real significance of the secondary role is to act as negotiator to the negotiator. In effect, the backup permits the negotiator to ventilate and share some of the stress. It should be pointed out that at no time do the two negotiators deal together with the criminal. If in fact they did, competition would be created and the outcome would be influenced negatively. Since no two hostage incidents are exactly alike, there is no standardized approach, but rather a general, passive stance designed to ease anxieties and tensions not only by what is said, but also through the use of time.

The selection of negotiators is one of the major considerations in forming hostage negotiating teams. The original selection procedures instituted by the New York City Police Department involved volunteers who expressed a belief in nonviolent methods and who were willing to undergo extensive training, which involved personal therapy and dealing with personal feelings. In addition to an intensive medical examination, there were psychiatric interviews and in-depth psychological testing. The tests used were group and individual, i.e., Minnesota multiphasic personality inventory (MMPI), thematic apperception test (TAT), Draw a Person (DAP), and Rorschach. In spite of all the testing and screening, we could not come up with a profile of the ideal negotiator. Experience has dictated that a variety of personalities do equally well. We also attempted to match the negotiator ethnically and by race to the criminal. In reality, this did not work out; no matter what combination was used, we were wrong and the criminal wanted somebody else. Current procedure provides that the first trained negotiator to arrive at the scene will be responsible for negotiating. The negotiators keep in mind the two basic objectives: (1) bargaining with the criminal in order to secure the release of hostages while not doing anything to make the situation worse than it is already; and (2) the ultimate surrender of the criminal. Other personnel at the scene are responsible for the general goals of law enforcement, namely, the maintenance of social order within constitutional limits, protection of life and property, and the enforcing of law. The members of the negotiating team generally have five activities that they must perform. The greater the number of members a team has available, the easier will be the stress upon each individual. The first activity consists of gathering basic information, such as the number of individuals involved, threats, types of weapons, etc. This is done on an ongoing basis; and a log is frequently kept by this negotiator. Depending upon the length of time the operation runs, the depth of information gathering will vary. The second activity involves a negotiator who will act as overall organizer, assigning work to individuals, and who generally is a supervisor in terms of organizational rank. In addition, the supervisor will perform the third, fourth, and fifth activities. These activities include coordination of hostage team with containment team, and maintaining an ongoing analysis of the information that he receives, which will lead to the fifth activity—planning strategy based on that analysis and on a continual assessment of the situation.

In summary, while we cannot specify a particular number of individuals needed to make up an ideal negotiating team, the concept that negotiations should utilize a team approach remains valid. By use of this approach, negotiating functions and tasks can be delegated for greater efficiency. Justification for expending manpower and funds to establish and train these teams is clearly found across the country in the daily news headlines. The incidents may not be of the dramatic international type, but every bank robbery, every family dispute, contains the elements of a nightmare that could sweep innocent people into the center. The problem for the authorities then becomes one of resolving the conflict without the loss of life.

THE DYNAMICS OF THE HOSTAGE TAKER: SOME MAJOR VARIANTS*

Jeanne N. Knutson

The Wright Institute
Berkeley, California 94704

As the phenomenon of terrorism has grown to be a continuing element in modern political behavior, the concurrent phenomenon of politically motivated hostage taking has increasingly impinged on the consciousness and even on the lives of many citizens. Certain categories of citizens are at special risk: government employees—especially those serving outside their country; top officials of transnational companies; individuals (like Patty Hearst) who may be abducted as symbols of political demands and politically motivated rage. Indeed, hostage taking in these high-risk categories has become a big business—not only for the terrorists, who have reaped considerable gains, but also for new transnational corporations selling insurance and security.

Yet, one need not be a member of this high-risk group to be imperiled by the hostage taker, for it is also possible to become an *inadvertent* hostage, someone whose hostage role is determined merely by the chance circumstance of being physically located where the action is. Citizens in this more general category become hostages because they are passengers on a hijacked airplane, because they are present in a government building during a terrorist incident (such as that led by the Hanaafi Muslims in Washington, D.C.), or simply because they are a secretary or a repairman auxiliary to a principal hostage (as in the OPEC raid in Vienna).

As the phenomenon of hostage taking is both discriminating and random, it is of more than academic interest to examine the psychodynamics of the terrorists behind the guns. Various books and papers have been written about negotiating with the hostage taker.[1-4] Other works have focused on the phenomenological experience of the captive.[5-8] However, an exhaustive literature review disclosed no papers that have examined the psychology of the hostage taker and *his* phenomenological view of his captives. Thus, the present paper stands alone and necessarily includes a degree of speculation unconfirmed by other sources. It will attempt to delineate two major types of politically motivated hostage takers and then will provide data to explicate their dynamics.

The data are derived from a long-range research project on terrorists (see Reference 9 for a detailed discussion), in which an attempt is being made to complete in-depth evaluations of all prisoners in U.S. federal

* This project has been supported in part by Dr. David Hubbard of the Aberrant Behavior Center (Dallas, Texas) and in part, through the efforts of Dr. Louis J. West, by USPHS Biomedical Research Support Grant RR05756 awarded to the Neuropsychiatric Institute, University of California, Los Angeles.

prisons who have been convicted of crimes that were politically motivated, and to gather a control sample from prisoners in several other countries. The taped interviews are being conducted in a standardized manner and include administration of both a Rorschach test and the Political Thematic Apperception Measure.[10] As the Symbionese Liberation Army (SLA) has conducted one of the few politically motivated kidnappings thus far in the United States of a specifically targeted, high-risk person, data from this research project have been supplemented by interviews with non–politically motivated prisoners who have taken specifically targeted individuals to achieve a particular goal.

Variants of Hostage Takers

It appears that only a small minority of politically motivated hostage takers are driven by pressing personal needs joined to inadequate psychological resources that cause them to lose an adequate hold on the reality of their personal problems as distinct from the problems of the political system.[11] This small group may seek forced emigration on a hijacked airplane or may make violent threats against the father-president as the solution to their own inner turmoil, or may deliberately abduct another who symbolizes their primitive rage. Because of their numerical insignificance, this paper will not deal with grossly psychologically impaired captors. Instead, it will seek to explicate the dynamics of captors whose actions are mediated by ego functions and directed toward the service of external goals.

Just as hostages can be placed in their captive role on either a deliberate or an inadvertent basis, so the politically motivated hostage taker dons his role of captor in either a deliberate manner (i.e., desiring a particular gain in exchange for his hostage) or casually, through a plan in which hostage taking is an inadvertent or minimal part of the overall scheme. It is the thesis of this paper that this difference in planning and anticipating the responsibility of having hostages reflects a psychological dissimilarity between the two types of captors.

The Reluctant Captor

In the United States, by far the predominant type of politically motivated hostage taking has been of the second, casual type. For example, terrorists have taken airplanes and, in so doing, have also taken hostages. When interviewed, these captors usually are quite aware that they were unwilling and, for most, unable to kill another human being. For them, it was important to take elaborate safeguards for the safety of their hostages and, additionally, to make efforts either to neutralize or, if possible, to convert their hostages to become supporters of their ideological view (and, hence, accomplices and no longer hostages).

These unwilling captors *never employ psychological processes to dehumanize their hostages*. Before, during, and after the event, they experience their hostages as people—with minds to win over; with emotions that may be assaulted by the terror of the event and may even go out of control, causing a dreaded act of violence to occur; with bodies that might fail and, in that way, burden the conscience of the hostage taker. These subjects experience their captor role as a psychologically stressful burden—a role that they undertook at great psychic jeopardy. They are not capable of seriously using another person's life as a poker chip in the pursuit of specific gains, nor are they capable of comfortably accepting responsibility for violence toward others or for the death of another human being.

These reluctant captors are motivated by the desire to publicize a cause, to underline a political demand, to dramatize a political injustice. Often in opposition to their personal psychology and personal beliefs, they act violently: they commandeer an airplane at gunpoint; they "expropriate" money from a bank for their revolutionary cause; they take over a public building. These subjects are principled individuals whose violence is really bravado—a facade of strength pressed into the service of what is deemed a critical political cause. Far from being characteristic of a "criminal personality," reluctant hostage takers usually have neither a criminal record nor a history of violence. This is not to say that such individuals do not at times inadvertently cause the death of other people,[9] but rather that they are not violence prone by nature or characterized by strong or uncontrolled aggressive impulses.†

In their role of hostage taker, these subjects handle the situation in ways that appear "stupid" or "dumb" to the deliberate hostage taker. If a passenger desires urgently to leave a hijacked airplane, the person is almost always allowed to deplane (so that, in an important sense, those remaining hostages could be described as volunteers). The reluctant hostage taker does not usually even have a weapon (although one is almost always feigned), trusting rather to his frequently charismatic personality and his powerful political vision to provide adequate hostage control, if control becomes a real issue.

While the reluctant hostage taker is not grossly impaired psychologically, several factors appear to operate frequently to facilitate his becoming a hostage taker. First, while he possesses considerable ideational resources, these resources are limited both by poor reality testing as well as by impaired ability to cognitively integrate, analyze, and make sense out of his ideational world. Thus, these reluctant hostage takers are frequently typified by lack of logical, systematically goal-directed thinking. Their interview material illustrates this illogical thinking and a lack of adequate consideration of possible alternatives. These subjects are dreamers—philosophers and ideologues—lacking adequate concreteness and present orientation in their thinking.

In addition, there is an overreliance on the power of their own will and

---

† For example, their Rorschach protocols do not include aggressive symbols and employ minimal, if any, color. The color that is employed is adequately form dominated.

that of their cause, which can shade over into a pathological degree of grandiosity. Frequently, these subjects are aware that at the time of their terroristic act, they felt themselves to be invincible and omnipotent. Thus, they felt that no hostage was going to grab for the gun or attempt to take control; and their thinking does not progress to a further consideration that asks, But what if? In the interview, these reluctant hostage takers are frequently asked by what psychological means they were able to avoid the anxiety that a hostage *might* attempt to subdue them or *might* die from a heart attack, or that the bomb *might* go off when someone was around to be harmed. With a measure of surprise, these subjects state that such alternatives had never seriously been considered, since they just *knew* that they could bring the situation to the desired conclusion by the sheer force of their will—a degree of faith unwarranted by the outcome of their actions in numerous cases.

Finally, while hostage takers as a whole are highly likely to have experienced a very close brush with death as a child—perhaps even having been declared dead or dying—this experience is dynamically important in a particular way to the reluctant hostage takers. For this group, a serious illness, the ingestion of rat poison, or long-term immobilization through an accident leads to a reaction formation[12] against feelings of weakness, fragility, or helplessness, which underlies both the bravado of their terroristic act and the lack of adequate plans for self-protection. Their stance involves both a desire to *look* tough and a protection against having to *be* tough (i.e., and thus to be found wanting).

The Deliberate Hostage Taker

Standing in stark contrast to the reluctant hostage taker is the person who purposefully sets out to control the life chances of another human being in order to achieve a desired goal. This person is perfectly willing to execute his hostage, with little or no psychic pain, should the hostage be unwilling or unable to serve as a totally controllable *implement*, an auxiliary facilitative of the hostage taker's threat. For the deliberate hostage taker, the essence of his act is the psychological dehumanization of his hostage, the stripping away of the hostage's human characteristics.

This psychological dehumanization does not imply a lack of awareness of the hostage's feelings and needs. To the contrary, the deliberate hostage taker is often a master of psychological insight, intuitively aware of those factors in his hostage that can be made to work for him, to ensure his control. What the psychological dehumanization does imply rather is a total orientation toward his goal, a total willingness to use psychological insight for purposes of manipulation and control, and a total inability for affective bonding. When push comes to shove, the heretofore friendly and nurturing deliberate hostage taker is quite able to callously sacrifice his victim's life. It is contended here that the well-known Palestinian terrorists, particularly the famed "Carlos,"[13] are the political prototypes of this deliberate hostage taker.

Such psychodynamics obviously contain a large element of psychopathology, particularly a lack of affect and conscience in dealing with others. Few of the deliberate hostage takers who have been interviewed, however, are true psychopaths. Most retain—though deeply buried—a measure of affect and of conscience. However, these characteristics are seen by these hostage takers as hindrances to their work. Therefore, to attempt to arouse their consciences and their caring feelings not only can be counterproductive, it also can be extremely dangerous. The deliberate hostage taker stresses emotional control: he wants his hostages to be in emotional control of themselves at all times, and he demands this of himself as well.

In practical terms, the deliberate hostage taker uses violence as a tool toward his ends. He may capture, execute, and maim—but in a controlled manner, to serve his purposes. As a rule, he is not typified by uncontrolled, violent impulses. He is the epitome of goal orientation. Opposed to the reluctant hostage taker, these subjects are pragmatists whose thinking lacks adequate ability to abstract and to orient to either past or future.

Compared to the complex personalities of the reluctant hostage takers, the deliberate captors' psychodynamics stand forth with simplicity. Lacking the historical experience and the present ability to trust another, to safely care for another, to depend upon another, the deliberate captor trusts only himself and his weapon. He may employ psychological controls ("I don't want to hurt you."; "Sure, you can fix some coffee, honey,"; "Why don't you just lie down now and get a little rest."), but he is constantly aware that it is force that is the key to his scenario. His hostages simply do not exist for him as people; their opinions of him, their children, their lives—all are subsumed under the attainment of his goal.

LET THE CAPTORS SPEAK

In this necessarily brief paper, only limited statements by captors can be given. However, in these brief words, the psychological differences between the majority group in each type is clear. Let us begin with the concerns of the reluctant hostage takers.‡

[S] Well, to tell you the truth, I—I was . . . concerned uh that people—that these particular uh *time* in their life would not uh *damage* them or would not scare them that much that—so that's why I—I went quite a few times from the cockpit to the plane *and* uh *talked* to them and they were drinking. I ordered the stewardess not to give any drinks to—to my—to these friends of mine who were with me nor to any passenger who would uh get himself drunk probably, because we might get into trouble. Other than that, I told these friends of mine, talk to them and uh try to get the situation as relaxed as possible and uh, believe me, that's what it uh—what—what the situation was.

[K] So it sounds like what you were feeling was worried—that every—

[S] Oh, definitely. I was concerned about their uh—their feelings and their being scared. I didn't want them to be scared.

---

‡ [S] is the subject; [K] is the author.

This subject was concerned about the emotional state of the passengers. He was also concerned about their minds. Literature for his cause was distributed, and various speeches were given. Further, he was concerned about their opinion of him as a person.

[S] I thought uh if everything went smoothly uh we would return from uh from Croatia and land up again somewhere in Europe and—on the way, right there and then I would give up uh and tell the passengers and Captain and everybody else that these things are not real and they—and I would *stand then* on the way ba—that's what I uh had in mind. I would be then at *their* mercy and uh I would try uh to give my message across to them, *now*, without their fearing me, and uh—to tell you the truth, I uh—I *pictured* that return to the United States as somehow uh—uh—happy ending of that dramatic situation, because they wouldn't be a-scared any—anymore. Now they would discover that I wasn't real uh—uh—such animal and or uh willing or uh—or being capable to harm them or kill them uh because I couldn't possibly do anything with those things I had on the plane. It's just uh—it's just uh—just uh—just uh—not explosive but kit—plat—kit—kits you play on uh—making all different kinds of . . .

Such a concern was general on the plane. One of this same band of captors subsequently wrote to each passenger from prison, saying in part:

Although I know this letter may not compensate for the feelings of fear and apprehension you suffered during the hijacking I am compelled to at least attempt to explain my seemingly brutal behavior during the hours spent in Paris . . .

And, at the end:

I pray that you can forgive me one day, if you haven't yet, and comprehend my state of mind at the time. As you may know, I will be paying dearly for my actions. During the long years that I will be spending in prison, it would be a great comfort to me to know that you understand that I meant no harm to anyone and am not a brute.

Let us consider the concerns of but one additional reluctant hostage taker:

[S] . . . first of all, let me say when I hijacked the plane to Vietnam, it wasn't a case—any kin—case where I was, you know, ransoming the passengers or attempting to hold hostage or anything like that.

What my intention was, was to take 'em to Vietnam, where they could have seen for themselves what was happening to that country and I figured that the Vietnamese would have showed them around, you know, different hospitals and places bombed and stuff like that and so it would have made not only the initial publicity of the hijacking but then I figured well, later the passengers will return to the United States and they will tell what they've seen, so I—I thought that was the best way—the most—the way that most publicity could be made against the war.

[K] So uh you intended to have your hostages really work with you?

[S] They did. They—well, they weren't hostages. I didn't consider 'em hostages. . . .

[K] Can you tell me a little bit more about what you mean when you say you didn't consider them as hostages?

[S] Well, I mean in the sense that I wasn't holding for any kind of ransom or any kind of demands, anything like that. I was never—there was never a question of threatening their—their—their lives for any type of demands whatsoever.

[K] A hostage is usually considered somebody who's not free to leave.

[S] Yeah, well, in that sense, they were hostages, but—

[K] Although they seemed to be free to leave. According to what I read, when they asked to go in Los Angeles and in Dallas, you let them go.

[S] Yes, ev—every, single person who asked to leave the plane I allowed them to leave the plane, *including* the crew.

The theme that unites all of the above quotations is clear: hostages are human beings whose lives, feelings, and opinions are of value. Never is violence seriously threatened or feigned threats of violence excused. Never is the responsibility for a successful outcome (idiosyncratically defined as an outcome in which all participants are alive, and experiencing mutual regard, and the political goal is accomplished) shifted from the captor.

The psychodynamics of the reluctant hostage taker are thrown into bold relief when we turn to the views of a deliberate hostage taker. The deliberate hostage taker, by definition, abducts a particular person (or persons) to employ his hostage's life and well-being as a bargaining tool. At the outset, the hostage taker clearly defines the options as "my goal or his life" and thus accepts responsibility, on some level, for the death of another. In the United States, the SLA's abduction of Patty Hearst stands out as an incident of politically motivated, deliberate hostage taking. Elsewhere, the deliberate hostage taker is *the* political prototype. As no politically motivated deliberate hostage taker has been interviewed to date, several interviews were arranged with subjects who had purposefully taken hostages in order to advance a particular goal (escape, ransom, etc.).

The subject whose views are quoted below is a very useful resource—intelligent, creative, and possessing considerable psychological insight into the dynamics of his hostages. His views of his hostages and his personal dynamics are strikingly similar to those of other deliberate hostage takers who have been interviewed. Over a period of time, he has taken a number of people hostage to achieve particular goals. At times, he has dealt considerable bodily harm to noncooperative hostages. It was clinically apparent that it has been favorable circumstances alone that have prevented this subject from killing a hostage.

To begin with, he *planned* to take hostages and to *use* them to advance his goals.

> [S] I know we all went over the plan differently. The way I went over it in my mind was that we would take this guy to a point and uh I never really anticipated a problem from him. Uh—
>
> [K] Tell me about that. Why didn't you anticipate a problem?
>
> [S] It's just not—it's just not the nature of, at least American people, to buck—when they've got a loaded gun pointed at 'em. And I figured if he was armed, we would have to get the drop first, so to speak. And uh—but we had continuously planned a backup man with a rifle, when we approached this guy, so we were perfectly safe there. We thought we were . . .
>
> [K] I'm interested in your saying American people anyway uh are very—if I remember the word you used—passive, submissive, when there's a gun, so you assumed that there was no trouble. It was almost like taking a suitcase.
>
> [S] Correct.

The view of *others as objects* pervades this subject's material. The dimensions of *projected responsibility* and *control maintenance* are also crucial to understanding his dynamics. He goes on to explain his modus operandi:

> . . . if I like now was to pull a weapon and tell you "don't make no noise; don't do nothin," you know. If somebody comes in this office and I'm u—unable to take them also, I'm gonna kill you, because it's gonna be your fault and—and I would just—

The subject was interrupted and questioned several times as to why if attention were called to him and his hostage by any means whatsoever, the captive would die. Why wouldn't his first impulse be self-protection—a look around to see what danger had been aroused? With growing frustration, he noted that he had a "contract" with his hostages on "a personal basis." In the hypothetical plan we discussed:

> [S] You're thinkin' about two things. You're thinkin' about gettin' out that back gate with your hostage, and you're thinkin' about gettin'—gettin'—n—away—or you're thinkin' about killin' him.
> [K] Well, what you're saying is, you're thinking about revenge. And I don't understand—
> [S] Oh, no; it's not revenge. That's a part of the plan. If I don't make it, I'm gonna kill him. If I don't make it, I *will* kill him. . . . I still have to go back to the thing that I have a plan; right? And a—a part of my plan is killin' him if it messes up.

After several other examples, the issue was joined:

> [K] But what you're saying, it seems to me, is the same thing, that what's *important* is that people obey you.
> [S] Absolutely. You—you have to have control. If I've got—if I've got six hostages and uh—and uh—and one of 'em is causin' dissension in the group, to sacrifice that one will draw the others into line.

The interviewer then noted that a number of terrorists, reluctantly finding themselves in possession of hostages, allowed the frightened or unwilling to leave. This subject commented:

> [S] Now, what I wouldn't do is—like you were talkin' about the terrorist—I wouldn't let *nobody* go . . . No, nobody. Anybody that went would go with a bullet.
> [K] Why?
> [S] Take this with you.
> [K] Why?
> [S] Because I'm not takin' hostages to let 'em go . . . I would let 'em go if my demands were met.
> [K] People I've talked to have let hostages go because they wanted, like you, to keep control of the situation. Like there was an hysterical woman or—
> [S] She's expendable; then she—she goes and takes a bullet with her. That's to enforce my demands.

Just as one would get rid of a malfunctioning appliance, an inedible piece of food, or an unmanageable pet, so the deliberate hostage taker grants his hostages conditional life: minimally, as long as they do not obstruct his plan or, optimally, as they are able to further it.

Like other deliberate hostage takers who have been interviewed, this subject is sensitive to those issues that motivate his captives to be "good" hostages, i.e., perfectly controllable and in control of themselves. One example will have to suffice. It relates to the abduction of a young couple:

> See, once you have a man and wife—'specially if they're young—you can control either one through the other . . . Whatever I want you to do, I can threaten your husband and you'll do it. Whatever I want him to do, I can threaten you, whatever—vice versa. And that was the situation there.

This deliberate hostage taker went on to offer an amazing insight—the obverse of the "Stockholm syndrome," the phenomenon in which hostages are found to become deeply emotionally attached to certain captors.[5,8]

[S] Like we had—we played the age-old game just like the police do, like one of us was uh—was the monster of the group, just growlin' and roarin' and cussin' and threatenin', and uh whoever was like guarding the hostages, one would be like the bad guy and the other one would be the soft-spoken good guy. . . .[Like the police do] The same thing with the hostages, like if you got one guy talkin' about "let's kill 'em, man. We can't wait. The police are gonna be here. Let's kill 'em. They're just gonna testify against us." The other guy sayin' "Man, you know, you don't wanna kill these—look at this little ol' gal. You know. Her and her husband ain't given' nobody no problem in the world." . . . "Man, let's *kill* 'em, you know." . . . "Look, just be cool, man; there ain't no need to hurt these people." And uh, you just become one with 'em.

[K] What purpose does it serve?

[S] As long as they think they got a champion, as long as there's any kind of straw held out to 'em that they can grasp, they're gonna grasp it, before they'll buck the gun.

Many government officials, publicly and privately, counsel potential hostages to "go along" with the Stockholm syndrome. Special note should be taken of the views of this expert captor. When asked if there was safety for the young wife who displayed trusting, dependent behavior, he replied:

No, I wouldn't hurt her . . . I mean, I wouldn't a let her run out the door, or I wouldn't a let her get on the phone, or scream out the window.

[K] So you wouldn't hurt her as long as she was a good hostage?

[S] Let's put it this way. I wouldn't a shot her. I would have dragged her down. I would of . . . maybe hit her with a pistol, if it became necessary.

And if a policeman was alerted by the woman?

[S] Then he would probably be killed immediately.

[K] What about her? What about your rule that if someone—

[S] Well, then—then she has put herself on the other side of the fence and uh she's just as much of a pig as he is then.

Critical Distinctions

For the deliberate hostage taker, his captive exists as an implement to be used or discarded on the basis of the furtherance of his goals. As a tool, the captive is stripped of those human qualities that normally give pause: psychic pain, personal attachments, weak body organs. These qualities exist in the awareness of the hostage taker, but they are divorced from any *affective* connection to remain only in the rational calculus of his overall plan. After the incident is concluded, the hostage ceases to exist in the memory of his captor as even a two-dimensional person, but only as an attribute of an externally perceived situation. It is thus inconceivable that the deliberate hostage taker would be troubled about the effect of his violence on his hostage, or that he could imaginably write a letter asking for forgiveness!

Further, the deliberate hostage taker is inordinately concerned with the issue of control. He *must* be in command at all times. His words *must* be respected. The urgency of this need for control surpasses the exigencies of the situation to reflect unmet intrapsychic needs of long standing. This is the child who almost died, the child who was never important to anyone, who holds the gun. To him, a "no" echoes with intolerable pain down the corridors of memory as a narcissistic[14,15] injury not to be borne.

The issue of control is not just one of control over the hostage; it is equally the issue of control over self. The deliberate hostage taker quoted above noted how most people instinctively appealed in the name of their children, their spouse, their family. This annoys him—as do tears—because such considerations obstruct the plan in which the hostage is an object. As he remarked, "In case somethin' happens later and I have to shoot this guy, I'd really feel bad, two little kids sittin' there and his wife."

In psychodynamic terms, the deliberate hostage taker is energized by two major forces. First, he is powerfully driven by needs to overcome feelings of weakness and inferiority. He must be tough. He must be consistent. Challenge him, and you will see a violent affirmation of his strength. Always, in his inner awareness, someone is watching whose approval has been painfully withheld because he wasn't tough enough. It is their standards—and not those to which a hostage may appeal—that he emulates in a constant search for affirmation of his worth. Second, he is energized by a need to deny dependency and trust. Here also, offers to act counter to this powerful need—to be soft, tender, trusting—are met with anger. In his psychic economy, the deliberate hostage taker *knows*—from historical experience and present conviction—that such offers are enveloped with pain and disappointment.

The reluctant hostage taker, on the other hand, is an obviously conflicted person, and the stress of his ever-present conflicts is readily apparent. He needs to be tough ("a freedom fighter"), to be brave ("I never know fear"), to take political actions beyond the approval of most. However, he also needs to be liked, to be accepted, to be seen as nonthreatening. He needs to manipulate and use people for his political goals, but he also needs their approval—their permission, as it were.

Thus, the reluctant hostage taker is burdened by an awesome sense of responsibility to appease both sides of his conflicted self. This need blurs actuality, practical considerations, and logical alternatives. In a pressing inner dialectic, he rapidly cycles from thesis to synthesis and bypasses awareness of the antithetical stance he plays out. His real punishment thus is internal, for whenever he wins (by being tough, by stating his cause dramatically), he necessarily loses (by frightening, hurting, and alienating others).

In the political world today, terrorists encompass both types of hostage takers, with the balance in any one society dependent upon the personal and societal values that they actualize. On the American political scene, idealism and humanitarianism are dominant political forces, and thus, almost all actors play with a very lively concern for acceptance by a liberal, humanitarian public that values the golden rule. Elsewhere (and in certain subsocieties in America), bitterness and intense narcissistic rage are rampant in selected publics and thus provide a tacit—though perhaps unconscious—acceptance of violence and retribution by violent, sociopathic actors. In these societies, the rule of the day is not golden but steel: an eye for an eye, a tooth for a tooth.

All terrorists—whether deliberate or reluctant hostage takers or employing entirely different means toward their political goals—are nurtured by and dependent upon public approval and support. As long as liberalism and humanism typify the American political ideology, the deliberate hostage takers are likely to play only a minor part in the cast of politically motivated captors here.

SUMMARY

This paper represents a unique effort to elucidate the dynamics of two major types of politically motivated hostage takers. The data presented are derived from an ongoing research project that is gathering extensive interview and psychological test materials from prisoners convicted of politically motivated crimes, both within the U.S. and several foreign prison systems. Data indicate that: (1) *the reluctant hostage taker*, who inadvertently or regretfully possesses hostages, is concerned with the opinions, emotional state, and safety of his captives and is burdened by a sense of responsibility; (2) *the deliberate hostage taker* experiences his hostages as nonhuman objects whose safety and existence are predicated on the furtherance of his goals, is concerned with the issue of control, and projects responsibility for violence onto others. Only a small subset of each type can be considered grossly psychologically impaired and unable to separate intra- and extrapsychic reality. The actions of the majority of each group are mediated generally by ego functions and directed toward the service of external goals.

ACKNOWLEDGMENTS

I wish to express sincere appreciation to Mr. Norman Carlson, Director of the United States Federal Bureau of Prisons, and to his staff throughout this large system who have been uniformly cooperative with my research requirements and supportive of the needs for confidentiality and protection of my subjects' rights of privacy. I would like to especially acknowledge the help at the Atlanta Federal Penitentiary of Mr. Ed Howard and Mr. Ed Watkins in gathering data for the present paper. Finally, I would like to express appreciation to Gail Hellstein and Sally Vamdiver for their patient editing of the research transcripts.

REFERENCES

1. CULLINANE, M. J. 1978. Terrorism—A new era of criminality. Terrorism 1(2): 119–124.
2. KOBETZ, R. W. & H. H. A. COOPER. 1978. Target Terrorism. Bureau of Operations and Research, International Association of Chiefs of Police. Gaithersburg, Md.
3. McKNIGHT, G. 1974. The Terrorist Mind. The Bobbs-Merrill Company. New York, N.Y.
4. MILLER, A. H. 1978. Negotiations for hostages: implications from the police experience. Terrorism 1(2): 125–146.
5. HACKER, F. J. 1976. Crusaders, Criminals, Crazies. Bantam Books. New York, N.Y.

6. JACKSON, G. 1973. Surviving the Long Night. The Vanguard Press, Inc. New York, N.Y.
7. JENKINS, B. 1976. Hostage Survival: Some Preliminary Observations. Report No. P-5637. The Rand Corporation. Santa Monica, Calif.
8. OCHBERG, F. 1977. The victim of terrorism: psychiatric considerations. Terrorism 1(1): 1–22.
9. KNUTSON, J. 1979. Social and psychodynamic pressures toward a negative identity: the case of an American revolutionary-terrorist. Paper presented at the Second Annual Meeting of the International Society of Political Psychology, Washington, D.C., May, 1979.
10. KNUTSON, J. 1973. The new frontier of projective techniques. In The Handbook of Political Psychology. J. Knutson, Ed.: 413–437. Jossey-Bass. San Francisco, Calif.
11. HUBBARD, D. G. 1978. The Skyjacker. Collier Books. New York, N.Y.
12. FREEDMAN, A. M., H. I. KAPLAN & B. J. SADOCK. 1972. Modern Synopsis of Psychiatry. The Williams & Wilkins Co. Baltimore, Md.
13. SMITH, C. 1976. Carlos, Portrait of a Terrorist. Holt, Rinehart and Winston, Inc. New York, N.Y.
14. KOHUT, H. 1971. The Analysis of the Self. International Universities Press. New York, N.Y.
15. KOHUT, H. 1977. The Restoration of the Self. International Universities Press, Inc. New York, N.Y.

VICTIM RESPONSES TO TERROR

Martin Symonds

Psychological Services
Health Services Division
New York City Police Department
New York, New York 10010

In this paper, I plan to share my knowledge and experience of victims' responses to criminally induced terror. Much of my understanding has been derived from my work with sudden, unexpected criminal violence. It is my hope and belief that the insights gained from the unfortunate experiences of these victims can be effectively used in understanding the responses of victims of terrorists.*

In 1971 when I first began my studies of victims of sudden, unexpected, violent crime, I included victims of crimes where there was generally no contact with the criminal, such as the crime of burglary; if violence did occur, it generally was to property and not to person. I also included victims of sudden, unexpected, violent crime where there was minimal contact with the criminal, such as street assault and robbery, popularly known as "mugging," and those victims of sudden, unexpected, violent crime where there was prolonged contact with the criminal—these were crimes of rape, robbery, kidnapping, and hostage taking.

When I reviewed the victims' behavior, I became aware that all victim responses regularly followed certain sequential phases regardless of what type of crime was involved. Only the duration and intensity of each phase was influenced by the nature and quality of contact with the criminal.

Briefly, all victims of sudden, unexpected, violent crime no matter of what kind respond initially with shock and disbelief. This first phase is the phase of denial. This is quickly followed by phase 2, when denial is overwhelmed by reality. These two phases form the acute response to sudden, unexpected violence.

After a varying period of time, the individual enters into phase 3. This is the phase of traumatic depression. It is characterized by circular bouts of apathy, anger, resignation, irritability, constipated rage, insomnia, startle reactions, and replay of the traumatic events through dreams, fantasies, and nightmares. It is also the phase of self-recrimination. Phase 3 can also be called the "I am stupid" phase, since the replay of the traumatic events is evaluated under peacetime conditions after the event is over and the criminal is gone and not under the conditions of criminal-induced terror. (Under the conditions of extensive contact with the criminal, such as prolonged hostage taking, it is highly unlikely that any significant behavior

---

* Much of the material described and quoted in this paper is from unpublished studies by the author.

seen in phase 3 would take place. These hostages would, in the active presence of criminal terror, still respond as if they were in phase 2. It is the responses of victims in phase 2 that I will develop in detail later on in this paper.)

It is in phase 3 that prior specific personality patterns and traits exert an influence on the victims' behavior. Those individuals who were excessively love oriented and dependent on others seem to be more prone to develop constricting, depressive behavior. Their fears increase, they develop phobic responses, and they often form hostile, dependent relationships with family and friends. Other individuals—those who were predominantly freedom oriented, detached from others, or power oriented and aggressive—tend to intensify their prior behavior. They may become more removed from people, develop reclusiveness and "short fuse" irritability. In effect they have said, "The world is a jungle and to hell with Mr. Goodguy." Phase 3 is similar to the "survivor syndrome" described by Niederland.[1]

As the individual attempts to integrate and adapt the traumatic experience into future behavior and life-style, he can be said to enter phase 4, which is the phase of resolution and integration. In this phase, the individual develops increased defensive alert patterns to minimize or prevent future victimization. Profound, permanent revision of values and attitudinal changes towards possessions and other people occur in this last phase.

* People whose homes have been burglarized reduce their personal investment and involvement in property, jewelry, watches, TV sets, etc. These items now become objects that can be replaced. No longer does the individual allow himself to be painfully vulnerable to loss by investing a personal sense of self in property.

* A woman ran screaming down the aisle of a plane that was just about to take off. She screamed, "Stop, stop the plane. I left my purse in the airport. Everything is in my purse. My life is in my purse."

These are individuals who are unable or unwilling to accept their victimization and integrate it into their future life-styles. These individuals experience their victimization as a personal affront to their pride compounded by their perceived indifference to their plight. They tenaciously hold on to their feelings of rage and injustice, seeking only reparations and revenge for their victimization, and thus remain psychologically disabled.[2]

In this paper, my focus will be on the acute psychological responses of victims to those crimes where there is prolonged contact with the criminal and thus the acute responses of the victims take place in the criminals' presence. These are the crimes of rape, robbery, and captive and hostage taking. I will particularly focus on the responses of victims to the crimes where the victim is used as instrumental leverage to pressure a third party to satisfy the criminals' demands. These are the crimes of kidnapping and hostage taking.

Criminals use violence or the dramatic threat of violence to induce extreme fright or terror in victims in order to render the victims helpless, powerless, and totally submissive. To fully understand victim responses to criminally induced terror, I found it helpful to explore reactions of people to terror in general. Terror is an affect that the dictionary defines as extreme fright. This past year, I asked a number of people—social acquaintances and colleagues—whether they had ever experienced terror and if so, when and how they had dealt with it. Everyone I asked—they numbered close to 100—said yes. Most recounted episodes related to unpredictable, frightening events and not to people.

- Awakening in a room and finding it filled with smoke.
- Developing a leg cramp while swimming and being unable to get back to shore.
- One person said that while flying to England during World War II, the pilot had announced that the plane was on fire and he didn't think he would be able to land the plane successfully. This man vividly recalled 37 years later that he had just sat still, reviewed his life, and hoped death would be sudden and he wouldn't suffer.

The popular concept that individuals respond to the terror of sudden, overwhelming danger by panicking, screaming, running, or going into a mindless, catatonic state is not supported by actual victim behavior, and not by the literature on catastrophes and disasters—man-made or natural. There are some individuals who exhibit panic terror in response to perceived sudden, overwhelming danger, with mindless running or acts of desperation. This panic-terror behavior generally occurs in situations where physical movement is not completely impeded and there exists the possibility of escape, whether it is realistic or not. Desperate, suicidal acts may occur after prolonged capture when the individual feels hopeless about release.

- Jumping out of a burning building.
- Frenzied behavior of an individual when a bee is in his car.
- Feeling hopeless and running into electrified barbed wire in concentration camps.

In the deliberate act of terror-inducing criminality, the criminal terrorist intends to hold the victim captive and prevent any possibility of his escape. In such situations, where the terrorized victims feel trapped with no exit, they respond to the sudden, overwhelming danger to their lives by a paralysis of affect that I have called "frozen fright."[5]

Years ago I became aware of the phenomenon of frozen fright when I interviewed an 8½-year-old victim of incest. During the interview, she was bright, vivacious, talkative, and very cooperative. At the end of the interview, I said she could go. This youngster took a deep breath, sighed heavily, and said, "I thought I would never get out of here alive." At that time, and even years later with further reflection, I did not see any evidence at all of fright bordering on terror. Since that time almost 20 years ago, after numerous interviews with victims of violent crime, I've been able to identify and confirm the presence of frozen fright behavior in these individuals. It superficially appears to be a cooperative and friendly behavior that confuses even the victim, the criminal, the family and friends of the victim, the police, and society in general. I must emphasize this point. Terrorized, trapped, held-captive individuals, whose only perceived hope of survival depends on the criminal, will exhibit the "cooperative behavior of frozen fright."

This paralysis of affect, with its pseudocalm behavior, is seen in most individuals. Sometimes, youngsters and some immature, dependent, and histrionic individuals will exhibit continual crying, shaking, clinging, and trembling behavior in the presence of the threat of overwhelming danger. Despite the active dramatic behavior, the victim's affect is frozen and unresponsive to any change except the external removal of danger.

• A youngster in a robbery cried, cried, and cried. Despite efforts to shut her up by other fellow victims or by the robbers, she persisted. One robber shot her to death.

• A common experience known to dog owners is their dogs' response to thunder. Many dogs shiver, shake, moan, and cling during a thunderstorm. No amount of assurance allays their response. As soon as the thunder ceases, the dogs stop responding.

Though the affect of the terrorized victims is frozen, the motor and cognitive functions are not. This dissociative phenomenon, which is normally seen in terrorized victims, differs from the splitting of affect from cognitive and motor functions that is seen in people, such as undercover agents, who are involved in dangerous-to-life, high-risk work. In these individuals, who voluntarily accept exceptionally hazardous work, there is a suspension of affect that allows for hyperawareness and hyperalertness. In terrorized individuals, the sudden threat to life causes an acute dissociative response. There is paralysis of affect with narrow constriction of cognitive and motor functions to serve purely one function, namely survival. In their frozen fright, the victims narrowly focus all their energy on survival, exclusively concentrating on the terrorist. This reaction is enhanced by the criminal terrorist's intent to totally dominate the victim. The terrorist creates a hostile environment and thwarts any efforts that would reduce this domination. The victim then feels isolated from others, powerless, and helpless.

The triad of being in a hostile environment, feeling isolated, and feeling helpless produces a profound reaction that Karen Horney has called "basic anxiety."[8] Under conditions of terror, this reaction causes the adult to lose the use of recently learned experience and to respond for survival with the early adaptive behavior of childhood. I have called this response in victims "traumatic psychological infantilism."[9]

This traumatic infantilism compels victims to cling to the very person who is endangering their lives. It accounts for the obedient, placid, compliant, and submissive behavior seen in frozen fright. Even the memory of terror, with the criminal not present, can produce the behavior of traumatic psychological infantilism.

• A supermarket manager was held up by criminals and placed into a meat freezer. He was released four hours later by the police. Six weeks following this incident, he received a phone call at work. He was told,

"Charlie, I am the cat that put you in the freezer. Do you want me to put you in their again?" Charlie said, "No." The criminal said, "O.K. You're a good boy, I want you to take the money from the safe and put it into a brown paper bag. Put it on the take out counter. I'll pick it up. Charlie, remember the freezer." The manager, a battle-honored veteran of World War II, did just that. The detectives couldn't understand how a guy could be robbed by telephone. Charlie, the manager, said, "You don't know what it is to be locked in a freezer and feel you are going to die."

If the atmosphere of terror still persists—and the psychologically traumatized victim perceives that the terrorist, who has the power of life and death over him, is letting him live—profound and persistent attitudinal and behavioral changes occur. He now sees the criminal as the "good guy." This phenomenon is called "pathological transference." I have seen this reaction repeatedly in men, women, and children under the conditions of perceived extreme threat to life.

• A detective undercover agent making a buy of narcotics was held captive for 3½ hours while the criminal gang deliberated whether to "waste him or not." However, the leader of the gang said, "No." Finally the detective's back-up team was able to figure out where he was and rescue him. I interviewed this detective two months later. He kept telling me what a good guy the leader was. For two hours he repeatedly stated, "He could have killed me and didn't." His superiors who were present kept on yelling at him [expletives deleted] what a mean bastard that crook was, but this undercover agent persisted in defending the criminal.

• In another situation, an off-duty detective was held captive when he walked in and interrupted a robbery. When the criminals found out he was a detective, two of the gunmen said, "We'll waste you, you mother fucker." They placed a bag over his head and made him go down on his knees. He later stated, "Silly as it may seem, I was glad it was going to be in the head because I thought it would be quick." He heard the robbers discussing him and then they left. He wasn't shot. Two of the robbers were caught months later. Jerry, the detective, was involved in their capture. The captured robber said to him, "You owe me something. I saved your life." The detective visited the man many times. A close relationship developed, and the detective said to the robber, "If you need me, I'm there for you because you were there for me at that time." When the second robber was caught, the detective related a conversation with his superior, "Chief, this guy has really changed." Jerry went out and bought lunch for him. The third robber is still at large. The detective fantasizes a conversation with him, "Listen Otis what went down, went down; turn yourself in. Believe me I'll work with you. I'm not looking for revenge."

Pathological transference only occurs when someone threatens your life, deliberates, and doesn't kill you. The victim no longer experiences the threat but feels he has been given life by the criminal. Pathological transference doesn't occur—or instantly evaporates—when the person is shot at.

Pathological transference is a consistent finding in individuals held hostage by criminal terrorists. Hostage victims are essentially instrumental victims. They are used and exploited by their captors to exert leverage on a third party, the family, the police, or the government to accede to the captors' demands. The captor expresses the threat of extreme violence to the victim primarily to the third party if the demands are not met. This creates the illusion for the victim that the terrorist captor would not harm him if the third party gave into the captor's demands. This use of the victim as leverage lays the grounds for intense pathological transference. This transference is both accelerated and heightened when the hostage has already been psychologically traumatized by terror. These two components—traumatic psychological infantilism and pathological transference—form the crucial elements in what has been called the Stockholm syndrome.

The Stockholm syndrome has often been viewed as the hostage's identifying with the terrorist. I think that concept doesn't adequately explain hostage behavior. I have found it more useful to view hostage behavior as an attempt to relate to an individual who has first captured the hostage by an act of terror and then used the victim as an instrument to obtain an objective from a third party.

The suffering of the victim is the leverage used for negotiations with a third party. Hostages, in their psychologically traumatized state, never view negotiations for their release as benevolent. The victim would immediately give all for his release, but he interprets and experiences any negotiation as endangering him. He then perceives negotiations, especially if protracted, as indifference, hostility, and rejection—nonloving and life-threatening behavior—by the very people who are negotiating for his release. This reinforces the pathological transference already developed by the prolonged exposure to the terrorist.

Up to now, I have presented the psychodynamics of behavior of victims held captive by criminal terror. An understanding of these dynamics is essential for the effective treatment of hostages from the moment of release. Since 1974, the Karen Horney Victim Treatment Center has utilized the following principles of "psychological first aid for victims of violent crime." They are based on reducing the feelings of isolation, helplessness, and powerlessness that have been induced by criminal terror.

1. Early restoration of power to the victim by asking permission to interview him, e.g., (a) Is this a good time to talk to you?; (b) Do you mind if I ask you some questions?

2. Reduction of isolation by nurturing behavior, thus diminishing the experience of the hostile environment that the victim was subjected to.

3. Diminishing the helpless, hopeless feelings of the victim by having him experience input into determination of his present and future behavior in terms of space and time.

4. To reduce the victim's feelings of having been subjected to the dominant behavior of the terrorist, we encourage the counselor to identify

himself to the victim's satisfaction, to ask for permission even to sit down in the victim's presence, to smoke, etc.

All the foregoing approaches to the victim are based on undoing and reversing the factors that brought about traumatic psychological infantilism.

The rescuers must remember that the sudden release of the victims reproduces an acute phase of crying, clinging, submissive behavior. They still are in the grip of traumatic infantilism. The above methods of nurturing and restoring power are crucial to prevent a second injury, which the rescuers may give the victims. It is important that the victims be allowed to clean up before being restored to familiar surroundings. Debriefing should be delayed. Victims should have privacy without isolation.

Essential both in the treatment of the acute responses after release and, most important, in the treatment of the delayed responses after release is the recognition of the need of the victim to ventilate his feelings of hostility towards the individuals involved in the negotiations for his release, as well as his feelings of the pathological transference towards the terrorist.

During the siege, while the victim is still being held hostage, it is important not to disturb the development of the pathological transference. It must be left alone. Disturbance of the pathological transference while the victim is held hostage would only activate the terror in the victim and may produce hopelessness, which may result in panic-terror behavior in the victim; he may do desperate acts, such as running out even into death. The negotiator must try to reinforce the pseudohelping efforts of the terrorist towards the victim. Rescuers must make no plans to utilize in any way the victim's cooperation in escape plans. Rescuers must remember that to victims of terror, "an open door is not perceived as an open door."

When the victim has been released, pathological transference is still present, and the victim is reluctant to express negative feelings towards his captors and even to participate in their later prosecution. It takes a while for this reaction to subside.

I believe the persistence of the behavior of pathological transference in the victims long after the victims' release is based on a primitive fear that any expression of negative feelings or behavior towards their former captors may result in awesome retaliation. Yet the victims are also aware of the captor's predatory use of their suffering to obtain his demands. This accounts for the persistent, impotent, constipated rage often seen in victims of violent crime. I have used the knowledge acquired from Nazi concentration camp victims who know that they cannot get revenge or even reparations for their suffering from the Nazis. I have encouraged victims to use the concept that "survival, living without fear, is getting even."

Finally, I feel it important to respond to victims of terror by continually reassuring them that their behavior during captivity was fully acceptable; "As long as they are alive, they did the right thing." They did nothing wrong; and it is important to welcome them back as we would a loved one who has recovered from a frightening and painful illness.

REFERENCES

1. NIEDERLAND, W. 1968. Post traumatic symptomatology. *In* Massive Psychic Trauma. H. Krystal, Ed.: 60-70. International Universities Press. New York, N.Y.
2. SYMONDS, M. 1980. Second injury to victims of violent crimes. Evaluation and Change Magazine. (Spring Issue.)
3. OCHBERG, F. 1978. The victim of terrorism. J. Terrorism 1(2): 147-168.
4. STRENTZ, T. 1980. The Stockholm syndrome: law enforcement policy and ego defenses of the hostage. Ann. N.Y. Acad. Sci. (This volume.)
5. SYMONDS, M. 1975. Victims of violence. Am. J. Psychoanal. 35(1): 19-26.
6. LANG, D. 1974. Swedish hostages. New Yorker (November 25): 56-126.
7. BUCKLEY, W. 1974. The kidnapper, the victim and society. Firing Line Program, WKPC-TV, May 15. SECA. Columbia, S.C.
8. HORNEY, K. 1950. Neurosis and Human Growth: 18-19. W. W. Norton and Co., Inc. New York, N.Y.
9. SYMONDS, M. 1976. The rape victim. Psychological patterns of response. Am. J. Psychoanal. 36(3): 27-34.

THE STOCKHOLM SYNDROME: LAW ENFORCEMENT POLICY AND EGO DEFENSES OF THE HOSTAGE

Thomas Strentz

FBI Academy
Quantico, Virginia 22135

THE BANK ROBBERY

At 10:15 A.M. on Thursday, August 23, 1973, the quiet early routine of the Sveriges Kreditbank in Stockholm, Sweden, was destroyed by the chatter of a submachine gun. As clouds of plaster and glass settled around the 60 stunned occupants, a heavily armed, lone gunman called out in English, "The party has just begun."[1]

The "party" was to continue for 131 hours, permanently affecting the lives of four young hostages and giving birth to a psychological phenomenon subsequently called the Stockholm syndrome.

During the 131 hours from 10:15 A.M. on August 23 until 9:00 P.M. on August 28, four employees of the Sveriges Kreditbank were held hostage. They were Elisabeth Oldgren, age 21, then an employee of 14 months working as a cashier in foreign exchange, now a nurse; Kristin Ehnmark, age 23, then a bank stenographer in the loan department, today a social worker; Brigitta Lundblad, age 31, an employee of the bank; and Sven Safstrom, age 25, a new employee, today employed by the Swedish government.[2] They were held by a 32-year-old thief, burglar, and prison escapee named Jan-Erik Olsson.[1] Their jail was an 11 x 47 foot, carpeted bank vault, which they came to share with another criminal and former cellmate of Olsson's—Clark Olofsson, age 26. Olofsson joined the group only after Olsson demanded his release from Norrkoping Penitentiary.[2]

This particular hostage situation gained long-lasting notoriety primarily because the electronic media exploited the fears of the victims as well as the sequence of events. Contrary to what had been expected, it was found that the victims feared the *police* more than they feared the robbers. In a telephone call to Prime Minister Olaf Palme, one of the hostages expressed these typical feelings of the group when she said, "The robbers are protecting us from the police." Upon release, other hostages puzzled over their feelings: "Why don't we hate the robbers?"[1]

For weeks after this incident, and while under the care of psychiatrists, some of the hostages experienced the paradox of nightmares over the possible escape of the jailed subjects and yet felt no hatred for these abductors. In fact, they felt the subjects had given them their lives back and were emotionally indebted to them for their generosity.

THE PHENOMENON

The Stockholm syndrome seems to be an automatic, probably unconscious, emotional response to the trauma of becoming a victim. Though some victims may think it through, this is not a rational choice by a victim who decides consciously that the most advantageous behavior in this predicament is to befriend his captor. This syndrome has been observed around the world and includes a high level of stress as participants are cast together in this life-threatening environment where each must achieve new levels of adaptation or regress to an earlier stage of ego development to stay alive. This phenomenon, this positive bond, affects the hostages and the hostage taker. This positive emotional bond—born in, or perhaps because of, the stress of the siege room—serves to unite its victims against the outsiders. A philosophy of "it's us against them" seems to develop. To date there is no evidence to indicate how long the syndrome lasts. Like the automatic reflex action of the knee, this bond seems to be beyond the control of the victim and the subject.

One definition of the Stockholm syndrome takes into account three phases of the experience and describes it as

> the positive feelings of the captives toward their captor(s) that are accompanied by negative feelings toward the police. These feelings are frequently reciprocated by the captor(s). To achieve a successful resolution of a hostage situation, law enforcement must encourage and tolerate the first two phases so as to induce the third and thus preserve the lives of all participants.[1]

Though this relationship is new in the experience of law enforcement officers, the psychological community has long been aware of the use of an emotional bond as a coping mechanism of the ego under stress.

Many years ago, Sigmund Freud forged the theory of personality and conceived three major systems, calling them the id, the ego, and the superego. Their functions are:

> The id is man's expression of instinctual drive without regard to reality or morality. It contains the drive for preservation and destruction, as well as the appetite for pleasure.[4]

> In the well-adjusted person the ego is the executive of the personality, controlling and governing the id and the superego and maintaining commerce with the external world in the interest of the total personality and its far-flung needs. When the ego is performing its executive functions wisely, harmony and adjustment prevail. Instead of the pleasure principle, the ego is governed by the reality principle.[4]

> The superego dictates to the ego how the demands of the id are to be satisfied. It is in effect the conscience and is usually developed by internalization of parental ideals and prohibitions formed during early childhood.[4]

Coping with reality is one function of the ego. The ego in the healthy personality is dynamic and resourceful. One of its functions is the use of defense mechanisms, a concept developed by Sigmund Freud in 1894 when he wrote "The Neuro-Psychoses of Defense." Freud conceived the defense mechanisms as the ego's struggle against painful or unendurable ideas or their effects.[5] The defense mechanisms have been discussed, explained, examined, and defined repeatedly since the last century. They vary in number depending upon the author. However, they all serve the same purpose—to protect the self from hurt and disorganization.[6]

When the self is threatened, the ego must cope under a great deal of stress. The ego enables the personality to continue to function, even during the most painful experiences—such as being taken hostage by an armed, anxious stranger. The hostage wants to survive, and the healthy ego is seeking a means to achieve survival.[7] One avenue open is the use of defense mechanisms. The mechanism used most frequently by hostages interviewed by the author has been regression, which Norman Cameron defines as a return to a less mature, less realistic level of experience and behavior.[8] Several theories have been advanced in an attempt to explain the observable symptoms that law enforcement officials and members of the psychiatric community have come to call the Stockholm syndrome.

In her book *The Ego and Its Mechanisms of Defense*, Anna Freud discusses the phenomenon of identification with the aggressor. This version of identification is called upon by the ego to protect itself against authority figures who have generated anxiety.[5] The purpose of this type of identification is to enable the ego to avoid the wrath—the potential punishment—of the enemy. The hostage identifies out of fear rather than out of love.[4] It would appear that the healthy ego evaluates the situation and selects from its arsenal of defenses that mechanism which served it best in the past when faced with trauma. The normal developing personality makes effective use of the defense mechanism of identification, generally out of love, when modeling itself after a parent.

> Identification often takes place in imitative learning, as when a boy identifies with his father and uses him as a model.[6]

Some authors have called this type of identification "introjection" and use the Nazi concentration camps as an example of people radically altering their norms and values.[9]

According to Coleman:

> Introjection is closely related to identification. As a defense reaction it involves the acceptance of others' *values and norms* as one's own even when they are contrary to one's previous assumptions [italics added].[6]

Coleman goes on to discuss the common occurrence of people adopting the values and beliefs of a new government to avoid social retaliation and punishment. The reaction seems to follow the principle, "If you can't beat 'em join 'em."[6]

Though identification with the aggressor is an attractive explanation for the Stockholm syndrome—and may indeed be a factor in some hostage situations—it is not a total explanation for the phenomenon. This reaction is commonly seen in children at about the age of five as they begin to develop a conscience and have resolved the Oedipus complex. They have given up the dream of being an adult and now begin to work on the reality of growing up. This is usually done by identifying with the parent of the same sex and is generally healthy. However, when this parent is abusive we see the identification serving the dual purpose of protection and of an ego ideal.

The Stockholm syndrome is viewed by this author as regression to a more elementary level of development than is seen in the five-year-old who identifies with a parent. The five-year-old is able to feed himself, speak for himself, and has locomotion. The hostage is more like the infant who must cry for food, cannot speak, and may be bound. Like the infant, the hostage is in a state of extreme dependence and fright. He is terrified of the outside world, like the child who learns to walk and achieves physical separation before he is ready for the emotional separation from the parent.

This infant is blessed with a mother figure who sees to his needs. As these needs are satisfactorily met by the mother figure, the child begins to love this person who is protecting him from the outside world. The adult is capable of caring and leading the infant from dependence and fear. So it is with the hostage—his extreme dependence, his every breath a gift from the subject. He is now as dependent as he was as an infant; the controlling, all-powerful adult is again present; the outside world is threatening once again. The weapons the police have deployed against the subject are also, in the mind of the hostage, deployed against him. Once again he is dependent, perhaps on the brink of death. Once again there is a powerful authority figure who can help. So the behavior that worked for the dependent infant surfaces again as a coping device, a defense mechanism, to lead the way to survival.

DOMESTIC HOSTAGE SITUATIONS

Since 1973, local law enforcement has been faced with many hostage situations. The subject-hostage bond is not always formed, yet case studies show that it is frequently a factor. As such, the Stockholm syndrome should be kept in mind by the police when they face such a situation, plan an attack, debrief former hostages,* and certainly when the subjects are prosecuted.

Hostage situations seem to be on the increase. Today, more than ever, police are responding to armed robberies in progress in a fraction of the time required a few years ago. This increased skill in incident response unfortunately promotes a perpetrator's need to take hostages. In the past, the armed robber was frequently gone before the employees felt safe enough to sound the alarm, but today silent alarms are triggered automatically. Computerized patrol techniques place police units in areas where they are more likely, statistically, to encounter an armed robbery. An analysis of past armed robberies dictates placement of patrol units to counter future at-

---

* In an attempt to gather intelligence about the subject, siege room, status and number of other hostages, etc., the police usually debrief, or carefully interview, victims in hostage situations.

tempts. Progress in one phase of law enforcement has created new demands in another.

The vast majority of hostage incidents are accidental. In cases such as these, it is likely the robber did not plan to take hostages. However, the police arrive sooner than anticipated, and as a new form of flight—a method of escape—the now trapped armed robber takes a hostage in order to bargain his way out.

In his desperation, the armed robber compounds his dilemma by adding kidnaping and assault charges. These considerations are initially minimal to him. His emotions are running high; he wants to buy time, and in this he succeeds. Research has shown that the leader among the abductors has a prior felony arrest.[10] Therefore, though desperate, the hostage taker is not ignorant or inexperienced in the ways of the criminal justice system and realizes the consequences of his new role.

The trapped subject is outgunned and outnumbered, and with each fleeting moment his situation becomes less tenable. Perhaps he takes hostages as a desperate offensive act, one of the few offensive acts available to him in his increasingly defensive position. Whatever his motivation, the subject is now linked with other individuals, usually strangers, who will come to sympathize and in some cases emphathize with him in a manner now recognized and understood.

The stranger—the victim—the law-abiding citizen—is forced into this life and death situation and is unprepared for this turn of events. Suddenly his routine world is turned around. The police, who should help, seem equally helpless. The hostage may feel that the police have let him down by allowing this to happen. It all seems so unreal.

STAGES OF HOSTAGE REACTION

Many hostages seek immediate psychological refuge in denial. According to Anna Freud:

> When we find denial, we know that it is a reaction to external danger; when repression takes place, the ego is struggling with instinctual stimuli.[5]

Hostages, in interviews with this author, frequently discuss their use of denial of reality. The findings of denial are not limited.

> As I continued to talk to victims of violence, I became aware that the general reactions of these victims were similar to the psychological response of an individual who experiences sudden and unexpected loss. Loss of any kind, particularly if sudden and unexpected, produces a certain sequence of response in all individuals. The first response is shock and denial.[11]

Hostages have also repressed their feelings of fear. Frequently these feelings of fear are transferred from fear of the hostage taker to fear of the police. Research has shown that most hostages die or are injured during the police assault phase.[12] This is not to say that the police kill them.

Denial is a primitive, but effective, psychological defense mechanism.

There are times when the mind is so overloaded with trauma that it cannot handle the situation.[11] To survive, the mind reacts as if the traumatic incident were not happening. The victims respond: "Oh no"; "No, not me"; "This must be a dream"; or "This is not happening."[11] These are all individually effective methods of dealing with excessively stressful situations.

Denial is but one stage of coping with the impossible turn of events. Each victim who copes effectively has a strong will to survive. One may deal with the stress by believing he is dreaming, that he will soon wake up and it will be all over. Some deal with the stress by sleeping; this author has interviewed hostages who have slept for over 48 hours while captive. Some have fainted, though this is rare.

Frequently, hostages gradually accept their situation but find a safety valve in the thought that their fate is not fixed. They view their situation as temporary, sure that the police will come to their rescue. This gradual change from denial to delusions of reprieve reflects a growing acceptance of the facts. Although the victim accepts that he is a hostage, he believes freedom will come soon.[13]

If freedom does not immediately relieve the stress, many hostages begin to engage in busywork, work they feel comfortable doing. Some knit, some methodically count and recount windows or other hostages, and some reflect upon their past life. This author has never interviewed a former hostage who had not taken stock of his life and vowed to change for the better, an attempt to take advantage of a second chance at life. The vast majority of hostages share this sequence of emotional events: denial, delusions of reprieve, busywork, and taking stock. The alliance that takes place between the hostage and the subject comes later.

TIME

Time is a factor in the development of the Stockholm syndrome. Its passage can produce a positive or negative bond, depending on the interaction of the subjects and hostages. If the hostage takers do not abuse their victims, hours spent together will most likely produce "positive" results. Time alone will not do so, but it may be the catalyst in nonabusive situations.

In September 1976, when five Croatian hijackers took a Boeing 727 carrying 95 people on a transatlantic flight from New York to Paris, another incidence of the Stockholm syndrome occurred. Attitudes toward the hijackers and their crime reflected the varying exposures of those involved in the situation.[14] The hostages were released at intervals. The first group was released after a few hours of captivity; the second group was released after a day. The debriefing of the victims in this situation has clearly indicated that the Stockholm syndrome is not a magical phenomenon, but a logical outgrowth of positive human interaction.

TWA flight 355, originally scheduled to fly from New York City to

Tucson, Arizona, via Chicago, on the evening of September 10, 1976, was diverted somewhere over western New York State to Montreal, Canada, where additional fuel was added. The hijackers then traveled to Gander, Newfoundland, where 34 passengers deplaned to lighten the aircraft for its flight to Europe via Keflavik, Iceland, with the remaining 54 passengers and a crew of seven. The subjects, primarily Julianna Eden Busic, selected passengers to deplane. She based her decisions on age and family responsibilities. The remaining passengers, plus the crew of seven, were those who were single, or married with no children, or those who had volunteered to remain on board, such as Bishop O'Rourke. After flying over London, the aircraft landed in Paris where it was surrounded by the police and not allowed to depart. After 13 hours the subjects surrendered to the French police. The episode lasted a total of 25 hours for most of the passengers and about 3 hours for those who deplaned at Gander.[14]

During the months of September and October of 1976, all but two of the hostages and all of the crew were interviewed. The initial hypothesis before the interviews was that those victims released after only a few hours would not express sympathy for the subjects, while those released later would react positively towards the subjects. In other words, time was viewed as the key factor.

The hypothesis was not proven. Instead, it seemed that the victims' attitudes toward the subjects varied from subject to subject and from victim to victim regardless of the amount of time they had spent as captives. Although this seemed illogical, interviews with the victims revealed understandable reasons. It was learned that those victims who had had negative contacts with the subjects did not evidence concern for them, regardless of time of release. Some of these victims had been physically abused by the subjects; they obviously did not like their abusers and advocated the maximum penalty be imposed.

Other victims had slept on and off for two days. This could be a form of defense mechanism of denial, a desperate ego-defensive means of coping with an otherwise intolerable event.[15] These victims had had minimal contact with the subjects and also advocated a maximum penalty. They may not have had distinctly negative contact, but they had experienced no positive association. Their only contact with the subjects had been on three occasions when hostage-taker Mark Vlasic awakened them in Paris as he ordered all of the passengers into the center of the aircraft where he threatened to detonate the explosives unless the French government allowed them to depart.

The other extreme was evidenced by victims, regardless of time of release, who felt great sympathy for their abductors. They had had positive contact with the subjects, which included discussing the hijackers' cause and understanding their motivation and suffering. Some of these victims told the press that they were going to take vacation time to attend the trial. Others began a defense fund for their former captors. Some recommended defense counsel to the subjects, and others refused to be interviewed by the law enforcement officers who had taken the subjects into custody.[14]

Perhaps one of the most self-revealing descriptions of the Stockholm syndrome was offered by one of these hijack victims:

> After it was over and we were safe, I recognized that they [the subjects] had put me through hell and had caused my parents and fiancé a great deal of trauma. Yet, I was alive. I was alive because they had let me live. You know only a few people, if any, who hold your life in their hands and then give it back to you. After it was over, and we were safe and they were in handcuffs, I walked over to them and kissed each one and said, "Thank you for giving me my life back." I know how foolish it sounds, but that is how I felt.[14]

Yet this feeling of affection seems to be a mask for a great inner trauma. Most victims, including those who felt considerable affection for the subjects, reported nightmares. These dreams expressed the fear of the subjects escaping from custody and recapturing them.[14] Dr. Ochberg reports similar findings,[16] as did the psychiatrist in Stockholm in 1973.[2]

Again, the hostages aboard the plane had developed a personal relationship with the criminals. The feelings of one hostage were expressed when she said, "They didn't have anything [the bombs were fakes], but they were really great guys. I really want to go to their trial."[17] This is a very different view from that of New York City Police Commissioner Michael Codd, who said in an interview, "What we have here is the work of madmen—murderers."[18] The interview with the commissioner followed an attempt to defuse a bomb left by the hijackers; the bomb killed one officer and seriously injured three others.[18]

The situation in 1973 in Stockholm was not unique. These same feelings were generated in the Croatian aircraft hijacking and, more recently, in the Japanese Red Army hijacking of JAL flight 472 in September/October 1977,[19] and also in the hostage situation that took place at the German consulate in August of 1978.[20]

ISOLATION

But the Stockholm syndrome relationship does not always develop. Sir Geoffrey Jackson, the British ambassador to Uruguay, was abducted and held by the Tupamaro terrorists for 244 days. He remained in thought and actions the ambassador, the queen's representative, and so impressed his captors with his dignity that they were forced to regularly change his guards and isolate him for fear he might convince them that his cause was just and theirs foolish.[21] Others, such as the American agronomist Dr. Claude Fly, held by the Tupamaros for 208 days in 1970, have also avoided identification with the abductor or his cause.[22] Dr. Fly accomplished this by writing a 600-page autobiography and by developing a 50-page "Christian Checklist," in which he analyzed the New Testament. Like Sir Geoffrey Jackson, Fly was able to create his own world and insulate himself against the hostile pressures around him.[22] According to Brooks McClure:

> In the case of both Dr. Fly and Sir Geoffrey Jackson, and other hostages as well, the terrorist organization found it necessary to remove the guards who were falling under their influence.[13]

In most situations, the Stockholm syndrome is a two-way street.

However, most victims of terrorist or criminal abductors are not individuals of the status of Dr. Fly or Ambassador Jackson, and do not retain an aura of aloofness during their captivity. As yet, there is no identified personality type more inclined to the Stockholm syndrome. The victims do share some common experiences, though.

POSITIVE CONTACT

The primary experience that victims of the syndrome share is positive contact with the subject. The positive contact is generated by *lack* of negative experiences, i.e., beatings, rapes, or physical abuse, rather than by an actual positive act on the part of the abductors. The few injured hostages who have evidenced the syndrome have been able to rationalize their abuse. They have convinced themselves that the abductor's show of force was necessary to take control of the situation, that perhaps their resistance precipitated the abductor's force. Self-blame on the part of the victims is very evident in these situations.

Stockholm syndrome victims share a second common experience; they sense and identify with the human quality of their captor. At times this quality is more imagined than real, as the victims of Fred Carrasco learned in Texas in August of 1974.[23]

On the afternoon of July 24, 1974, at the Texas Penitentiary in Huntsville, Fred Carrasco and two associates took approximately 70 hostages in the prison library. In the course of the 11 day siege, most of the hostages were released. However, the drama was played out on the steps of the library between 9:30 and 10:00 on the night of August 3, 1974. It was during this time that Carrasco executed the remaining hostages.[23] This execution took place in spite of his letters of affection to other hostages who had been released earlier due to medical problems.[24]

Some hostages expressed sympathy for Carrasco.[25] A Texas Ranger— who had been at the scene and had subsequently spoken to victims—stated to the author that there was evidence of the Stockholm syndrome.[26] Though the hostages' emotions did not reflect the depth of those in Sweden a year before, the hostages admitted affectionate feelings toward a person they thought they should hate. They saw their captor as a human being with problems similar to their own. Law enforcement has long recognized that the trapped armed robber believes he is a victim of the police. We now realize that the hostage tends to share his opinion.

When a robber is caught in a bank by quick police response, his dilemma is clear. He wants out with the money and his life. The police are preventing his escape by their presence and are demanding his surrender. The hostage—an innocent customer or employee of the bank—is also inside. His dilemma is similar to that of the robber—he wants to get out and cannot. He has seen the arrogant robber slowly become "a person" with a problem just like his own. The police on the outside correctly perceive the freedom of the hostages as the prerogative of the robber. However, the hostages perceive that the police weapons are pointed at them; the threat of tear gas makes them uncomfortable. The police insistence on the surrender of the subject is also keeping them hostage. Hostages begin to develop the idea that "if the police would go away, I could go home. If they would let him go, I would be free"[20]—and so the bond begins.

HOSTAGE TAKER REACTION

As time passes and positive contact between the hostage and hostage taker begins, the Stockholm syndrome also begins to take its effect upon the subject. This was evident at Entebbe in July of 1976. At least one of the terrorists, one who had engaged in conversations with the hostages from Air France flight 139, elected at the moment of the attack to shoot at the Israeli commandos rather than execute hostages.[27]

A moving account of this relationship is presented by Dr. Frank Ochberg as he recounts the experience of one hostage of the South Moluccans in December of 1975. Mr. Gerard Vaders, a newspaper editor in his 50s, has related his experience to Dr. Ochberg:

> On the second night they tied me again to be a living shield and left me in that position for seven hours. The one who was most psychopathic kept telling me, "your time has come. Say your prayers." They had selected me for the third execution. . . . In the morning when I knew I was going to be executed, I asked to talk to Prins [another hostage] to give him a message to take to my family. I wanted to explain my family situation. My foster child, whose parents had been killed, did not get along too well with my wife, and I had at the time a crisis in my marriage just behind me. . . . There were others things, too. Somewhere I had the feeling that I had failed as a human being. I explained all this and the terrorists insisted on listening.[16]

When Mr. Vaders completed his conversation with Mr. Prins and announced his readiness to die, the South Moluccans said, "No, someone else goes first."[16]

Dr. Ochberg observes that Mr. Vaders was no longer a faceless symbol. He was human. In the presence of his executioners, he made the transition from a symbol to be executed to a human to be spared. Tragically, the Moluccans selected another passenger, Mr. Bierling, led him away, and executed him before they had the opportunity to know him.[16]

Mr. Vaders goes on to explain his intrapsychic experience, his Stockholm syndrome:

> And you had to fight a certain feeling of compassion for the Moluccans. I know this is not natural, but in some way they come over human. They gave us cigarettes. They gave us blankets. But we also realize that they were killers. You try to suppress that in your consciousness. And I knew I was suppressing that. I also knew that they were victims, too. In the long run they would be as much victims as we. Even more. You saw the morale crumbling. You experienced the disintegration of their personalities. The growing of despair. Things dripping through their fingers. You couldn't help but feel a certain pity. For people at the beginning with egos like gods—impregnable, invincible—they end up small, desperate, feeling that all was in vain.[16]

Most people cannot inflict pain on another unless their victim remains dehumanized.[28] When the subject and his hostages are locked together in a vault, a building, a train, or an airplane, a process of humanization apparently does take place. When a person—a hostage—can build empathy while maintaining dignity, he or she can lessen the aggression of a captor.[28] The exception to this is the subject who is antisocial, as Fred Carrasco demonstrated in August of 1974. Fortunately, the Fred Carrascos of the world are in a minority, and in most situations the Stockholm syndrome is a two-way street. With the passage of time and the occurrence of positive experiences, the victims' chances of survival increase. However, isolation of the victims precludes the forming of this positive bond.

In some hostage situations, the victims have been locked in another room, or they have been in the same room but have been hooded or tied, gagged, and forced to face the wall away from the subject.[29] Consciously or unconsciously, the subject has dehumanized his hostage, thereby making it easier to kill him. As long as the hostage is isolated, time is not a factor. The Stockholm syndrome will not be a force that may save the life of the victim.

INDIVIDUALIZED REACTIONS

Additionally, it has been observed that even though some of the hostages responded positively toward their captors, they did not necessarily evidence Stockholm syndrome reactions toward all of the subjects. It was learned, logically, that most of the victims reacted positively toward those subjects who had treated them—in the words of the victims—"fairly." Those hostages who gave glowing accounts of the gentlemanly conduct of some subjects did not generalize to all subjects. They evidenced dislike, even hatred, toward one hostage taker whom they called an animal.

A hypothetical question was posed to determine the depth of victims' feelings toward their captors. Each former hostage was asked what he would do in the following situation: A person immediately recognizable as a law enforcement officer, armed with a shoulder weapon, would order him to lie down. At that same instant, one of his former captors would order him to stand up. When asked what he would do, the victim's response varied according to the identity of the captor giving the "order." If a captor who had treated him fairly hypothetically yelled, "Stand up," he would stand up. Conversely, if he thought it was the command of the subject who had verbally abused him, he would obey the law enforcement officer. This would indicate that the strength of the syndrome is considerable. Even in the face of an armed officer of the law, the victim would offer himself as a human shield for his abductor. As absurd as this may seem, such behavior has been observed by law enforcement officers throughout the world.†

---

† This was observed in the hijacking of a Philippine Airlines flight on September 17, 1978; during a hostage situation in Oceanside, Calif., February 3, 1975; during an aborted bank robbery in Toronto, Canada, in November 1977; and during a hostage situation that grew out of an aborted bank robbery in New York City in August 1976, which was later made into a movie entitled "Dog Day Afternoon."

Whether the incident is a bank robbery in Stockholm, Sweden, a hijacking of an American aircraft over western New York, a kidnaping in South America, or an attempted prison break in Texas, there are behavioral similarities despite geographic and motivational differences. In each situation, a relationship—a healthy relationship (healthy because those involved were alive to talk about it)—seems to develop between people caught in circumstances beyond their control and not of their making, a relationship that reflects the use of ego defense mechanisms by the hostage. This relationship seems to help victims cope with excessive stress and, at the same time, enables them to survive—a little worse for wear, but alive. The Stockholm syndrome is not a magical relationship of a blanket affection for the subject. This bond, though strong, does have its limits. It has logical limits. If a person is nice to another, a positive feeling toward this person develops, even if this person is an armed robber, a hijacker of an aircraft, a kidnaper, or a prisoner attempting to escape.

The victim's need to survive is stronger than his impulse to hate the person who has created his dilemma. It is his ability to survive, to cope, that has enabled man to survive and claw his way to the top of the evolutionary ladder. His ego is functioning and has functioned well, and has performed its primary task of enabling the self to survive. At an unconscious level, the ego has activated the proper defense mechanisms in the correct sequence—denial, regression, identification, or introjection—to achieve survival. The Stockholm syndrome is just another example of the ability of the ego, the healthy ego, to cope and adjust to difficult stress brought about by a traumatic situation.

The application for law enforcement is clear, though it does involve a trade-off. The priority in dealing with hostage situations is the survival of all participants. This means the survival of the hostage, the crowd that has gathered, the police officers, and the subject. To accomplish this end, various police procedures have been instituted. Establishing inner and outer perimeters is a long-standing procedure designed to keep crowds at a safe distance.‡ Police training, discipline, and proper equipment save officers' lives. The development of the Stockholm syndrome may save the life of the hostage as well as the subject. The life of the subject is preserved, as it is highly unlikely that deadly force will be used by the police unless the subject makes a precipitous move. The life of the hostage may also be saved by the Stockholm syndrome, the experience of positive contact, thus setting the stage for regression, identification, and/or introjection. The subject is less likely to injure a hostage he has come to know and, on occasion, to love.[28]

It is suggested that the Stockholm syndrome can be fostered while negotiating with the subject by asking him to allow the hostage to talk on the telephone; by asking him to check on the health of a hostage; or by discussing with him the family responsibilities of the hostages. Any action

‡ Perimeters are zones of controlled access. The inner perimeter would be set up to keep out everyone except certain police officials; the outer perimeter would be a zone restricted to police.

the negotiator can take to emphasize the hostage's human qualities to the subject should be considered by the negotiator.

The police negotiator must pay a personal price for this induced relationship. Hostages will curse him, as they did in Stockholm in August of 1973. They will call the police cowards and actively side with the subject in trying to achieve a solution to their plight, a solution not necessarily in their best interest or in the best interest of the community.

Unfortunately, it may not end there. Victims of the Stockholm syndrome may remain hostile toward the police after the siege has ended. The "original" victims in Stockholm still visit their abductors, and one former hostage is engaged to Olofsson.[30] South American victims visit their former captors in jail.§ Others have begun defense funds for them.[14] A hostile hostage is a price that law enforcement must pay for a living hostage. Anti-law enforcement feelings are not new to the police. But this may be the first time it has been suggested that law enforcement seek to encourage hostility, hostility from people whose lives law enforcement has mustered its resources to save. However, a human life is an irreplaceable treasure and worth some hostility. A poor or hostile witness for the prosecution is a small price to pay for this life.

REFERENCES

1. LANG, D. 1974. A reporter at large. New Yorker (November): 56–126.
2. Police Officers. 1978. Interviews with police officers from Stockholm, Sweden, on March 22 and November 8. FBI Academy. Quantico, Va. (Unpublished.)
3. OCHBERG, F. M. 1968. Interview on November 2 with Dr. Ochberg, Acting Director, National Institute of Mental Health, Rockville, Md. (Unpublished.)
4. HALL, C. 1954. A Primer of Freudian Psychology. World Publishing Co. New York, N.Y.
5. FREUD, A. 1966. The Writings of Anna Freud. II. The Ego and the Mechanisms of Defense. revised edit. International Universities Press, Inc. New York, N.Y.
6. COLEMAN, J. C. 1972. Abnormal Psychology and Modern Life. 5th edit. Scott Foresman Co. Glenview, Ill.
7. BELLAK, L., M. HURVICH & H. K. GEDIMAN. 1973. Ego Functions in Schizophrenics, Neurotics and Normals. John Wiley and Sons, Inc. New York, N.Y.
8. CAMERON, N. 1963. Personality Development and Psychopathology: A Dynamic Approach. Houghton Mifflin Co. Boston, Mass.
9. BLUHM, H. O. 1948. How did they survive? Mechanisms of defense in Nazi concentration camps. Am. J. Psychotherapy 2: 3–32.
10. GRAVES, B. & T. STRENTZ. 1977. The Kidnaper: His Crime and His Background. Research Paper. Special Operations and Research Staff. FBI Academy. Quantico, Va.
11. MCCLURE, B. 1968. Hostage Survival. U.S. Department of State. Washington, D.C. (Unpublished research material.)
12. JENKINS, B. M., J. JOHNSON & D. RONFELDT. 1977. Numbered Lives: Some Statistical Observations from Seventy-Seven International Hostage Episodes. Report No. P-5905. Rand Corporation. Santa Monica. Calif.
13. Committee on the Judiciary. 1975. Terrorist Activity; Hostage Defense Measures. Hearings before the subcommittee to investigate the administration of the Internal Security Act and other internal security laws of the Committee on the Judiciary. Senate, U. S. Congress. Part 5. 94th Cong., 1st Sess., 1975.

§ This was evident during the hostage situations in Cleveland, Ohio, on October 29, 1975 and in Chicago, Illinois, on August 18, 1978.

14. Victims of Hijacking. 1976. Interviews with victims of hijacking of Trans World Airlines flight 355. New York, Chicago, and Tucson. (Unpublished.)
15. LAUGHLIN, H. P. 1970. The Ego and Its Defenses. Appleton-Century-Crofts, Inc. New York, N.Y.
16. OCHBERG, F. 1978. The victim of terrorism: psychiatric considerations. Terrorism 1(2); 147-168.
17. ALPERN, D. M. 1976. A skyjacking for Croatia. Newsweek (September 20): 25.
18. New York Times. 1976. Skyjackers are charged with murder. September 12: 3.
19. Victims of Hijacking. 1977. Interviews with victims (American citizens) of hijacking of Japanese Airlines flight 472. San Francisco, Los Angeles, and Tokyo. (Unpublished.)
20. Victims of Hostage Situation. 1968. Interviews on August 19 with victims of a hostage situation at the German consulate. Chicago, Ill.
21. JACKSON, SIR GEOFFREY. 1973. Surviving the Long Night. Vanguard Press, Inc. New York, N.Y.
22. FLY, C. L. 1973. No Hope But God. Hawthorn Books, Inc. New York, N.Y.
23. Houston Post. 1974. Murder suicide found in Huntsville case. September 4: 1.
24. HOUSE, A. 1975. The Carrasco Tragedy. Texian Press. Waco, Tex.
25. COOPER, L. 1974. Hostage freed by Carrasco aided prison officials in assault plan. Houston Chronicle (August 5): 4.
26. BURKS, G. W. 1975. Interview in December with Captain Burks of the Texas Rangers. Austin, Tex. (Unpublished.)
27. STEVENSON, W. 1976. Ninety Minutes at Entebbe. Bantam Books. New York, N.Y.
28. ARONSON, E. 1972. Social Animal. W. H. Freeman Co. San Francisco, Calif.
29. Victims of Hostage Situation. 1978. Interviews in March with victims of the Hanafi Muslim siege. Washington, D.C. (Unpublished.)
30. Washington Post. 1976. Swedish Robin Hood. Parade Magazine Supplement, November 14.
31. EITINGER, L. 1964. Concentration Camp Survivors in Norway and Israel. Allen and Unwin. London, England.
32. HACKER, F. J. 1976. Crusaders, Criminals, Crazies. Terror and Terrorism in Our Time. W. W. Norton Co. New York, N.Y.
33. MIRON, M. S. & A. P. GOLDSTEIN. 1978. Hostage. Behaviordelia, Inc. Kalamazoo, Mich.
34. PARRY, A. 1976. Terrorism from Robespierre to Arafat. Vanguard Press, Inc. New York, N.Y.
35. SARGANT, W. W. 1957. Battle for the Mind. Greenwood Press. Westport, Conn.
36. Conference on Terrorism. 1977. Final Report on Dimensions of Victimization in the Context of Terrorist Acts. Proceedings of the Conference, Evian, France, June 3-5.
37. FATTAH, E. Z. Some Reflections of the Victimology of Terrorism. Simon Fraser University. Vancouver, B.C., Canada.
38. HOWELL, A. C. 1975. The hidden crime. Ph.D. Dissertation. Temple University. Philadelphia, Penn.
39. JENKINS, B. M. 1976. Hostage Survival: Some Preliminary Observations. Report No. P-5627. Rand Corporation. Santa Monica, Calif.
40. OCHBERG, F. M. 1978. Terrorism—Is There an Answer? Practical Suggestions to Potential Hostages and to Those Working to Rescue Victims: How to Lead from Strength. Institute of Psychiatry. London, England (Unpublished.)
41. WOLK, R. L. 1977. Psychoanalytical Conceptualization of Hostage Symptoms and Their Treatment. Forensic Services, New York Department of Mental Hygiene. Eastern New York Correctional Facility. Napanoch, N.Y.
42. BROCKMAN, R. 1976. Notes while being hijacked. Atlantic Monthly (December): 68-75.
43. LUNDE, D. T. & T. E. WILSON. 1977. Brainwashing as a defense to criminal liability. Crim. Law Bull. 13(November): 341-382.
44. MILLER, A. H. 1978. Negotiations for hostages: implications from the police experience. Terrorism 1(2): 125-146.
45. SEGAL, J., E. J. HUNTER & Z. SEGAL. 1976. Universal consequences of captivity: stress reactions among divergent populations of prisoners of war and their families Int. Social Sci. J. 28(3): 593-609.
46. SYMONDS, M. 1975. Victims of violence: psychological effects and after effects. Am. J. Phychoanal. 35: 19-26.

HOSTAGE TAKING—THE TAKERS, THE TAKEN, AND THE CONTEXT: DISCUSSION

Discussant: Charles Bahn*

Temple University
Philadelphia, Pennsylvania 19122

Let us begin with the distinction that Dr. Knutson makes between *reluctant* hostage takers and *deliberate* hostage takers. Since we are in the infancy of understanding the phenomenon of hostage taking, the dynamics of the hostage taker, and the dynamics of the hostage, it may very well be helpful to begin with the hypothesis that they are separate phenomena. The circumstances that we're trying to analyze range from a situation in which a crime is in progress, and the perpetrator, the criminal—perhaps even without a weapon and simply by a threat of physical violence—forces a victim to accompany him as part of his escape, to that situation in which a group of people—highly trained, quite deliberate in their actions, assigning roles to each member—set out to and succeed in taking hostages. A significant point that has begun to emerge from the evidence that Agent Strentz presented is that the deliberate hostage taker appears to have a great deal of insight into the dynamics of the situation with regard to the effects of the interaction between hostage taker and victim, whereas the reluctant hostage taker seems to act with a lack of insight into those effects.

Nevertheless, one wonders, for example, where the classical kidnapper would be placed with regard to this distinction. One other point with regard to reluctant hostage takers is that this may be another instance of the factor of contagion in crime. That is, some crimes become fashionable during given periods, perhaps due to the influence of the mass media, perhaps for other reasons as well. Dr. Schlossberg's comments about the craving for attention on the part of the hostage taker—particularly the reluctant hostage taker, who is problem solving and really trying both to solve his problem and gain attention in this way—imply that this really becomes an advantageous tool for such a person, but not a deliberately chosen one. The principal distinction between deliberate and reluctant hostage taking would involve the extent of deliberate and planned depersonalization of the victim from the beginning of the hostage event.

From the victim's perspective, it is not clear that the difference that Dr. Knutson suggested is meaningful. Whether the hostage taker is reluctant or deliberate, I would suggest that from the victim's perspective, the central issue is whether in fact a credible threat to life has been made. More likely, of course, when a deliberate hostage event transpires—particularly a deliberate hostage event with political motivation—we observe that the event generally begins with a kind of initial brutal signature act that makes

* Present affiliation: Department of Psychology, John Jay College of Criminal Justice, New York, N.Y. 10019.

the threat to life fully credible and is undoubtedly intended to bring about the Stockholm syndrome, or victim compliance behavior. This initial terrorization is not unknown in the commission of other violent crimes; studies on the specific interactions between criminals and victims—for example, on what robbers and muggers first say to their victims—show a deliberate terrorization.

Quite often, the first communication is not only depersonalizing, but also a vile insult and an extremely violent threat. For example, "Keep quiet or I'll kill you, mother fucker." Now, in the case of hostage situations, we have something that goes beyond mere terror and is a highly credible threat to life; and once that happens, from the moment that it's not carried out, we have the beginning of the gratitude that builds up on the return of one's life from the individual who made a credible threat and nevertheless is not acting upon it.

So, with some caution, I would identify the possible dichotomy of hostage situations as heuristic, that is, worthy of further analysis and the basis of specific hypotheses to be tested. The general hypothesis is that both the different outcomes in hostage situations and the differing responses by victims, perhaps even the levels of depersonalization, stem from the interaction function of the personalities involved, the specific social interaction that transpires, the extent of conversation or isolation between the hostage taker and the hostage, and perhaps the duration of the incidents.

In other countries, there are studies of the political hostage situations that are retrospective longitudinal studies trying to identify the effects of duration on the dynamics of the hostage situation.

Making the distinction between the reluctant and deliberate hostage taker will help us to respond more clearly as well to those hostage situations that are related to international terrorism. International terrorism usually begins with maximum initial brutality, equalling or surpassing the brutality involved in ordinary crimes.

It is obvious both from a review of the literature and from the papers given by my colleagues that our concentration has been focused primarily on developing an understanding of the psychological state of the hostage taker and secondarily on analyzing the psychological effects of being taken hostage.

We have made studies in both areas, uncovering the need for attention on the part of the hostage taker, the suicidal aspects of his act, and the process of depersonalization of the hostage that enables the hostage taker to exercise control over the hostage and, in some cases, ultimately to kill the hostage.

The more complete description of the Stockholm syndrome that has now begun to emerge points up not only the regressive dependency that dominates the behavior of the hostage, but also the manifold effects on any human being of facing a credible threat of immediate and arbitrary death. Truly, hostages are victims of terror, for a credible death threat is the ultimate terror.

What has been given less attention is the social psychology of hostage taking, and its psychopolitical implications.

To begin with, we must distinguish between those situations in which an individual takes a hostage in the course of committing a crime or during temporary mental derangement and situations in which hostage taking is a tactical component of a terroristic thrust.

In the latter situation, hostage taking is simply one more extreme tactic, often the dominant tactic, used by those who would advance their political cause by means of terror. Other tactics in their array have included bombings, bombings of public places, suicide missions of wholesale killing, and assassinations.

Within this context, hostages taking and the other tactics of terror have in common the fact that they are directed either against innocent people or against those who symbolize the opposing political force. Rather than being directed against the actual foe—against a police force or an army—the terror is directed against a secondary, symbolic target, usually a target that is unprotected and defenseless.

Terror tactics also tend to be carried out with maximum initial brutality, equalling or surpassing the brutality involved in ordinary crimes.

Now, these characteristics of terrorism play a significant role in the way in which terrorism is perceived. Due to its quasi-suicidal nature, political sympathizers view the terrorist as one willing to make even the extreme sacrifice of giving his own life in order to advance the common cause. It thus becomes imperative that sympathizers do not dare to question or criticize the tactics employed because they are, ipso facto, not as committed to the cause as the terrorists, since they have not publicly demonstrated their willingness to lay down their lives for it. They must instead support the activities of the terrorists and provide rationalizations both to themselves and to others that will explain the brutality directed against the innocent.

The general public has a similar imperative problem with terrorism. The tactics of terrorism are so harsh—so much a contradiction to the basic tenets of decency in human relationships, particularly in face-to-face encounters—that the uninvolved observer feels compelled to adduce some extraordinary motivation to explain the act. Thus, because terrorism appears to be spontaneous in nature and to demonstrate an indifference to personal safety, the public is more than willing to believe that the terrorist act is committed by a desperate individual who has no other alternative but death to committing the deed. This quickly becomes elaborated into a belief that the terrorist's desperation undoubtedly derives from grievances that he sees as legitimate, that have been consistently ignored and shunted aside. The terrorist's frustration and desperation have thus driven him to acts beyond the bounds of acceptable social behavior, which will at the very least guarantee the terrorist a hearing, if not actually bring about the amelioration of intolerable conditions.

It is this response by the public, often including members of the government against which the terrorism is directed, that makes terrorism effective. The audience, to make sense of a terroristic act, assumes the terrorist's deep-lying frustration and ultimate desperation.

No doubt, many terrorists are, in fact, people in just such a state. Whether we identify someone as a terrorist or as a freedom fighter is, in some measure, a reflection of our own political position.

However, there are many situations in which other alternatives have not been explored by the terrorists and found useless, and in which the apparent spontaneity of the terroristic acts belies not only an extensive period of planning and training (a preparation not inconsistent with a stance of desperation), but also the involvement of other groups or forces who have no immediate share in the grievance and who are neither desperate nor frustrated but simply malevolent and manipulative.

Surprisingly, even when evidence of funding or training by such Machiavellian outsiders is introduced, the force of the initial explanation of the terrorism as spontaneous outbursts of desperation is so great that the contradictory information becomes difficult to assimilate.

During the past year, we have been confronted with increasingly detailed evidence of linkages between a number of insurgent terrorist movements and the Soviet Union. These linkages go beyond the provision of funding, equipment, and weapons; they are based on common training undertaken on Soviet soil by members of various insurgent groups from different countries, who don't necessarily share a common political ideology or even a common perception of motivating grievances. Two respected former intelligence officials—Dr. Ray Cline, director of the Center for Strategic Studies at Georgetown University, and Robert Moss, editor, The Economist Foreign Report—have testified about Russian training of terrorists, as part of their presentation at the recent Jonathan Institute Conference on International Terrorism (July 1979). They described Russian training camps, one conducted at a base near Moscow, and one at another base in the vicinity of the city of Simperofol in the Black Sea region. These camps were for members of such diverse terrorist groups as the Palestine Liberation Organization, the Popular Front for the Liberation of Palestine, the People's Democratic Front for the Liberation of Palestine, and the Universal Red Army. The course of study included the use of regular and electric detonators, chemical and biological warfare, production of incendiary devices, a study of fuse types, and preparation of antipersonnel minefields.

Nevertheless, in the first issue of the journal *Terrorism* in 1977, when this above-mentioned training was being established, there is an article by (ironically enough) the then "permanent" representative of Iran to the United Nations, in which he approvingly cites a Saudi Arabian statement that contributed to the downfall of a proposed United Nations condemnation of terrorism.

The Saudi amendment suggested that the title of the proposal be amended to include the words,

and study of the underlying causes of those forms of terrorism and acts of violence which lie in misery, frustration, grievance and despair and which cause some people to sacrifice human lives, including their own, in attempts to effect radical change.[1]

This is an almost classical statement of the rationale of terrorism that comes to our minds when we encounter this behavior phenomenon, which seems to violate the most basic tenets of human decency.

Were we able to fully assimilate the meaning of the training programs in which partisans of diverse groups are encouraged to suppress their ideological differences so that they can learn the techniques of hijacking, skyjacking, forays against civilian targets, and bombing of random victims, we should then realize that we have been engaged in what Brian Crozier, director of the London-based Institute for the Study of Conflict, has called "low-intensity" warfare—a secret warfare, sporadic and unpredictable, carried out by zealots who direct their attacks toward random targets, often randomly chosen innocent targets.

In the United Nations debate that led to the downfall of the proposal to condemn terrorism, much was made of the fact that it is difficult to identify the "innocent" in the contemporary political world. Several nations, including Russia, objected to the assumption that some people were innocent and others were not. There are soldiers, they pointed out, without malevolent intentions, while civilians, including women and the aged, may be deeply committed, implacable adversaries of the cause for which terroristic war is being waged.

This semantic debate highlights the difference between spontaneous acts of desperation and covertly developed acts of low-intensity warfare. When a cause eliminates neutrality as a possible stance, it moves beyond just grievance into an area of imposed and rigid ideas of what is right and fair.

The spontancity of the acts becomes vitiated with the months of intensive training in a foreign country, where only the most rigid fanatic could fail to notice that the host country, in addition to affirming the grievances of the terrorists, is also using their activities to further its own self-interest.

The desperate and almost suicidal quality of the acts, while an implicit aspect of terrorism, fails to explain or illuminate the vast majority of cases. Not only can the terrorist reasonably expect that he will successfully coerce safe pasage away from the scene of his criminal acts to a country where he can find refuge and even acclaim, but he has the added assurance that even if he is caught by one of the western countries—one with a fair judicial and penal system—his compatriots will mount a subsequent terroristic attack whose objective will be to obtain his freedom and safe return.

The existence of countries that provide sanctuary and a hero's welcome to terrorists—and the likelihood that, through a hostage exchange or some other extreme action, an incarcerated convicted terrorist can look forward to release—makes it much easier to contemplate terror without any thought of sacrificing one's life.

It is important for us to understand the individual psychology of the terrorist if we are to deal with it in hostage negotiation. Our comprehension of the plight of the victims of terror, particularly of hostages, can help us both to obtain their freedom and to assuage some of the trauma resulting from their experience.

A deeper understanding of our own need to rationalize terrorism—to understand it and, if possible, to explain it away—can help us to keep both our moral and political balance. If we suspect that our rationalizations are based on inaccurate beliefs, we may be less concerned with vain attempts to redress deeply felt grievances and may admit the possibility that the grievances have been shaped and reinforced by forces whose apparent objectives are the achievement not of justice but of disruption.

REFERENCES

1. 1977. Terrorism **1** (1): 71–85.
2. BURTON, A. 1975. Urban Terrorism. Leo Cooper. London, England.
3. CLUTTERBUCK, R. 1975. Living with Terrorism. Faber and Faber. London, England.
4. ELIOT, J. D. & E. GIBSON, Eds. 1978. Contemporary Terrorism: Selected Readings. International Society of Chiefs of Police. Gaithersburg, Md.
5. LIVINGSTON, M. H., L. B. KRESS & M. G. WANER, Eds. 1978. International Terrorism in the Contemporary World. Greenwood Press. Westport, Conn.
6. SCHREIBER, J. 1978. The Ultimate Weapon, Terrorists and World Order. William Morrow and Co., Inc. New York, N.Y.

THE PLACE OF PSYCHOTHERAPY IN PROBATION AND PAROLE: THE PATIENT AS OFFENDER

Alexander B. Smith and Louis Berlin

Department of Sociology
John Jay College of Criminal Justice
New York, New York 10019

In the past three decades, our evaluation of psychotherapy as a treatment approach in probation and parole has undergone an appreciable change. When the authors began their careers in probation and parole, the prevailing view was that offenders were people suffering from a disturbance in their self-concepts, in their attitudes toward peers and authority, and in their grasp of reality. It followed, therefore, that the basic role of the probation and parole officer was that of corrector of erroneous and unrealistic concepts so that the offender might be put in a position to effect a better adjustment. In this connection, administrators sought out officers who had earned their master's degrees in social work and/or people who had had experience and training in psychotherapy.

A basic assumption of the above orientation was

> the concept that the offense is a symptom; the court must be concerned with treatment of the person. This would involve all that can be learned about his mental and physical condition and the attitudes and external influences which condition his personality and behavior,[1]

After such an in-depth study, the officer classified the offender—who was considered sick—into such categories as neurotic, psychotic, and character disordered. This latter type frustrated the probation and parole officers in their psychotherapeutic endeavors. These offenders were characterized by

> . . . one, an absence of severe neurotic or psychotic symptomotology; two, a lack of development of the superego (the self-control that one expects in an adult is lacking); three, an extremely low frustration tolerance (demands must be met immediately, regardless of future consequences). . . . Unlike the neurotic who may be motivated by his anxiety to seek help, the character disorder tends to "act out" (commits some physical act, usually anti-social), and alleviate his anxiety in this manner.[2]

The faith and confidence in psychotherapy during the decades mentioned were enormous. The one-to-one technique was applied universally and without discrimination. Failures and rejections by the offenders were ascribed to their "resistance" to getting well. When a variation of therapy—such as the Rogerian nondirective approach—was used, the results were frequently disheartening. Particularly was this the case with the so-called character disorders. As a result of the failures expressed in recidivism rates, the reasons were sought not in the nature of the clients, but in the therapists themselves. The literature of the period reflected this self-searching. The one-to-one technique was ineffective because

> the techniques of psychotherapy used today were formulated on a middle-class neurotic

157

population whose goals, values, and anxieties are entirely different than those of the repetitive offender. . . . The attempt to translate techniques and methods which have been successful on neurotics to the character disorder, including the persistent offender, have been almost a total failure.[2]

Faced with failures of psychoanalytically oriented therapy with its emphasis on the genesis of symptoms, interpretation of dynamics, and imparting of insight, a new orientation towards treatment—disregarding the origin of the condition and concentrating on the way to change behavior—was offered. This psychological modality is behavior modification. Eysenck and Rachman, exponents and practitioners of behavior modification, explain:

Given that a particular behavior pattern, whether neurotic or criminal, has in fact developed, our approach would now be quite ahistorical. We are not particularly concerned, in the majority of cases, with the particular reasons for the emergence of this pattern, but we are virtually concerned with the problem of how this pattern is to be changed. Such change must clearly take the form of deconditioning in the case of dysthymic disorders, and one of reconditioning in the case of the criminal and psychopathic disorders. We do not postulate any underlying complexes or even "neuroses"; in our account, these are unnecessary hypotheses not called for by the facts in question. Thus, our theory and our treatment are purely symptomatic; the symptom in each case is a conditioned, unadapting autonomic or skeletal response, and our task is to abolish this particular, maladaptive pattern of behavior. Once this is accomplished our task is over; there is no anticipation of any recrudescence of the symptom itself, or any emergence of new symptoms, as would be expected if there were any hypothetical complex or underlying cause for the behavior outside the field of conditioning. It is here that the facts must pronounce their judgment as to the adequacy of these two hypotheses.[3]

Introduced into the lexicon of treatment were such terms as behavior modification, operant conditioning, aversive therapy, contractual psychology, and commitment. Probation, parole, and prison workers attempted to utilize this orientation with some successes as well as failures. This orientation was hailed with enthusiasm by probation and parole officers who were not too comfortable or enthusiastic about probing feelings, psychoanalytically or otherwise.

The influx of minorities into probation and parole caseloads—and into the correctional institutions in the 1950s, 1960s, and today—has brought about changes in orientations and techniques in treatment. These offenders were disadvantaged people who needed jobs, housing, health care, and some voice in solving community problems. The primary need of these offenders was for community services. The emphasis in corrections shifted from treating the personality of the offenders to changing the institutions under which they lived.

This new view transforms the way workers assess their clients. The client is now a person whose future depends not only on how well he adjusts and adapts to the environment, but additionally on how well he is linked to social institutions.[4]

Commenting on priorities, the authors of the above take an extreme position regarding concrete services versus counseling: "As members of the helping professions, we have special responsibilities for the delivery of urgently needed services to our clients. Often what they least need is counseling."[4] In addition, these authors express today's view:

Most offenders are not pathologically ill, therefore, the medical (casework) model is

inappropriate. . . . Most probation and parole officers are not equipped by education
and experience to provide casework counseling even if it is needed.[4]

Though we might accept the assertion that most offenders are not
"pathologically ill," counseling is not *thereby* ruled out. One does not have
to be "pathologically ill" to need counseling. It is sufficient reason that one
has acted out his impulses in an antisocial way, in order for him to be a can-
didate for counseling aimed at changes in behavior and attitudes. Meeting
such needs as jobs, housing, medical treatment, and other concrete needs
does not, per se, insure miraculous changes in behavior and attitudes.

Entertaining such views of the nonpathological client and of the
psychotherapeutically inept officer, current sociologically oriented correctional theorists assign the officers priority to acting as community resource
managers. Some authorities go so far as to encourage officers to become involved in changing institutions:

> The most important activity in which a probation agency can be engaged is, therefore,
> to provide leadership in the direction of vital social change. Without social change . . . ,
> the most progressive programs will have little effect.[5]

The pendulum has swung to the opposite extreme. The impact of the
sociologists, however, has not eliminated the role of counseling but has
assigned to it a low priority as compared to the role of resource manager,
advocate, and community worker, striving to create new resources and/or
helping to coordinate existing resources.

The sociologists, though, have not completely rejected the psychiatric
interpretation of crime. However, before presenting their views, it will be
helpful to present the classic Freudian view of crime and mental illness. A
lucid psychoanalytic presentation of the relationship of mental illness to
crime is given by Philip Q. Roche, a Pennsylvania psychiatrist in private
practice:

> In meeting stress all of us attempt to maintain a balance and in so doing exhibit what
> are called symptoms. When such devices are ineffective the balance is shifted and we
> experience what is called mental illness in some degree. In some persons who have had
> poor life training, symptoms become fixed in patterns which are called character defor-
> mations. We apply various names to them such as "psychopathic personality,"
> "constitutional psychopathic inferior" . . . sociopath. In others we observe symptoms
> of such intensity and at such variance with common-sense values that we regard and
> accept the person exhibiting them as psychotically incapacitated. Again, a large number
> of persons are incapacitated to a degree less than psychotic—we regard them as neu-
> rotic. All have in common a tendency to repetitive symbolic destructive behavior
> directed both outwardly and toward themselves.[6]

Roche notes that the individual who absorbs his antisocial impulses instead
of acting them out pays for it in terms of mental illness. "In this light the
criminal insures his sanity and maintains an isolation from an awareness of
his own 'mental illness.' "[6]

Sociologists generally agree with their colleague Edwin Schur, who
holds that deviance does *not* necessarily mean mental illness. He asserts that

> sociologists have often complained that psychiatric interpretations of delinquency
> and crime have failed to take adequate account of the variation in outlook and behavior
> patterns that are given social approval in the different socioeconomic strata of our

society. What is considered "normal" in one social class context may be adjudged "pathological" in another. . . . This kind of perspective is increasingly recognized by the more sociologically sophisticated psychiatrists, who nowadays often take into account that the antisocial behavior and outlooks of even a hardened-offender—in terms of the social milieu out of which they developed—are not always evidence of psychic abnormality. Accordingly, new types of psychiatric treatment programs have arisen in which an effort is made to grapple with the group and cultural sources of the antisocial patterns and to create a "therapeutic milieu"—rather than simply attempting to utilize conventional forms of one-to-one psychotherapy.[7]

In this view, sociologists recognize the need to change personal values and attitudes engendered by the group and cultural milieu from which the offender sprang.

In spite of the tide downgrading counseling and other psychotherapeutic approaches, there have been sufficient sober influences to encourage federal funding for community mental health resources. For the officer to engage in therapy while such resources exist is considered a wasteful duplication of services. Probation and parole officers referred their subjects to local city, state, and private psychiatric facilities for evaluation and consultation even at the time when facilities were scarce; but at present, there is greater use of such community mental health facilities. These current practices are helpful to both client and officer. Some corrections agencies boast full-time psychiatrists attached to a court clinic. Others have a "resident psychiatrist" who devotes several days a week to examining and evaluating clients referred to him by the officers. In addition, the psychiatrists meet with probation and parole officers not only for consultation on cases, but to train them "in the techniques of fact gathering, counseling, interpretation and understanding of psychodynamics, as well as providing support for the officers as they developed their own interpretive capabililties."[8] By means of such close cooperation, the clients are serviced and the officers' treatment skills are enhanced. "But by and large, it is the function of the resident psychiatrist to explain to the probation officer what type of mental or emotional disorder the probationer or parolee has, and to offer suggestions as to the best techniques and therapy to be used in effective supervision."[8]

In spite of all the criticisms of the ineffectiveness of psychotherapy in probation and parole, we are of the opinion that psychotherapy and the basic dynamic concepts underlying it can and should be applied in the three basic phases of probation activity—namely, presentence investigation, supervision, and intake—as well as in the precommitment, prerelease, and postcommitment phases of placement on parole. There are various levels of psychotherapy: educating a client about vital facts, such as sex and hygiene information; counseling a client regarding the merits and drawbacks of options in solving problems in family matters and job situations; encouraging a client to ventilate stressful feelings; and lending support to a client in a new and critical situation. These are all forms of psychotherapy in which the probation and parole officer can engage with his clients in a meaningful and helpful way. The officer, during a presentence or preparole interview, is provided with ample opportunity to practice this type of intervention on the various levels mentioned, exclusive of depth analysis. For example, an offender's patent lack of self-confidence may be buttressed by the officer's supportive comments. In addition, an alert, sensitive officer, detecting some confusion in regard to matters of sex and family relationships, may and should utilize the psychotherapeutic technique of clarification and educational exposition. Finally, the offender's conduct and vocational and educational goals can and should be the subject of counseling by the probation and parole officer.

Another way in which psychiatric concepts can and should be applied in this phase of probation activity is the interpretation of the meaning of the offender's act and antisocial behavior. It is not enough for an officer to describe a subject's repeated bickering with his or her employers without the officer's suggesting that such behavior is possibly the acting out of a deep hostility to authority figures. Similarly, misbehavior in school may be attention getting on the part of an offender whose parents were rejecting or neglecting of him or her. If such insights and interpretations were tactfully revealed to the offender, they might contribute to a therapeutic control of his or her future behavior. Most certainly such comments in a presentence report are helpful to the judge in obtaining a deeper understanding of the offender, thus enabling the judge to arrive at a proper sentence.

A sensitive and compassionate description of how trying it is for an offender at his or her referral for a presentence investigation and the role of the officer is contained in this excerpt:

> The appearance before the court, both at the time of referral for presentence investigation, and for sentencing, is a trying and emotional experience for the defendant. It is a time of personal crisis and the role of the probation officer is a significant one. Often he is in court as a reassuring figure and almost always he interviews the defendant immediately after he is placed on probation.[9]

The basic purpose of the precommitment interview is to prepare and lend support to the offender for the new situation with which he or she is confronted. The postcommitment counseling with families most certainly is concerned with counseling on problems rising from incarceration, lending support, and alleviating in a practical manner stresses resulting from the interrupted family relationships. Prerelease counseling is educational in that its purpose is to acquaint the inmate with the conditions of parole supervision, and it is supportive in that the inmate's ventilation of his or her fears and anxieties is encouraged and confronted, and ways of handling these fears are suggested.

Supervision of probationers and parolees provides opportunities for therapy on the levels already mentioned. Differential treatment in terms of counseling to meet differing needs of offenders is desirable.

> A young drug offender, involved in the drug culture as a palliative for family disinterest or rejection, can certainly be assisted by sensitive, supportive counseling by the probation officer. Other offenders, including those with sociopathic tendencies, can and do respond favorably to the more forthright approaches of reality therapy. With additional officers of high capabilities, we have the opportunity to evaluate the effectiveness of different types of counseling with differing offenders.[10]

An interesting question raised by doctrinaire libertarians in regard to probation and parole supervision is, Who has the right to tell anyone what he shall do and how he shall live his life? Such liberals would permit drug addicts and suicidal persons to gratify their needs without coercive restraint by any authority. These same liberals point out that historically, treatment and counseling have been effective only in the absence of authority and coercion.

> The therapist, it was felt, could only operate within a voluntary, permissive framework which included client freedom to accept or reject treatment. Inasmuch as this approach is appropriate to virtually all "helping" situations, treatment in the correctional and juvenile justice field followed suit up until the recent past.[11]

The results were frustrating to the helpers, hence they adopted such techniques as the reality therapy approach of the psychiatrist William Glasser (a technique with which many probation and parole officers are comfortable); the guided group interaction approach devised by the penologist Lloyd McCorkle (a modality adopted by many agencies handling adolescent offenders); and the concepts of positive peer culture; all integrated within an authoritative framework. Another psychiatrist who uses behavioral techniques with sociopaths (antisocial personalities) affirms the authoritative approach, asserting:

> Our Day Treatment Program regularly includes probationers and parolees on an involuntary basis because of our experience that people who break the law usually need to be coerced into treatment initially if meaningful involvement is to be achieved.[12]

Another resolution of the problem of coercion versus self-determination regarding treatment is that of determining whether an offender's crime was related to, let us say, his or her alcoholism and/or mental or emotional problem.[13] If there is this relationship of offense to personal problem, then it would be just and relevant for the court and probation and parole to coerce the offender into treatment. Failure of the offender to heed this condition of probation and parole would then be adequate grounds for citation of a violation.

The officer may use any of several different therapeutic systems on a one-to-one basis. He may practice Rogerian nondirective therapy, Albert Ellis' rational emotive therapy, or Glasser's reality therapy; he may utilize Freudian concepts, such as masculine-feminine conflict, sibling rivalry, identification with parents, severe superego, and others that may be appropriate and understood and accepted by the supervisee. If the officer is trained and skilled, he or she may organize groups and practice the above therapies in a group situation. Further, if the officer is truly creative and experienced, behavior modification principles and operant conditioning may also be used.

Also in supervision, an officer making a referral to another agency (family, job, medical, psychiatric, educational) must utilize therapeutic skills in discussing the offender's need for such community service, and must counsel the offender on what to expect and how to get the most out of the designated program. However, if the supervisee fails to follow through, then the ensuing interviews must and should cover the offender's emotional reaction to the program, some clarification of the realities involved, and some counseling as to alternatives.

In the New York City Family Court, Juvenile Term, there is an intake service where all delinquents are interviewed in an attempt to save them from court action. If either the complainant or the juvenile insists on court action, then the delinquent is moved out of intake. However, if the offender remains in intake, the officer may undertake therapeutic servicing of the youth or make a referral to a community agency. Some considerations entering into such a decision are the case load at the time; the availability of skilled and experienced officers; and the willingness of the delinquent and his or her family to become involved in therapy.

There are probationers and parolees who are so emotionally disturbed as to merit institutionalization or involvement in an intensive therapeutic program with a psychiatrist. Such individuals can be found in any supervision probation and parole case load. These disturbed persons not only require close surveillance, but also some form of therapy, such as supportive counseling. However, should these individuals begin to manifest psychotic symptoms, such as paranoia, hallucinations, or radical mood swings weakening their grasp of reality, the officer must work with members of the family, exercising the therapeutic skills of educating the family members as to the meaning of the erratic behavior, counseling them to the course of action most beneficial to the offender and the family, and, in many cases, working through with them their feelings of guilt, shame, and anger engendered by having a psychotic person in the family. Parolees and probationers who are emotionally disturbed tend to indulge in behavior that violates the conditions of probation or parole. Such behavior may be failure to report, running away from the court's or parole agency's jurisdiction, and acting out of aggressive behavior toward family members or spouses. Though each case is to be treated on an individual basis, the general attitude of the officer is one of interpreting to the court or to the parole agency the deeper, more subtle meaning of the behavior; and where the officer feels the direction of the offender's efforts was generally positive, a recommendation may be made to retain the offender on probation or parole.

An officer who has effected a voluntary or court commitment of a disturbed offender to a mental hospital eagerly awaits the report that will provide him or her with meaningful information on dynamic behavior patterns or significant psychological factors throwing light on the offender's general conduct or criminality. However, in all too many cases, the documents are stereotyped and repeat the information already submitted by the officer in the referral letter. Currently, there are many federally financed community organizations that solicit probationers and parolees who show behavioral and/or emotional problems. Many of these organizations originally focused on drug addicts. With the diminishing number of addicts utilizing their services, these organizations are expanding their target populations, offering in some cases psychiatrists, psychiatric social workers, group therapists, and educational programs to appeal to this emotionally disturbed group. The probation or parole officer, harried by a large case load, may refer his or her charges to these organizations. Some of these therapists send monthly reports and work closely with the officers. Where that is the case, the officer's therapeutic activities are marginal and mainly supportive.

The patient (probationer or parolee) who is undergoing therapy with a private psychiatrist can still become involved, on a lesser level, in a therapeutic relationship with his or her officer. Again, the officer may be supportive and reenforce the insights provided by the psychiatrist. Such intervention depends on the cooperation and sharing of information between the psychiatrist and the officer. Unfortunately, some psychiatrists refuse to work with the officer and accept the offender as a patient on the condition that the psychiatrist will not be "bothered" by the court or parole agency in any way.

The attitude of many psychiatrists treating sex offenders on probation is exemplified by the following:

> Populations convicted of antisocial offenses are generally avoided by most treatment agencies when the persons are paroled from prison into the community or are on probation. Poor motivation for treatment or lack of desire to change generally head the list of reasons why psychotherapy is not offered.[14]

An explanation for this attitude contends that

> most psychiatrists evolve from a culture and training background which emphasizes scholastic achievement as measured by verbal skills. Their dynamic psychotherapy has usually evolved from psychoanalytic concepts developed in a sophisticated verbal culture and attain greatest relevance when the patient and practitioner enjoy a common educational background.[14]

Drawing the obvious conclusions, these psychiatrists organized a group of offender peers from a common background, thus facilitating verbal and nonverbal communication, problem solving, and combating of social isolation more effectively than the one-to-one psychotherapeutic approach.

It is our feeling that a specialized case load in probation and/or parole consisting of between 20 and 30 selected psychiatrically disturbed supervisees would be an effective rehabilitative tool. Such a case load was established in the 1950s in the Kings County Court in Brooklyn, New York. Milton Nechemias, a probation officer, delineated the rationale, problems, and results of intensive casework with the offenders and their families.[15] Establishment of such case loads in probation and parole agencies, especially in urban centers, would drain off these troublesome cases from the run-of-the-mill case loads, enabling the officers to render better services to their regular, nonpsychiatric cases, while the specially trained, skilled officer concentrates on meeting the needs of the disturbed offenders. This arrangement does not rule out referrals to available community resources but will retain the advantage of unfragmented services.

Philadelphia's Adult Probation operates a project known as the Intensive Services Unit. Sex offenders and persons in need of "psychiatric probation" are placed in this unit. Case loads in this project number near 50. An evaluation team from the Georgia Institute of Technology, working with Law Enforcement Assistance Administration funds, noted:

A comparison of rearrest rates between a sample of project clients and a sample of similar clients in caseloads exceeding 100 showed statistically significant lower rates for project clients. However, the project concept calls for a different quality as well as quantity of supervision than that experienced in regular caseloads. In particular, the Intensive Services Unit seeks to take a more psychological psychiatric approach to probation, including a heavy emphasis on assessment.[16]

As indicated above, psychotherapy, though much maligned, is still practiced by correction authorities in probation and parole. Though much faith was invested in the psychological/psychiatric approach for several decades (30s, 40s, and 50s), a disillusioned reaction has set in, severely critical of the medical model and its lack of effectiveness.

Yet, while these assaults on psychotherapy were being mounted, agencies still continued referrals to psychiatrists and encouraged the latter to train probation and parole officers to understand the classical Freudian psychodynamics of behavior and to sharpen their treatment skills. The reason for the persistent life of psychotherapy is that it is useful in corrections. At its best, psychotherapy is effective in changing behavior and attitudes in certain cases; and at its least practical level, it is effective in changing personality. In addition, psychotherapy is humane and helpful in easing stresses and tensions in troubled people who happen to have been placed on probation or parole. Hopefully, in this anxiety-free state of mind, the offenders will refrain from committing other crimes. Probation and parole evolved out of social currents of compassion, and it is only just and right that they utilize techniques of counseling, support, ventilation, and clarification to lighten the burdens of unhappy people caught in the web of the criminal justice system. Psychotherapeutic techniques are not only used in the officer's role of counselor, but can and should be used in his or her roles of community resource manager, advocate, and community worker. It is our feeling that probation and parole agencies should train their officers in the basic tools of psychotherapy so that they will be more competent in using them in all the roles that the officers must fulfill today.

REFERENCES

1. KAWIN, I. 1967. Swing of the pendulum. Federal Probation 31(1): 31.
2. VON WEST, A. 1964. Cultural background and treatment of the persistent offender. Federal Probation 28(2): 17.
3. EYESENCK, H. J. & S. RACHMAN. 1965. The Causes and Cures of Neurosis: 58–59. Robert R. Knapp. San Diego, Calif.
4. DELL'APA, F., W. T. ADAMS, J. D. JORGENSEN & H. R. SIGURDSON. 1976. Advocacy, brokerage, community: the ABC's of probation and parole. Federal Probation 30(4): 41.
5. MACPHERSON, D. P. 1971. Probation and corrections in the seventies. Federal Probation 35(1): 15.
6. ROCHE, P. Q. 1965. Mental health and criminal behavior. Federal Probation 29(3): 15.

7. SCHUR, E. M. 1969. Our Criminal Society: 72. Prentice-Hall, Inc. Englewood Cliffs, N.J.
8. WILKERSON, W. W. 1969. Psychiatric consultation with probationers and parolees. Federal Probation 33(2): 47.
9. GRONEWALD, D. H. 1964. Supervision practices in the federal probation system. Federal Probation 28(3): 20.
10. McLAUGHLIN, C. 1975. The federal probation system: an inside view. Federal Probation 39(2): 35.
11. STOLLERY, P. L. 1977. Searching for the magic answer to juvenile delinquency. Federal Probation 31(4): 29.
12. PARLOUR, R. R. 1975. Behavioral techniques for sociopathic clients. Federal Probation 39(1): 3.
13. SMITH, A. B. & L. BERLIN. 1979. Introduction to Probation and Parole. 2nd edit.: 163–182. West Publishing. St. Paul, Minn.
14. PETERS, J. J. & R. L. SADOFF. 1971. Psychiatric services for sex offenders on probation. Federal Probation 35(3): 33.
15. NECHEMIAS, M. 1957. Probation supervision of a specialized caseload. Federal Probation 21(2): 23–29.
16. BANKS, J., T. R. SILER & R. L. RADIN. 1977. Past and present findings in intensive adult probation. Federal Probation 41(2): 22.

GROUP TREATMENT OF DELINQUENTS:
A REVIEW OF GUIDED GROUP INTERACTION

Albert Elias

New Jersey Department of Corrections
Trenton, New Jersey 08628

The concept of the primary group, especially the peer group, which plays a significant role in the socialization of children, has been integrated into programs that provide planned, intensive group experiences for juvenile delinquents. In fact, in a relatively brief span of time, this type of experience, in the form of group treatment, has emerged as a major therapeutic tool. It ranks with psychotherapy, behavior modification, and chemotherapy among the major developments in the care of young people with problems.

The peer group, a potentially powerful force in the lives of young people, provides the context for normal growth and development and social and psychological support during a period of rapid physiological and psychological change, role experimentation, and the emergence of a sense of identity. It serves, also, as a testing ground for the adolescent in relation to others, as a source of one's self-image, and as a framework within which to strive for autonomy and independence from parents.[1,2]

Among all of the influences assumed to create delinquency, the peer group has emerged as probably the single most important factor in determining the presence or absence of delinquent behavior.[3] It is not surprising, therefore, that therapists have developed techniques for utilizing the peer group as a corrective experience for many juvenile delinquents.

This article will provide a brief examination of a few of the major approaches to the group treatment of juvenile offenders and a more extensive review of one of these approaches, namely, guided group interaction. Also, this paper will define some of the principal issues that should be addressed by practitioners and others in the field.

Although the concept of treating adolescents in group settings has been in use for many years, it was not until after the Second World War that it gained acceptance on a broad scale in many countries.[4] Currently, group treatment is a principal approach to the problems of a widening range of young people with highly diverse problems. This situation has been accompanied by the development of many different group therapeutic approaches, which vary not only in their underlying philosophies, but also with respect to the planning and conduct of treatment.

Each of the approaches is designed to deal with delinquents who have varying developmental capabilities and problems. Each one in the universe of group treatment methods offers advantages and limitations in working with different groups of juveniles.

One of the most widely used approaches is group counseling. This technique focuses on a particular type of problem—social, educational, vocational, or personal—usually in schools, human service agencies, clinics, and institutional settings. It deals primarily with conscious problems and is oriented toward the resolution of specific, short-term issues.

Group psychotherapy with delinquents, on the other hand, is designed to promote personality and behavior change through interaction in a carefully structured environment that is influenced strongly by the therapist. Delinquent behavior is assumed to arise from serious distortions of family relationships that are treatable on the level of conscious ego functioning. The focus is on the individual intrapsychic conflicts of the juvenile, in a group setting. This approach is heavily dependent on communication and is supplemented with individual sessions. Kaplan and Sadock have labeled it "structured interactional group psychotherapy."[4] There are a number of variations of this approach, depending on the age and the presenting problem of the delinquent, such as activity group therapy, activity interview group therapy, play therapy, and others.[5] Also, the approach presupposes a relatively lengthy period of treatment.

A third major category of group treatment approaches is the behavior therapy model. A basic assumption underlying this model and its variations is that all behavior is learned through reinforcement and that the principles of social learning can be applied to individuals to produce behavioral changes. The focus is on the specific targets for behavioral change that are reflected in the delinquent acts of the juvenile. The treatment method involves defining goals in terms of clearly identifiable, manageable objectives for each group member. Progress is monitored through self-recording and observation of specific behaviors by group members. The group process is used to facilitate change by the establishment of behavioral objectives for the group as a whole, mediation of positive and negative reinforcers by the group, and the modeling function of individual members.[6]

A variant of the behavior therapy model is reality therapy, a system that was developed in a training school for girls.[7] Like other behavioral approaches, it rejects the medical model of mental illness. The core concept of this method is that delinquents are personally responsible for their own behavior and that, by examining it and making value judgments about it, they can achieve a "success identity." The group leader assists by establishing a personal relationship with the group members and by not accepting excuses for irresponsible behavior. The treatment involves the identification of specific behavioral changes that must be made, formulating plans for change, carrying out the change, and evaluating the results.

Guided group interaction, which incorporates some of the elements in the approaches mentioned above, emerged relatively early in the development of group methods. McCorkle, who originated this technique, traces the influence of Wolf, Abrahams, and others on guided group interaction. Like reality therapy, guided group interaction was developed during World War II for use with delinquents in an Army disciplinary center.[8] After the war, McCorkle introduced this approach in the New Jersey correctional system. At that time, it was described by Bixby and McCorkle as follows:

To avoid confusion with the use of group psychotherapy as practiced by psychiatrists, and to avoid any implications that all inmates are mentally abnormal and unbalanced, we decided to call the application of group therapy principles to inmates, Guided Group Interaction.[9]

Pilnick has suggested a more recent definition of this technique as follows:

Guided Group Interaction is a process of group treatment which directs the dynamics and strengths of the peer group toward constructively altering and developing the behavior of the group members.[10]

Like other approaches to group treatment, variations of the original guided group interaction model have been developed, including positive peer culture and peer group counseling.[11,12] However, since the differences between them are essentially operational and the basic assumptions and core concepts are similar to the original formulation, the discussion that follows will apply to all of them.

Although guided group interaction approaches were developed initially in institutional settings with older male adolescent delinquents, especially at the Highfields Residential Group Center in New Jersey, they have been adopted for use with male and female, early adolescents and young adults as well. Also, the settings have varied from clinics, nonresidential programs, schools, and probation and parole offices to halfway houses, group homes, camps, job corps centers, and others.[13,14] Moreover, the size of the treatment group is fairly constant in each of these settings, in that each group consists, on the average, of 10 members. Larger groups usually develop subgroups, which establish their own goals, norms, and relationships without reference to the objectives of the program.

Another distinguishing feature of this model is the length of participation, which is usually about four to six months. The rationale for selecting this period is based largely on the experience of the practitioners. It appears that prolonged participation in this type of program encourages the development of ritualistic behavior and serves to isolate the group members from stable, routine contacts with the community. Also, release from the program is usually a function of several variables, including (1) an assessment of the member's career in the program by the peer group and the staff; (2) an estimate of the member's ability to function effectively in the community; (3) a review of the member's role in assisting other members with their problems; and (4) a decision by the group and the leader that optimal gains have been achieved at a particular time.[15]

The type of juvenile offender referred to programs employing the group method includes a wide range of offense types. However, the limited available research evidence suggests that the adaptive offender, the individual who gets involved in delinquency in association with others, is best suited to this method. Unsocialized personalities and delinquents who are diagnosed as severe neurotics might not participate profitably in this treatment model.[16,17]

Group structure can facilitate or inhibit group development and the accomplishment of group purposes. Aspects of structure that are important to group treatment approaches, including guided group interaction, are (1) the number of group meetings; (2) how often the group will meet; (3) how long each meeting will last; (4) whether the group will be open-ended or closed;

(5) what degree of control will be retained by the therapist; and (6) the format the meetings will have.[18]

Although it is traditional for other group treatment approaches to meet once a week, in guided group interaction programs, the meetings are held from three to five times each week. However, as in other therapy group situations where the 1- to 1½-hour group meeting has become a standard practice, this method employs the same procedure. Ideally, the duration of group meetings should be related to the problems of the members, the purposes for which the group meets, the format of the meetings, and the capacity of the members to cope with the time span.

The issue of employing an open-ended structure or a closed structure is often related to the interest of the agency that sponsors the group or the therapist. In guided group interaction programs, closed group structure is employed. The basis for assignment is usually determined by the date of admission. It is not necessarily related to any other factors, so that a new member is usually assigned to a group that is in the process of forming. The groups are closed to admissions when there are about 10 members. In this manner, each group develops a history and a culture of its own. Generally, new members are assigned to a group that is beginning to release members. The assignment of new admissions to a functioning group provides them with opportunities to experience the ways in which older members deal with their problems as a group and to learn how to communicate with their peers and the group leader. In many respects, the new admissions learn about the functioning and the format of the group meetings through a process of participant observation. This experience serves also to transmit the culture of the old group, a nondelinquent culture, to the new group.

The issue of control and authority in the group is a crucial one because it determines the climate of the group. Some forms of group treatment require a high degree of control by the therapist, others a low degree, as in client-centered therapy where the leader is viewed as a facilitator and the assumption is made that the group can find its own direction. In guided group interaction settings, as in other settings, an attempt is made to establish sufficient levels of control by the leader to help get the group started and then to transfer power and authority, progressively, as the group is ready to assume it. The role of the leader depends on the nature of the problems confronting the group at a particular time. Generally, however, the leader's role varies from providing support to making interpretations, confronting the group or individual members, and summarizing the interactions.

With reference to the format of the meetings, this is usually related to the intended goals of the group, the problems of the members, the number, frequency, and duration of the meetings, and the degree of capacity of the members for interaction. In some variations of guided group interaction, there is a strict agenda, which includes reporting problems, awarding the meeting to a particular member, attempting to resolve problems, and summarizing the meeting; summaries are made by the group leader, an individual member, or several members. In the original model, however, the agenda varies depending on the stage in the group process at which a group finds itself. The agenda is more flexible and is related to the nature of the problems facing the group or the leader at the time. In either case, the themes that are discussed revolve around "here and now" problems of the members.

Implicit in the structure of this group method are the major assumptions that underlie it. The central assumption is that delinquency is learned behavior that results principally from association with other delinquents in a peer group. Consequently, it follows that the delinquent will change his behavior, in a prosocial direction, only if such conduct is acceptable to the peer group. A second assumption is that change can be achieved effectively if the entire peer group, not just the individual member, is the target of change. In other words, change is most acceptable not only when it receives the confirmation of the peer group, but also when the peer group becomes the major vehicle by which nondelinquent standards are established and problems are solved. A third assumption is that the change will occur through a process of interaction with others who are also changing. If the delinquent can see others changing, then he is more likely to change himself. In a very real sense, a group member changes by helping others to change, not by seeking private solutions to personal and group problems.

A fourth major assumption is that opportunities for reality testing through sharing "here and now" experiences with others provide a means for validating changes that are alleged to have occurred in the group meetings. In total institutions, the social roles played by the inmate represent a serious departure from the roles played before the incarceration. In guided group interaction programs, the opportunity to duplicate delinquent roles learned in the community and to attempt new social roles is crucial for change to occur.[19]

In group treatment approaches, the group process is an important factor in influencing the nature of each member's experience and the role of the leader. It is important, therefore, to have an understanding of this process and its meaning for changing behavior.[20]

The group process can be viewed in terms of a number of dimensions, including the amount and type of participation by the group leader; the themes discussed in the group; the extent to which these themes are introduced by the group leader or emerge from the members; the definition of the group operations in terms of whether the group is individually oriented or group oriented; the degree of analytic orientation that occurs in the group interaction as opposed to concern with current behavior; and the degree to which an accepting climate is generated and maintained or confrontation is emphasized.

The group process that occurs in guided group interaction can be viewed in terms of these dimensions. The developmental process is divided into four phases. Each phase is described in terms of the major problems confronting the group and the characteristic behavior that is found at each phase. In stating that groups have distinct patterns that are observable and predictable, I am making an assumption that is essentially untested—

although it is based to some degree on research evidence and my own and others' participation in and observation of many group meetings.

The first phase can be characterized as a search for structure. Since the members have no common past and no common present relationships outside of the group, there is no identification with each other or with the group leader. The members engage in a considerable amount of random, hostile behavior that involves testing one another and the leader. Each member is involved in a private world in which he is searching for meaning. There is no structure because the members do not know very much about each other, and know even less about the leader. Their problem is to develop a structure, and they do it in a variety of ways. In fact, some groups will attempt to invent a structure by suggesting that a president, vice-president, and secretary be appointed. The themes that emerge are short-lived and almost never discussed in depth. There are long moments of silence and much smoking, whispering, and asking for information from the group leader. Also, there are outbursts of shouting, even laughter, and movements in and out of the meeting.

Later during this phase, the group members communicate by relating stories of how they got into trouble, by describing their escapades, and in other safe, nonthreatening ways. In effect, they are seeking ways to relate to each other. Also, some members take risks and attempt to assume the leadership role.

The objectives of this first stage are to foster and reward interaction, to teach the members that the level of group performance depends heavily on them, to instill confidence in the group, to introduce substantive problems, and to gather information on the members.

The group leader is fairly active in that he poses problems for which solutions must be found and refuses to accept all responsibility for the operation of the meeting. He or she does not provide conclusive answers but encourages discussion of matters of interest to the group.

From the point of view of the individual member, this stage has enabled him or her to introduce to the group substantive problems that exist in the family, the school, and the street; to become aware of differences and problems the members share with each other; to begin to learn to trust the group leader and other group members; and to tell the truth.

The second stage involves principally the formation of subgroupings and friendship pairs. The members of each subgroup sit together, support each other, and attempt to control the discussions of the meetings or perhaps refuse to attend meetings. This is an important experience because it is the point at which the group problems are being identified by the members. Also, they are now in the process of attempting to relate to each other, to take risks, and to begin to trust each other by telling the truth about themselves and their involvement with each other in the daily activities. At the same time, there is a continual struggle among the subgroups for control of the meeting. In effect, there is a public awareness of the existence of each other member since almost everyone belongs to a subgroup that is clearly identified by all.

The group leader, during this stage, is usually stereotyped by the members as all-knowing and omnipotent. The leader attempts to crystallize dilemmas, to encourage the group to explore alternative modes of interaction and behavior, to teach the group to examine problems, and to develop concern for the welfare of the group.

The third stage is concerned with a struggle for survival. This is a crucial period in the careers of the group members because, at this point, they are struggling to survive as a group. They begin to recognize the fact that they are not helping each other by contending for power. Once again, much hostility is expressed. The subgroups begin to fall apart because, in analyzing the bases for their relationships, the members discover that their relationships are not rooted in trust or concern for one another's welfare. In fact, there emerges an awareness of the tenuous character of the clique relationship and that, unless the issue is confronted, the members will not be able to cope with their other problems.

It is interesting to observe the tremendous amount of hostility that is generated between members of subgroups that may have been together for several weeks. Initially, during this third stage, they distrust each other, steal from each other, argue, and even fight on occasion. Unlike the second stage when the discussion is more mechanical and intellectualized, the emotional content in the third stage is very high. It is at this point that a considerable amount of acting out occurs. Hostility is clearly directed toward former friends and the group leader as well. Moreover, group problems are clearly defined at this stage, for there emerges a recognition of the fact that, unless members join together as a total group, they will not be able to address their problems openly, honestly, and directly.

The group leader plays a fairly active role during the third stage, partly because much of the hostility in the group is directed toward him. Also, he plays more of a teaching role at this point. His objectives are principally to help the members understand the group structure and the process, to increase the capacity of the members to see themselves in relation to the group structure, and to help the group become aware of the consequences of factionalism. Also, interestingly enough, at the end of this stage, the power and authority of the leader decreases and begins to be assumed by the group.

The fourth stage is characterized by group solidarity and decision making. During this period, the total group is seen as a special entity, since the subgroups have broken up and the members have reorganized as a cohesive unit. This integration provides the group with the capacity to undertake any of the problems of their members, of the group itself, and of new admissions to the group. The group engages in quiet, deliberate, rational discussions of problems, solutions to problems, and decision making. Also, it is at this point that the group members become the culture bearers for new admissions and share power with the leader in discussions about release from the program and other important issues. Also, the group leader is seen as more of a group member, since others have assumed the leadership role. It is a period of highly cooperative and motivated problem solving. There is greater trust and communication than at earlier stages, and certainly great concern for the group as a whole.

The ultimate test of any group treatment approach is whether changes in attitude and behavior in the group setting will result in long-term, overt behavioral changes in the life-style of the participants. This is a key issue; yet there appears to be relatively little research directed toward it. One of the reasons may be that treatment outcomes cannot be empirically determined by currently available measurement techniques. In the case of guided group interaction, the results of several evaluations generally have neither confirmed nor denied its effectiveness. However, Weeks reported in his study of the Highfields program in New Jersey that recidivism rates for the graduates of this program compare favorably with those for graduates of a state reformatory where guided group interaction was not employed.[16] Furthermore, Stephenson and Scarpetti, in a review of several institutional and community-based programs, found that on the whole, guided group interaction graduates fared better than parolees but not as well as probationers.[21]*

A related issue is the extent to which a group treatment approach lends itself to replication, apart from the therapist who uses it. The systematic character of the method itself to a great extent determines the degree to which the method may be transferred intact under varying conditions. This is an issue that has not been addressed in a systematic way in this field. An attempt was made to replicate guided group interaction programs by providing internships and training experiences for interested persons, many of whom subsequently implemented this approach in other settings. Another technique involved the use of graduates of one program to help establish another one.[23]

A third key issue involves the question of how well group approaches incorporate a thorough understanding of the use of the group process. A major objective of group development is to integrate the dynamics of the individual and the group. In many instances, the potential of the group is either underutilized or neglected.[24] The guided group interaction approach, in contrast to other methods, uses the group as a means for treatment, rather than as the context for treatment, by working on problems through the group process.

Group treatment approaches appear to have great potential for assisting juvenile delinquents with their problems. Each of the several methods that have been developed can contribute to that end. No single approach is the most appropriate therapeutic tool for all types of delinquents. However, when used with awareness of their strengths and limitations, each of the methods presented in this paper has some demonstrated potential for contributing to the resolution of a difficult social problem, namely, the treatment of the juvenile delinquent.

---

*Other evidence indicates that guided group interaction has a positive effect on reducing incidents of school violence and reduces school absenteeism (see References 12 and 22).

REFERENCES

1. JOSSELYN, I. M. 1971. Adolescence. Harper and Row Publishers. New York, N.Y.
2. ERICKSON, E. H. 1968. Identity: Youth and Crisis. W. W. Norton & Co., Inc. New York, N.Y.
3. BERGER, A. 1977. Study of Juvenile Delinquent Behavior. Institute of Juvenile Research. Illinois Department of Mental Health. Chicago, Ill. (Unpublished manuscript.)
4. KAPLAN, H. I. & B. J. SADOCK, Eds. 1972. New Models for Group Therapy. E. P. Dutton and Co., Inc. New York, N.Y.
5. SLAVSON, S. R. & M. SCHIFFER. 1975. Group Psychotherapies for Children. International Universities Press. New York, N.Y.
6. SARRI, R. C. 1964. Behavioral theory and group work. In Individual Change through Small Groups. P. Glasser, R. C. Sarri & R. D. Vinter, Eds.: 50-71. Free Press. New York, N.Y.
7. GLASSER, W. 1965. Reality Therapy. Harper and Row, Publishers. New York, N.Y.
8. ABRAHAMS, J. & L. W. MCCORKLE. 1946. Group psychotherapy of military offenders. Am. J. Sociology 51(5): 455-464.
9. BIXBY, F. L. & L. W. MCCORKLE. 1948. A recorded presentation of a program of Guided Group Interaction in New Jersey correctional institutions. Proceedings of the 78th Annual Congress of Correction. American Correctional Association. College Park, Md.
10. PILNICK, S. 1971. Guided Group Interaction. In Encyclopedia of Social Work. R. Morris, Ed. 1: 181. National Association of Social Workers. New York, N.Y.
11. VORRATH, H. & L. K. BRENDTHRO. 1974. Positive Peer Culture. Aldine Publishing Co. Chicago, Ill.
12. HOWLETT, F. W. & R. G. BOEHM. 1975. School-Based Delinquency Prevention: The Rock Island Experience: 12-14, 40. Justice Systems, Inc. Austin, Tex.
13. MCCORKLE, L. W., A. ELIAS & F. L. BIXBY. 1958. The Highfields Story. Holt, Rhinehart and Winston. New York, N.Y.
14. PILNICK, S. & A. ELIAS. 1966. The Essexfields group rehabilitation project for youthful offenders. In Corrections in the Community 4. California Board of Corrections. Sacramento, Calif.
15. ELIAS, A. 1968. Group treatment programs for juvenile delinquents in New Jersey. Child Welfare 47(S): 286.
16. WEEKS, H. A. 1959. Youthful Offenders at Highfields. University of Michigan Press. Ann Arbor, Mich.
17. WARREN, R. 1965. The Community Treatment Project. Presented at the Annual Conference of the Illinois Academy of Criminology, Chicago, Ill., May 14.
18. LEVINE, B. 1979. Group Psychotherapy. Prentice Hall, Inc. Englewood Cliffs. N.J.
19. RABOW, J. & A. ELIAS. 1969. Organizational boundaries, inmate roles and rehabilitation. J. Res. in Crime and Delinquency (January): 8-16.
20. WHITAKER, D. S. & M. A. LIEBERMAN. 1964. Group Psychotherapy through Group Process: 1. Atherton Press. New York, N.Y.
21. STEPHENSON, R. M. & F. R. SCARPETTI. 1974. Group Interaction as Therapy: 189. Greenwood Press. Westport, Conn.
22. HANNON, J. P. & J. W. WICKS. 1977. Program Evaluation—Peer Culture Development: 5. Report No. 77-114-15. Board of Education. Chicago, Ill.
23. ALLEN, R. F. et al. 1965. Collegefields: 14-15. Special Child Publications, Inc. Seattle, Wash.
24. LEVINSON, H. M. 1973. Use and misuse of groups. Social Work (January): 66-72.

THE VIOLENT PATIENT IN THE COMMUNITY

Maurice R. Green

*Columbia University Physicians
and Surgeons at St. Luke's
New York, New York 10024*

I shall begin with a discussion of violence in America in general, and then proceed to the various categories of patients wherein violent behavior is more frequent and conspicuous; although it must be stressed that most surveys of civil and criminal violence show that less than 20% is associated with a diagnosable mental illness of either a psychotic or neurotic type.[1]

Violence seems to have been increasing steadily over the past several decades, not only in America, but throughout the Western world. The nature of violence, too, seems to have grown more vicious, impersonal, and almost random—such as impulsively pushing someone off a subway platform, or killing someone old and helpless after robbing them. This increased violence has risen in all areas of the country and in all social strata. Certainly it pervades the consciousness of everyone to become a profoundly disturbing social concern. This concern weighs heavily on the raw edge of our consciousness, bidding us to bar our windows, to look warily over our shoulders, and to keep to well-lighted streets when we are out at night.

This ambience of fearful anticipation of violence pervades all our conversation, plans, outings to restaurant and theatre, and even our walking the dog at night. Churches have begun to provide escorts to the elderly for security during their shopping for food and necessities. Violence conditions our lives and social behavior in ways inconceivable to earlier generations. Our drama, popular literature, press, podium, and pulpit and the powerfully persuasive mass media of film, radio, and television all bring the spectre of epidemic irrational violence home to us. Youngsters today apparently take this for granted—not familiar with any other atmosphere. Older folks share nostalgic memories of times, just a few decades past, when no one locked his door in suburbs or rural areas; when no one thought twice about cavorting in Central Park after midnight; when crime and violence seemed far away and sharply limited to the poor, culturally deprived, and politically disinherited population areas of slums and shantytowns. Today violence knows no boundaries; it is in the marketplace, the schools and suburbs, the farms and villages, just around any corner, in our home and community. It is clear now from recent statistical research that the increase is actual and not simply derivative of more thorough record keeping, sampling, and accounting; although for family violence between spouses, parents and children, or siblings, there may be no actual increase, but rather a lessened tolerance for it as reflected in the laws regarding spouse abuse and child abuse.

The complex causes of violence change, to be sure, with the social matrix; with demographic shifts, immigration, urbanization, and the conflicts of subculture; with the alterations in the distribution of wealth and opportunity and the consequent rise of new aspirations and expectations, creating new frustrations and a changed sense of social status and deprivation.[2]

Social attitudes and their subsequent representation in law show a parallel development. New categories of violence, new definitions of crime, come into being with changes in the norms. The legitimate corporal punishment of one era becomes the censurable or punishable abuse of another, properly recorded in the statistics of violence. The kick, cuff, or punch in the nose that was the ordinary accent to an altercation in one era or milieu becomes a reportable assault in another. Only a generation ago, violence between spouses was a popular subject of humor in movies, radio, and the vulgar comic strip. When Jiggs in business suit and spats went drinking with his former working-class cronies, Maggie, the status-hungry, nouveau riche matron, was waiting for him with a "blue collar" rolling pin that said "Pow!" This was considered funny then and not too great an exaggeration of the mores and conflicts of the urban ethnic-immigrant working class. Our sensibilities have changed, the diligent women's movement has flowered, and increasing social and forensic intervention into the affairs of families is providing new insight.

Traditionally, the child-rearing function was the responsibility and near-sacred preserve of the parents: extended family, neighbors, and the church provided supervision and correction, insuring social and moral conformity. Increasingly, with the changes brought about by the human consequences of urban industrial development, the extended family shrank to the nuclear family and, more recently, to the "floating couple" of serial monogamy or the relatively isolated "single parent." Neighborhood and community faded away to a considerable degree in the increasing flux of movement from one place to another, and with the rapid changes in the architecture and character of cities and suburbs. Increasingly, through the 19th century and into the 20th, schools have assumed more and more of the physical, intellectual, and social training of children—and to some extent of parents themselves. And increasingly, throughout the Western world, the authority and influence of the family were weakened as parents became subject to the suasion of educators, social theorists, and the indoctrinating complex of interests and influence that constitute organized public opinion. The Oedipal-incest theories of the Freudians, the writings of the sometimes misguided followers of the great John Dewey, the developmental charts of Dr. Spock, and the stepladder social achievement scale of Eric Erickson have all had their effect—sometimes for the better, often adverse—on the rearing of children and therefore on the integrity of family life. Feminism and the massive entrance of women into the labor force have played their obvious part. So has the army of behavioral scientists marching under the banners of antiauthoritarianism and family democracy.

This egalitarianism, as de Toqueville predicted over a hundred years ago, has become embedded in official and professional rhetoric and has penetrated the family fortress; it feeds the fires of rancorous generational struggles that now reach downward from the college campus to the cradle. Children of all ages today have "rights," asserted by themselves and more convincingly by the attorneys, agencies, and sociopolitical groups that speak for them. Family courts listen, legislation is proposed and adopted, and now the rights of children are respected in due process, however furiously at cross purposes they may be with the wishes, intentions, or requirements of the adults who are called upon to nurture, educate, and somehow govern their children. In the past year I have seen several cases where parents seeking help from the court in coping with a defiant, hostile youngster are met with a counter action by the youngster and the youngster's attorney (paid for by the parents' taxes) of alleged child abuse.

There is little literature on the actual incidence of violence against parents other than the sensational, dramatic accounts of matricide and patricide, which occur relatively rarely. (Although they seemed to be of frequency in the ancient royal families, where these acts were more of a political grab for power than anything else.) An informal survey in the family court in New York City recently showed that about 10% of the family offenses that came to the court were charges against children for assaulting and threatening their parents.

However, most of the participants in these cases of assault never became patients. The population of psychiatric patients as a whole is less violent than the general population. The incidence of violent (or for that matter of *any*) offenses among the discharged-patient population is much less than the incidence among the nonpatient population in the community at large. (A recent survey at Bellevue shows a reversal of this statistic under the so-called revolving door policy of brief hospitalization and early discharge to inadequate or nonexistent community resources.)

During 10 years at Bellevue, Dr. Grace Frank and I studied several children under the age of 11 years who had murdered other children; most of these children showed psychotic signs and symptoms at the time of admission. But children who commit murder do not necessarily show evidence of psychosis or insanity. Many of the children we studied recovered with no further incidence of violent offense or psychosis during a 10-year follow-up. They were treated with medication, individual and family therapy, and supportive guidance in the community and at school.

Of course, since ancient times children under 7 years have been considered incapable of intent, and those between 7 and 12–14 have been held accountable only if proof of intention was very clear and certain. In New York City today, as you all know, the age has been recently lowered to 13 years. Despairing of rehabilitation and treatment, the community is demanding harsher legislation, not only in New York, but throughout the country.

Although most mentally retarded people in the community are not involved with violent or sexually offensive behavior, they are as vulnerable as the rest of the population—a little more so when they are not protected or supported, perhaps. About 30 years ago, I did a random sampling at a center for the retarded and found that out of 100 chosen, the majority of boys were brought to the attention of authorities for help when their aggressive behavior became intolerable to the parents, and the majority of girls were brought for help when their sexual behavior disturbed the family or community. With the increased provision for services obtained by the now-proverbial lobby for the retarded, this situation must be much improved. However, in spite of the improvement, there is still inadequate service for retarded adolescents who, although less than 3% of the general population, make up 10.5% of the delinquent population.

The most commonly diagnosed disorder among violence-prone school children is the attention deficit disorder with hyperactivity. In fact, although learning disorders show no causal link to juvenile delinquency, there is a disquieting statistic that 50% of adjudicated juvenile delinquents manifest a history of learning disability. At any rate, this disorder—previously described under the label of minimal brain dysfunction—responds very well in most instances to medication, psychotherapy, and other treatment when available. A recent study shows that the same group of children not treated with ritalin show the same delay in growth and maturation as evidenced by those receiving it, suggesting a systemic congenital developmental disorder for at least a significant part of this patient population.[3] Special corrective education is required for these children, many of whom show varying signs of mild organic brain impairment. Archie Silver[4] has shown in a seven-year follow-up on children with attention deficit disorders both with and without hyperactivity, and with as well as without any organicity, that corrective educational intervention in the first and second grades was very effective. In fact, in a sizeable sample (150), Silver found a very sharp drop in the incidence of delinquency among the teenage follow-up group.

Another sizeable population of children and youths who become involved in violence in the family and/or the community fall under the rubric of conduct disorders (undersocialized aggressive type and socialized aggressive type), which begin in the primary grades and increase in frequency as these children approach the high school years. This includes the antisocial personality—what sometimes even today is called the psychopath. Walker and McCuble—in Rieber and Vetter's recent book, *The Psychological Foundations of Criminal Justice*—trace the history of the concept back to the 17th century.[5] The concept itself refers to a disorder or group of disorders that does not meet the criteria for more definite forms of mental disorder and is always associated with antisocial conduct. This type of disorder was earlier called moral insanity or moral imbecility. The term psychopathy, which originally meant all mental disorders, came to be used in this restricted way when the German physician Koch used the term "constitutional psychopathic inferiority" because these criminals showed no evidence of insanity in the strict sense. At first, this term included neurasthenia, obsessive-compulsive neurosis, and all sexual deviance.

Sir David Henderson, a Scottish disciple of Adolf Meyer, began the present usage of the term psychopathic disorder—which is more or less synonymous with antisocial personality disorder—which Henderson divided into aggressive and inadequate types.

The other frequent personality disorder of violent aggression, but of a noncriminal type, is the explosive personality disorder in which perfectly law-abiding, conventional, well-mannered people suffer outbursts of exaggerated rage and temper tantrums in response to relatively modest provocation. This diagnostic category has been removed from the category of personality disorders in the third *Diagnostic and Statistical Manual* and placed in the new category of impulse disorders. This category describes individuals who have recurrent and paroxysmal episodes of significant loss of control of aggressive impulses that result in serious assault on another person or destruction of property. There is always genuine regret and self-reproach. Alcohol seems to be a frequent predisposing agent, and there is often a history of hyperactivity in childhood. Using a special activating technique for electroencephalograph (EEG) examination, Russell Monroe found EEG abnormalities among 80% of these episodic impulsive patients.[6] Forty-two of the 70 patients showed aggressive dyscontrol acts towards themselves or others. The epileptoid groups of episodic dyscontrol respond well to a combination of anticonvulsant medication and psychotherapy. The others tend to resent engagement in treatment but need a thorough diagnostic evaluation. Some may do well on lithium; others may do better on benzodiazepines.

Out of 416 patients presenting to a large urban psychiatric emergency service in a two-week period, 62 were classified as violent because of outwardly directed aggressive ideation or behavior, and 63 showed suicidal impulses only.[7] Twenty-five of the 62 were classified as schizophrenic; 18 were classified in a combined category of neuroses, personality and character disorders, and situational disturbances; 7 were alcoholic; 4 were affective disorder with psychosis. Sixty-five percent of the total violent sample showed a major disturbance in perception, cognition, and reality testing that resulted from either psychosis, organicity, or intoxicants.

The criteria for dangerousness—a history of fighting, of the use of weapons, repeated expression of intention to hurt, etc.[8]—were met by most of the violent patients seen. The 65% showing psychosis, organicity, or intoxication could profit from an emergency commitment or voluntary hospitalization. Crisis intervention, short-term hospitalization, environmental manipulation, supportive psychotherapy, and the appropriate medical and psychopharmacological treatments could restore control and help the patient integrate himself safely into the family and community. However, for the group labeled personality and character disorders, or impulse disorders, there may be no treatment or no response or interest in whatever treatment may be available. Such persons may need to be managed within the judicial or penal system. However imperfect these institutions may be, they are more appropriate than psychiatric modes that are inappropriate or ineffective.

Even in institutions, nonpsychotic patients with certain personality and character traits are at a higher risk for assaultive behavior than psychotic patients. The common elements in the violent groups are an intense affect, hostile or depressed; impulsive tendencies with poor capacity for restraint; manipulative behavior with frequent testing of the limits; and regressive childish behavior associated with immaturity, poor judgment, and intolerance of frustration and stress. Transient, very brief psychotic[9] episodes may occur, as well as unpredictable stress-related defensive violence in the form of property destruction and fights with other patients.

A recent study in British Columbia of violent men who raped little girls revealed that very few of these men showed any signs of psychosis, but, like the group above, these men showed neurotic symptoms and personality and character disorders.[10] In general, these violent rapists were characterized by personality traits of hidden inadequacy and impotence, with compensatory violent displays manifested in their cruel sexual assaults on young girls as well as in a fast, reckless, violent life-style associated with excessive drinking, reckless driving of cars and motorcycles, excessive debts, sexual promiscuity, and preoccupation with pornographic materials and fantasy. Incidentally, rapists usually have a history of violent and/or criminal behavior, whereas exhibitionists do not.

In spite of the increase in extrafamilial violence between strangers, by far the greatest amount of violent behavior still occurs between intimates—immediate family, relatives, and neighbors. Although a small percentage, the violent patients who suffer from a manic-depressive illness make up a significant number. It is especially important to recognize this group because treatment is so successful with the use of lithium.

It is useful at this point to have some perspective on the incidence and prevalence of mental disorders among the population of those who commit offenses. Rosner, Wiederlight, Horner-Rosner, and Wieczorek[11] at the New York Criminal and Supreme Courts examined 140 adolescent offenders aged 16–18 and found, as suggested by studies already cited, that by far most (54.9%) were in the category of personality disorders. Eighteen-and-three-tenths percent were found to suffer from schizophrenia, which is about 10 times the incidence and prevalence of this disorder among the same age and socioeconomic group in the general population. However, the Midtown Home Survey[12] reported that about 17.2% of the population in the poverty section were markedly impaired psychiatrically although most had had no contact with a health facility. Nonetheless, 30% of the offenders described by Rosner et al. had had some previous psychiatric hospitalization and/or neurological problems.[11] Robins has shown that 25% of children referred for antisocial behavior were later diagnosed as adult antisocial personalities.[13] Incidentally, a New York State investigative committee showed a high incidence of child abuse in the history of delinquent youths.[14]

Dorothy O. Lewis and her coworkers found that sexual violence among young men is very much a part of a generally violent pattern of behavior:

sexually assaultive children had been behaving in a variety of violent antisocial ways since early childhood . . . prevalence of psychotic symptoms, major neurological abnormalities, minor neurological impairment and learning disabilities was approximately equal.[15]

Her observations confirm the findings in British Columbia and elsewhere that sexual violence is not a specific entity but simply another manifestation of a generally violent pattern of behavior and life-style.

In contrast to these violent, antisocial adolescents, most violent husbands of battered wives do *not* show antisocial behavior. For most of these men, seen by Janet Geller,[16] there was no evidence of impairment in any area of their lives apart from the marital relationship. All these men were steadily employed, homeowners, good neighbors, and respected, well-liked citizens from a middle-class background. In spite of initial severe resistance, most of them seemed to have profited markedly from a 10-session all-male group experience.

Offer, Marohan, and Ostrov, in Chicago, did a very thorough study of 55 juvenile delinquents referred principally from the juvenile justice system.[17] They screened out all those who exhibited organic brain syndromes, epilepsy, mental retardation, and psychotic or schizophrenic states and selected only chronic offenders who had performed serious offenses, excluding the one-time offender or those who had committed only minor offenses. Hence, the chosen groups were characterized by violent acts against others, associated with attempted murder, armed robbery, burglary, theft, drugs, prostitution, larceny, and property destruction. They found that this group of delinquents would be divided into four subtypes:

1. The impulsive, who is the most violent and antisocial type, has little tolerance for delay and tends to be disliked by teachers and staff.

2. The narcissistic—resistant to any form of psychotherapy—is defensive, denies all problems, and depresses the staff.

3. The empty borderline, always seeking some kind of merger with a parental figure, seems hopelessly passive and incapable of orienting herself to the future.

4. The depressed borderline—trying to evade the painful depressive affect by self-destructive and antisocial behavior—suffers severe superego guilt, has strong internalized values, and was well liked and admired by the staff.

It is clear from the above that any factors that contribute to the following cluster will probably increase the incidence and prevalence of violent behavior in the community: a sense of entrapment; a poor sense of identity, particularly gender identity; sudden loss of status; isolation; and organic impairment of foresight and control due to drugs, infection, heredity, trauma, or alcohol. Therefore, it is practically impossible to predict violent behavior *out of context* for a particular given individual.

Norval Morris has pointed out that the law and psychiatry have failed to come up with actuarial tables—such as the insurance companies have—for categorizing violence.[18] Such an effort would improve the capacity within existing powers better to protect the community from violent recidivists and would lessen the frequency of assimilating all criminals to the prototype of the violent ones.

In actual practice, this assimilation is what is done when we define any particular patient or offender as dangerous. In effect we are saying that this person meets the criteria for membership in the dangerous category. This judgment cannot be made lightly but it must be made—as it is made on inpatient services over and over again when precautions are ordered because a patient is believed to be becoming dangerous to himself or to others. Under the haste to protect innocent patients from undue restriction or detention, the courts were once inclined to insist that an overt violent act or attempted act first must have been made. Evidence beyond a reasonable doubt was insisted upon, as several studies had suggested that 60-70% of those predicted to become violent would not become so. However, clear and convincing evidence is now becoming established as a standard of proof. In *Addington* v. *Texas*,[19] the judge indicated that the protection of the community dictated the sufficiency of clear and convincing evidence, with all regard for due process and judicial review within a reasonable period indicating that there were sufficient safeguards to avoid injustice.

Loren Roth, separating the issue of protecting the community from that of mandating treatment, has proposed a new model commitment law (1979).[20] He urges that brief periods of mental health commitment be permitted on the basis of *parens patria,* the interest of the state in caring for persons unable to care for themselves. However, he insists on the provision that only patients with a specific adjudication of incompetency to consent to or refuse treatment be committed, and for six weeks or less.

This differs from the dangerousness-to-self-or-others type of commitment. When dangerous patients—who are at the same time perfectly competent to consent to or refuse treatment—are forced to have treatment, the physician's identity is degraded and distorted (apart, of course, from emergency situations of imminent danger). Roth insists that dangerousness then must be proved beyond a reasonable doubt, ignoring the *Addington* v. *Texas* ruling; and once proved—and the patient committed as a dangerous, but competent, person—the patient has the right to refuse any or all treatments. Roth envisions the creation of a new type of quasi-penal institution for the long-term detention of dangerous, mentally ill patients who are competent to refuse treatment.

The patient who is dangerous to self falls under both the *parens patria* and the police power of the state, and is not permitted to refuse treatment necessary for his health. Such cases occur in the categories of chronic schizophrenia, alcoholic dementia, and senile dementia with psychosis. The dangerous-to-self approach can also be implemented by effective community care and treatment for the chronically disabled patient.

In conclusion, we see that violence among patients in the community—like violence among the nonpatients of the community—is a community problem, a social problem, as much as it is a psychiatric and legal problem. Patients fall into categories, some of which show a high incidence of violent behavior, as we have reported. Once cooperation is secured, relatively effective modes of treatment are available that are appropriate to the diagnosis of the individual patient—a medically informed, biosocial diagnosis. A large category of character and personality disorders, showing no symptoms or signs of neurosis or psychosis and little, if any, interest in treatment, might respond to innovative approaches or even to some kind of coerced learning experience, as Smith and Berlin indicate.[21] However, there are scant data to warrant much optimism in this area. The majority of violent offenders, like the majority of violent nonoffenders, suffer no diagnosable mental disorder and never become patients. The violence we suffer, fear, and inflict on each other is part of the values, mores, and way of life that most of our population live by.

REFERENCES

1. GUTTMACHER, M. 1960. The Mind of the Murderer. Farrer, Strauss & Cudahy. New York, N.Y.
2. STORR, A. 1968. Human Aggression. Atheneum Publishers. New York, N.Y.
3. OETTINGER, J. R., L. V. MAJOVSKI & W. H. WRIGHT. 1979. Minimal Brain Dysfunction: Effect of Stimulants on Maturation and Growth. Pamphlet No. 175-92174.
4. SILVER, A. A., R. A. HAGEN & R. BEECHER. 1978. Scanning, diagnosis and intervention in the prevention of reading disabilities. J. Learn. Disabil. 2(7): 439-448.
5. WALKER, N. & S. McCUBLE. 1979. In Psychological Foundations of Criminal Justice. R. Rieber & H. Vetter, Eds.1: 144. John Jay Press. New York, N.Y.
6. MONROE, R. 1970. Episodic Behavioral Disorders: 238-246. Harvard University Press. Cambridge, Mass.
7. SKODAL, E. A. & T. B. KARESU. 1978. Emergency psychiatry and the assaultive patient. Am. J. Psychiatry 13(2): 202-205.
8. NANGLE, O. 1976. Dangerousness, reasonable doubt and preconviction psychopath legislation. Southern Ill. Univ. Law J.: 218-236.
9. SOLOFF, P. H. 1979. Physical restraint and the nonpsychotic patient. J. Clin. Psychiatry 40: 302-305.
10. WEST, D. J. 1978. Understanding Sexual Attacks. Heineman. Exeter, N.H.
11. ROSNER, R., M. WIEDERLIGHT, M. B. HORNER-ROSNER & R. R. WIECZOREK. 1976. An analysis of demographic variables in adolescent defendants in a forensic psychiatry clinic. Bull. Am. Acad. Psychiatry Law 4: 251-257.
12. SROLE, L., T. S. LANGNER, S. T. MICHAEL, M. K. OPLER & T. A. C. RENNIE. 1962. Mental Health in the Metropolis 1. McGraw Hill Book Co. New York, N.Y.
13. ROBINS, L. 1966. Deviant Children Grown Up. Williams and Wilkins Co. Baltimore, Md.
14. Pisani Report. 1978. Report on the Relationship between Child Abuse and Neglect and Later Socially Deviant Behavior. Select Committee on Child Abuse. New York State Assembly. Albany, N.Y.
15. LEWIS, O., S. S. SHANOK, J. H. PINCUS & G. H. GLASER. 1979. Violent juvenile delinquents: psychiatric, neurological, psychological and abuse factors. J. Am. Acad. Child Psychiatry 18: 2, 307-319.
16. GELLER, J. 1978. Reaching the battering husband. In Social Work with Groups 1: 1-19.
17. OFFER, D., R. D. MAROHN & E. OSTROV. 1979. The Psychological World of the Juvenile Delinquent: 51-80. Basic Books. New York, N.Y.
18. MORRIS, N. 1969. Should law students encounter the new research techniques. In Law and the Social Order. Ariz. St. Law J.: 55-67.
19. Addington v. Texas, 60 L. Ed. 2d 323 (U. S. Supreme Ct., 1979).
20. ROTH, L. 1979. A commitment law for patients, doctors and lawyers. Am. J. Psychiatry 136: 1121-1127.
21. SMITH, A. & L. BERLIN. 1974. Treating the Criminal Offender. Oceana Publications, Inc. Dobbs Ferry, N.Y.

THE INSANITY DEFENSE, THE MENTALLY DISTURBED OFFENDER, AND SENTENCING DISCRETION

Thomas R. Litwack

Department of Psychology
John Jay College of Criminal Justice
New York, New York 10019

In recent years, proposals for reforming the adjudicatory aspect of our criminal justice system have increasingly stressed two suggestions: (a) that the insanity defense be abolished; and (b) that sentencing discretion on the part of judges be likewise abolished, or at least severely circumscribed.

For example, in New York State, the Department of Mental Hygiene has officially adopted the position that "mental disease or defect" should be abolished as a complete defense to a criminal charge;[1] and a special commission headed by Manhattan District Attorney Robert Morgenthau has advocated significantly curtailing the sentencing discretion now wielded by criminal court judges in New York. Similar proposals have accompanied bills to codify, and amend, the federal criminal code.

Proposals to abolish the insanity defense and sentencing discretion are obviously related in that they both are aimed at reducing the arbitrariness and capacity for error of our criminal justice system and, conversely, at enhancing both the actual fairness and the *perceived* fairness of that system. Indeed, both proposals attack very real and serious problems and, taken individually, have much merit. The points I wish to argue here, however, are (1) that the insanity defense—though it may be very narrowly circumscribed and divorced from the term "insanity"—cannot be completely abolished under the Constitution of the United States; and (2) that in any event, proposals to limit—if not abolish—the insanity defense and proposals to limit sentencing discretion seek to obtain goals that, however laudable, are incompatible with one another. For one of the aims of abolishing the insanity defense is to gain greater flexibility in our capacity to deal with mentally disturbed offenders; but to the extent that limits upon sentencing discretion were rigidly mandated and enforced, much of this sought-after flexibility would be lost.

I shall return to the issue of sentencing discretion and the mentally disturbed offender later in this presentation. For now, however, I would like to amplify upon my first point—that the insanity defense cannot, constitutionally, be totally abolished. This is so, I believe, for a simple reason: the Supreme Court has clearly indicated that it would be unconstitutional to subject to criminal penalties one who has violated the law without *mens rea*, that is, without any awareness of wrongdoing or the ability to control one's wrongdoing.

Consider the example of an individual who genuinely believes that he has heard God speak to him and that God has ordered him to kill another person. Or consider the example of someone who kills another in the delu-

sional (and objectively unreasonable) belief that his victim was about to attack him with deadly force. Both these individuals have violated the law, to
be sure. They have committed unjustified homicide; but they have done so
without any sense or awareness of wrongdoing—without, that is, what the
common law referred to as mens rea, or an "evil state of mind."

Under the common law, mens rea was a prerequisite to any conviction
for a crime. As one English judge observed during the last century:

> [A] criminal mind, or mens rea, must . . . ultimately be found by the jury in order to
> justify a conviction, . . . [although] in some cases the proof of the committal of the acts
> may prima facie, . . . by reason of their own nature, . . . import the proof of mens rea.
> But even in these cases it is open to the prisoner to rebut the prima facie evidence, so
> that if, in the end, the jury are satisfied that there was no criminal mind, or mens rea,
> there cannot be a conviction in England for that which is by the law considered to be a
> crime.[2]

Or, as one American authority has put it: "An evil deed, without more,
does not constitute a crime; a crime is committed only if an evil doer harbored an evil mind."[3]

The Supreme Court of the United States, by its own admission, "has
never articulated a general constitutional doctrine of mens rea."[4] I believe,
however, that the Court has clearly indicated that mens rea is a constitutionally required element of all offenses defined as criminal and that it
would be unconstitutional to punish or label as criminals those offenders
who, when they committed their offense(s), wholly lacked mens rea.

For example, in *Powell* v. *Texas,*[4] a case decided in1968, the Court held
that public drunkenness *could,* constitutionally, be subjected to criminal
penalties. However, a clear majority of the Court (including three of its
present members—Justices Brennan, Stewart, and White) stated that if such
behavior were truly uncontrollable, or the result of an "irresistable urge,"
rather than merely *difficult* to control, then to criminalize such behavior
would run afoul of the Constitution's prohibition against cruel and unusual
punishment. As the four justices who would have overturned the
appellant's conviction explicitly stated in *Powell:* "Criminal penalities may
not be inflicted upon a person for being in a condition he is powerless to
change."[4] Those justices who affirmed Powell's conviction did so only
because they could *not* conclude on the evidence that Powell's compulsions
were "completely overpowering." To be sure, a person who commits an act
such as murder has done more than just suffer from a condition. But it
seems to me that the underlying principle behind the just-quoted statement
would apply to our hypothetical cases as well: criminal penalties may not be
inflicted upon a person for having acted without having chosen, knowingly,
to do evil. After all, the defendant in *Powell* clearly did more than suffer
from a condition; he was not only an alcoholic, he appeared while drunk in
public places. Yet four judges voted to reverse Powell's conviction, and
Justice White—and, apparently, at least two other justices in the majority—refused to do so only because he could not conclude upon the
evidence that the defendant "could not prevent himself from appearing in
public places," i.e., that his public drunkenness resulted from "completely
overpowering urges."

That should hardly be surprising. The notion that individuals should be punished only when they choose to act wrongfully is deeply ingrained in our heritage and traditions. As the Court of Appeals for the District of Columbia stated in the well-known *Brawner* decision (which replaced the Durham rule of insanity in the District of Columbia with the American Law Institute test):

> "free will" is the postulate of responsibility under our jurisprudence. . . . Criminal responsibility is assessed when through "free will" a man elects to do evil.[5]

And since mens rea is an essential element of every crime, defendants are constitutionally entitled to a jury determination of whether or not they acted with mens rea. Thus, proposals that would allow insanity plea defendants a jury trial only on the issue of whether or not they committed the charged act, while leaving it to judges to determine issues regarding the defendant's mental state, likewise run afoul of the Constitution—at least insofar as defendants have a mens rea defense.

The concept of mens rea, it is important to stress, refers to a particular state of mind. It means more than electing to do an act that society views as evil; it means electing to do an act—or, in the case of criminal negligence, not to do an act—with some awareness that society would view that choice as morally wrong. Thus, though a psychopath may commit crimes without any subjective sense of guilt or remorse, he still has acted with mens rea, for he knows fully well that such acts are considered wrong by society. Similarly, if one kills in a premeditative fashion to avenge a previous harm, that murder is committed with mens rea no matter how justified the murderer may feel about having taken the law into his or her own hands. As long as the vengeful perpetrator realizes that society disapproves of such action, mens rea exists. (In such cases, of course, a sympathetic jury might nevertheless find the offender not guilty by reason of insanity.)

But when a crime is committed without such an awareness of wrongdoing, mens rea does not exist. To use our previous examples, if a paranoid individual kills in the delusional belief that he is about to be attacked with deadly force, he has no awareness of wrongdoing. In fact our society would sanction his behavior if his premises were true. Similarly, if one acts illegally in response to the commands of God, one has acted without mens rea, for our society teaches that the word of God is supposed to take precedence over the law of man.

Mens rea must also be distinguished from the words "intentional" and "knowingly" as they are often used in the criminal law. In New York, for example, crimes require conduct to be performed "intentionally," "knowingly," "recklessly," or with "criminal negligence." And, in New York, a person acts *intentionally* with respect to a result or to conduct described by a statute defining an offense "when his conscious objective is to cause such a result or to engage in such conduct";[6] and "*knowingly* . . . when he is aware that his conduct" is violating the law or will cause an illegal result.[7] Thus, a person can "intentionally" commit homicide within the meaning of the New York Penal Law and still lack mens rea, as would be the case with the individual who plans and commits a murder—with intent to kill and with awareness of the consequences of his acts—in accordance with instructions from God.

On the other hand, one can act with less of an evil mind than is conveyed by the words "intentionally" or "knowingly" and still possess mens rea. As Justice Black observed in *Powell* v. *Texas*, states have "wide freedom to determine the extent to which moral culpability should be a prerequisite to conviction of a crime."[4] Indeed, the Supreme Court has upheld convictions that were based upon actions that could only be described as "negligent" or irresponsible.[8] To my knowledge, however, the Supreme Court has never upheld a criminal conviction based upon strict liability, that is, without *any* element of conscious wrongdoing on the part of the offender. Indeed, in *Lambert* v. *California,* the Supreme Court ruled that consistent with due process, an ex-felon could not be convicted for failure to register herself as an ex-felon, under an ordinance requiring her to do so, without proof that she knew of the duty to register or without the probability of such knowledge.[9] Thus, while it is true that "there is no one . . . state of mind which constitutes mens rea,"[10] mens rea requires at least a negligent, that is, an irresponsible, failure to act when one should have acted. To subject an offender who has acted without any mens rea to criminal punishment would appear to violate both the due process clauses and the Eighth Amendment.

Does this mean that some insanity defense is constitutionally required to take into account those offenders who, as a result of a "mental disease or defect," have violated the law without any mens rea? The answer, I believe, is yes. But a very strict insanity test—stricter even than the McNaughton test—would suffice. Specifically, the only insanity test that would seem to be constitutionally required is one that would provide for those defendants who wholly lacked mens rea—those defendants who committed their criminal act without any awareness that what they were doing was wrong and without recklessness or negligence and those defendants who, if they did know what they were doing was wrong, were nevertheless simply unable (and not just "substantially" unable) to conform their conduct to the requirements of the law.

A few things should be noted about this suggestion. To begin with, there is no reason—and no constitutional justification—for limiting this defense to those who have suffered from a diagnosable "mental disease or defect." While that might be one cause of an absence of mens rea, it need not be the only one. I am thinking, for example, of the Torsney case, in which a police officer shot and killed an unarmed youth who, the officer claimed, *appeared* to be drawing a gun.[11] At his trial, Torsney was able to present psychiatric testimony to the effect that he suffered from unusual epileptic attacks and that it was, in part, as a result of one of these episodes that he believed he saw his victim draw a gun. Torsney, of course, was found not guilty by reason of insanity—to the chagrin of many who believed that his claim of insanity was a farce. (And, indeed, during his subsequent commitment for over a year to various civil mental hospitals, no evidence of epilepsy was ever observed or discovered.) But the point is this:

What if, under very trying and frightening circumstances (I believe Torsney was called to the scene of the crime with information that there was an armed and dangerous individual about), Torsney simply panicked? What if he killed his victim because he indeed thought he saw a gun, but his perception was a result of his fright rather than a psychotic "mental disease or defect"? If those were indeed the circumstances, was he any more blameworthy than he would have been if epilepsy, rather than overwhelming fear, caused his misperception? In fact, perhaps so! If Torsney was at all aware of his nervousness or excitability—or of any racial prejudices he was harboring that might have influenced his performance as a policeman—then it may well have been negligent or reckless for him to have continued to work as a policeman and he might well have been legitimately convicted of reckless or negligent homicide.

Thus, while we must have an insanity defense, we need not—and should not—call it the "insanity" defense. Rather we should call this constitutionally required defense the "mens rea defense"—not only because it would be a more accurate description of the defense, but also because it would remove the outdated and confusing term "insanity" from our jurisprudence. Such a step might also forestall the negative misperceptions about the "mentally ill" in general that the public might otherwise derive from reading about cases in which very violent individuals are claiming the "insanity defense." Moreover, I believe it would be wise policy for states to limit their insanity defense to a mens rea defense. For one thing, the more narrow, or strict, the "insanity " defense, the less likely it will be that offenders will be able to successfully feign "insanity." It is one thing to feign having, or having had, a "mental disease or defect," and it is another matter entirely to feign having been completely unable to distinguish between right and wrong or to control one's criminal tendencies.

Similarly, a mens rea defense does not suffer from the vagueness and ambiguity that characterize most other insanity defenses and that make the applicability of such other defenses to particular cases a source of such confusion and disagreement among lay persons and professionals alike. It should be far easier to agree upon the issue of whether a defendant *wholly* lacked mens rea than upon the question of whether he or she "substantially" lacked mens rea—the formulation of the increasingly prevalent American Law Institute test.* I recognize that some sympathetic defendants—for example, wives who have murdered their husbands after having suffered years of physical abuse, and certain police officers—may obtain jury acquittals though they rather clearly did not lack mens rea. However, a basic premise of our society is—and should be—that if one can control one's inclinations toward criminality, then one should exercise such control, however difficult that may be. By adopting a strict mens rea defense in place

---

* Under the American Law Institute test, a "person is not responsible for criminal conduct if at the time of such conduct as a result of a mental disease or defect he lacks substantial capacity either to appreciate the criminality (wrongfulness) of his conduct or to conform his conduct to the requirements of the law."

of the more broadly conceived defenses of "insanity," we may even serve to prevent criminality by reinforcing the notion that the ability to control our criminal tendencies exists and that society expects us to exercise such control, at least whenever possible. (Even if the assumption of the ability for self-control is, in fact, false—even if all our actions are, in fact, determined by forces beyond our control despite our illusion of "free will"—the reinforcement of that illusion via our criminal law may nevertheless be a determinant of behavior, directing behavior towards socially acceptable channels.)

Another major advantage of adopting a mens rea defense in place of the insanity defense is that, by limiting the breadth and ambiguity of the insanity defense, it would more fairly limit the actual and perceived role of psychiatry in the determination of the defendant's guilt.

Actually, the role of psychiatrists in the determination of the claims of insanity has been unfairly criticized. Whatever insanity defense we adopt—and I have argued that we must have at least somewhat of an insanity defense (the mens rea defense)—someone must present to the trier of fact the relevant evidence regarding the mental and emotional state of the accused at the time of her or his crime, i.e., evidence that would allow the trier of fact to determine whether or not a finding of not guilty by reason of insanity would be appropriate. The fact that it is difficult to know how someone thought and felt in the past does not change the fact that we are obligated to do the best we can. Fifth Amendment problems aside (an issue to which I shall return), it would be unfair to require the defendant himself—who may well be barely articulate—to alone present his case to the trier of fact. Therefore, as I said, someone (other than the defendant) must present this information to the jury. While there is no reason in the world why that someone must be a psychiatrist (or even a mental health professional—though the data adduced by a nonprofessional interviewer might well be given less weight than the data adduced by a "professional" interviewer), it is unfair to criticize psychiatrists because they cannot describe more precisely inherently ambiguous psychological processes or because they cannot, in good conscience, make judgments that are beyond their competency. Indeed, it seems to me, psychiatric witnesses get into trouble precisely when they seek to move beyond their range of competency—which is to unveil and describe the relevant mental and emotional state of the interviewee as best they can—and attempt to decide questions that are for the trier of fact to decide. Thus, for example, psychiatrists should *never* be willing to state conclusively whether or not a defendant had or lacked "the capacity to conform his or her conduct to the requirements of the law." Given our present state of knowledge, psychiatrists have no special expertise in making that determination. But, as one court suggested, the psychiatrist should still be free "to describe the defendant's mental condition and symptoms, his pathological beliefs and motivations, if he was thus afflicted, and to explain how these influenced or could have influenced his behavior, particularly his capacity [to] knowingly [commit the crime charged],"[12] while largely leaving it to the trier of fact to determine the ultimate issue of guilt or innocence.

Indeed, even those who would abolish the insanity defense—for example, the authors of the New York State Department of Mental Hygiene Report[1]—often support in its place a rule of "diminished capacity," under which "evidence of abnormal mental condition would be admissible to affect the degree of crime for which the accused could be convicted." Though the authors of that report state that under such a rule, "a psychiatrist would be limited to testimony and documentary evidence of an accused's capacity for culpable conduct,"[1] it seems to me that all the problems with psychiatric testimony that supposedly adhere to the availability and use of the insanity defense would also adhere to the determination of the issue of diminished capacity. The only thing that would be different under the proposed rule is that psychiatric testimony would no longer be able to eventuate in the complete exculpation of defendants.

Perhaps that is what much of the shouting is really about: fear on the part of the public that the existence of the insanity defense allows psychiatrists to convince juries that bad and dangerous people should be treated leniently—too leniently for the public's taste; and fear on the part of the psychiatric profession that that perception will diminish the public's respect for psychiatry and psychiatrists. As I have already suggested, however, that problem largely can be resolved by limiting the insanity defense to a strict mens rea defense. Under such a strict test, the psychiatric witness would not have to engage in determining such ambiguous issues as whether or not a defendant's crime was the "product" of a mental illness (the Durham rule), whether or not the defendant could "appreciate" the wrongfulness of his or her conduct, or whether the defendant was "substantially" unable to conform his or her conduct to the requirements of the law. Under a mens rea test, such vague terms would be abandoned and the only issue regarding the defendant's knowledge would be whether or not the defendant was unaware that he or she was acting in a manner condemned by society. I submit that the answer to that question will almost always be clear from the facts of the case (e.g., whether or not the defendant planned an escape or an alibi) and from the results of the psychiatric interviews. While the question of whether a defendant lacked the capacity to conform his or her conduct to the requirements of the law inherently calls for a more subjective determination, the psychiatric witness always can—and should—make it clear that, while certain apparent facts may have led him or her, for particular reasons, to a particular conclusion on that issue, the issue of when free will is overborne by fear, anger, or desire is essentially a philosophical issue regarding which psychiatrists, as a group, have no special expertise. (That would not prevent the witness—or, during the summation, the sponsoring attorney—from arguing that given the evidence he has adduced regarding the defendant's mental state at the time of the crime, the reasons for crediting that evidence, the other facts of the case, the reasonableness of the witness' basic assumptions about human nature, and the cogency and logic of the witness' integration of all those elements, the witness' conclusion in this particular instance is meritorious and worthy of being adhered to by the trier of fact.)

There is an additional way to ensure that witnesses with professional credentials do not overly sway jurors in cases in which defendants seek to exculpate themselves, in whole or in part, by offering psychiatric testimony regarding their state of mind. Or, looked at from the perspective of the profession, there is another way to get psychiatry off the hook without foreswearing its responsibilities—and its legitimate claims to expertise—altogether. That way is simply for prosecutors to call the defendant himself to the stand for cross-examination when the defendant has offered exculpatory state-of-mind testimony via psychiatrists who have interviewed the defendant subsequent to the alleged crime (unless strategic consideration would make such a move inadvisable). Though at first glance such a policy would appear to violate the defendant's constitutional privilege against self-incrimination, and though I have not had the opportunity to research the issue thoroughly, I wish to argue that such a policy would *not* violate the Fifth Amendment. Consider, first of all, the fact that a criminal defendant waives the privilege when he takes the stand on his own behalf. When a mental health professional testifies, on behalf of a defendant, as to the defendant's state of mind at the time of the crime charged, the mental health professional is often doing little more than repeating to the jury—though perhaps in a more articulate form—the defendant's *own* description of his state of mind. There is nothing wrong with that. However, as the United States Court of Appeals for the Second Circuit has observed, under these circumstances the defendant "is able to get the effective benefit of testifying without doing so by having his experts testify at length as to what he said to them."[13] Thus, why shouldn't the prosecution have the same privilege it would clearly have if the defendant were to testify directly to the court? Indeed, the law is clear in most states that defendants who enter psychiatric testimony on their own behalf *do* waive their Fifth Amendment privilege to the extent that they must then submit to psychiatric examinations by the prosecution's professionals, who are then fully entitled to describe their transactions with the defendant—including the defendant's statements to them—to the trier of fact.[14] Why should that waiver stop at the courtroom door? Looked at from another perspective, What values protected by the Fifth Amendment[15] are served by allowing such defendants *not* to testify? The defendant's right to the privacy of his own thoughts that is protected by the Fifth Amendment is already vitiated by virtue of the fact that prosecution psychiatrists have the right to interview—indeed, interrogate—the defendant and present their findings, including the defendant's verbatim statements, to the trier of fact. Just as the prosecution cannot now use evidence obtained during psychiatric examinations to prove its case that the defendant committed the acts for which he is charged,[16,17] the prosecution would still have to prove its case-in-chief without resort to interrogating the defendant. Thus, the Fifth Amendment's protections against coerced (false) confessions would remain. Moreover, just as the defendant may now present evidence of his insanity and yet refuse to undergo a psychiatric examination, as long as the evidence produced is other than that of a post-offense psychiatric examination,[16] so too defendants should remain able to present nonpsychiatric exculpatory mental-state evidence without having to testify themselves. However, once the defendant does enter into evidence what is essentially his own version of his relevant mental state, he should stand no different from a defendant who directly testifies in his own behalf. To be sure, some truly disturbed defendants will be unable to maintain sufficient composure and coherence under the rigors of cross-examination to be able to adequately defend themselves; some might even suffer breakdowns. Some truly disturbed defendants may be all too willing to admit to powers of reasoning and control that were, in fact, absent at the time of their crimes. But such possibilities go to the issue of the defendant's *competence* to stand trial—as the trial is likely to be conducted. We can all think of defendants who claim a state-of-mind defense—e.g., Dan White, who recently murdered the mayor of San Francisco—who are nevertheless sufficiently capable of undergoing the rigors of cross-examination and sufficiently free of self-punitive motivations to be competent to stand trial even if they would be cross-examined. (If the defendant's competency is in question, the prosecution would have to decide, prior to trial, whether or not to call the defendant to the stand so that the defendant's competence can be determined accordingly. In any event, it would ill behoove the prosecution to call a truly disturbed defendant to the stand; the defendant's behavior on the stand would only argue for the validity of his claim of severe disturbance.)

Finally, a strict insanity test would yield the result that offenders who are seriously disturbed but not wholly lacking in mens rea would not automatically be confined to civil mental hospitals (whether or not that disposition was best for them, for the hospitals, or for the community), as must be the case if such individuals, under a broad or broadly interpreted insanity defense, are found not guilty by reason of insanity. Rather, if such individuals are effectively precluded from entirely exculpating themselves through the defense of insanity, they could be sentenced—if found guilty of some crime—with the flexibility required for reconciling their needs with the legitimate interests of society—to a hospital or community facility, if that is appropriate; to a prison, if the defendant cannot be safely managed elsewhere; and, most important, from one facility to another—within the time limits of the defendant's sentence—as the defendant's behavior and amenability to treatment dictate.

This brings us to the issue of sentencing discretion and the difficulty of reconciling the goals of limiting sentencing discretion with the goal of treating mentally disturbed offenders humanely and therapeutically.

The problem can be simply stated. To the extent that sentencing discretion is abolished, the judiciary will lose the flexibility that is required to deal with mentally disturbed offenders as humanely and intelligently as possible. This problem will be exacerbated if we severely circumscribe the insanity defense (as I have suggested we should), because fewer mentally disturbed defendants than ever will be able to avoid the harshness of criminal sanctions entirely by virtue of a successful plea of not guilty by reason of insanity. Indeed, proposals to abolish the insanity defense are often accompanied by proposals to treat mentally disturbed offenders at the sentencing stage with the flexibility and humanity that their condition deserves and requires.[18] However, to the extent that we allow judges to exercise such discretion in determining an offender's sentence, one of the prime goals of the sentencing reform movement must be sacrificed—the goal of ensuring that an offender's sentence will not be severely affected by the luck (good or ill) of the judicial draw and that similarly situated defendants will not be treated very differently simply because they come before judges of very different temperaments and philosophies. If judges have the flexibility to treat some offenders especially leniently, they also have the discretion to treat offenders unduly harshly; a disturbed offender's fate may then turn more upon the idiosyncracies of the sentencing judge than upon objective, or at least articulated, considerations.

Unfortunately, there is no simple solution to this problem, although it should be noted that even proposals to abolish sentencing discretion would permit judges to sentence offenders to the most appropriate facility available. What would be abolished would be the judge's ability to determine the *length* of the offender's sentence. Still, I think we would all agree that there are offenders who—though not legally insane (or lacking in mens rea)—have committed crimes largely in response to acute emotional stress (rather than out of hardened indifference to the rights of others) and that such offenders should not, and need not, be sentenced to long periods of incarceration, especially when such sentences may have no relation to the likelihood of when such disturbed offenders can be safely returned to the community. Thus, mental health professionals who are concerned with the fair and therapeutic treatment of the mentally disturbed should be wary of proposals to limit sentencing discretion.

Such proposals need not be unduly rigid, however. Indeed, I believe that the Morgenthau commission proposal strikes a proper balance between the goal of limiting sentencing discretion and the goal of allowing judges sufficient flexibility to deal fairly and helpfully with the mentally disturbed offender. Under the commission's proposal, the state legislature would continue to set maximum penalties for each category of crime, but an independent commission would establish guidelines (emphasizing the severity of the offense and the defendant's prior criminal history) that, within a narrow range, would indicate what sentence the judge should hand out in each case. However, and most important, the sentencing judge would be free to depart from the guidelines in unusual circumstances; though when sentencing outside the guideline range, the judge would have to make, on the record, findings of fact justifying his or her deviation from the guidelines, and the sentence would then be subject to appellate review (at the behest of either the defense or the prosecution). Thus, under the Morgenthau commission's proposal, judges would presumably be free to depart from the sentencing guidelines when an offender's criminal behavior was apparently the result of a severe or acute psychological disturbance and when an unusual sentence would best serve to "rehabilitate" the defendant (while still protecting the community).

This leads me to my final topic—the implications of the adoption of such a proposal for the utilization of professional psychological and psychiatric input into the sentencing process.

One thing seems clear to me: the adoption of the Morgenthau commission proposal would increase judicial requests for presentence psychiatric examinations in New York. This is because judges who would be inclined to depart from the sentencing guidelines in the direction of greater leniency, when faced with an apparently disturbed offender, will likely want to obtain professional support for their observations and decision to justify their departure from the sentencing guidelines and to avoid being reversed upon appellate review. (At present, sentencing judges rarely need justify their sentences—however harsh or lenient—to anyone.)

But can mental health professionals genuinely improve the rationality of sentencing decisions? More specifically, Can they determine any better than can judges when confinement is necessary to rehabilitate, or at least deter, particular offenders?; and if so, Can they determine how long such confinement need be? Can they determine—again, any better than judges can without their help—which offenders need to be confined to protect the community and, if so, for how long? These are the hard questions that must be answered before a thoughtful sentence can be imposed. It seems to me that the mental health profession has yet to demonstrate any special competence in answering these questions.

That pessimistic appraisal of the usefulness of presentence psychiatric reports seems, in any event, to be prevalent among judges themselves. Having attempted at least to survey the literature on judicial utilization of presentence psychiatric reports, the findings I have been able to uncover are that while judges frequently request such reports, they are rarely satisfied with the results. Even when judges do find such reports useful, it is usually only because the report has confirmed judicial conclusions about the defendant that were independently indicated by the circumstances of the defendant's crime and by the facts of the defendant's history. As one study concluded:

> It appear[s] that judges hope that psychiatry can tell them which defendants they can safely release to society, which of them will benefit from psychiatric or other rehabilitative treatment, and which are so dangerous that they will need prolonged incarceration. Most judges recognize that they are not given this type of guidance in the psychiatric reports they receive. [Many] judges complained that the reports they receive are too technical, unclear, conclusory, or perfunctory. In fact, there seems to be a widespread feeling that many psychiatric reports merely tell a judge the name of the defendant's mental illness, if any, but do not suggest to him what he should do with the defendant. The dissatisfactions with these evaluations may be due to the unavailability of first rate psychiatric services in some counties. However, it is more likely that the judges' dissatisfaction arises from the fact that the questions they want answered, those concerned with the defendant's dangerousness or potential for rehabilitation, are generally not questions that can be answered by psychiatric evaluation.[19]

It is hardly worth harping on the fact, at this late date, that it is indeed the case that psychiatrists have no special expertise in predicting violence. Indeed, that is now the official position of the American Psychiatric Association. It is not strictly accurate to state, however, that psychiatrists have no ability to predict violent behavior. The studies demonstrating the erroneousness of psychiatric prediction of violence all involved individuals who had not committed violence or threatened violence in the recent past. In such circumstances, presumably, *no one* can accurately predict who will and who will not be violent in the future. In other circumstances, however—for example, when an individual has a recent history of violence, is currently threatening violence, or still harbors delusional beliefs that led to violence in the past—more accurate predictions may be possible. It remains to be demonstrated, however, even in such circumstances, or in any circumstances, that mental health professionals can *better* predict violence or nonviolence than can laymen—including judges.

Probably the most intensive study to date of the use of presentence psychiatric reports is that conducted by Bohmer,[20,21] although her study was limited to the use of such reports in sex offense cases. In any event, she concluded that psychiatric reports had very little effect upon sentencing decisions, though she did find that judges were more appreciative of psychiatric reports that recommended long periods of incarceration than of reports that suggested more risky dispositions. Obviously, such harsher recommendations allowed the judge to impose a long prison sentence with a clear conscience, thus completely taking the judge off the hook. However, it appeared that such sentences were recommended and meted out in cases in which the defendant had a long and/or lurid history of offensive behavior, thus justifying a long period of incarceration (whether in a hospital or a prison) without regard to psychiatric input.

Along the same lines, (former) Judge Marvin Frankel has related the following experience with psychiatric presentence advice:

> An obviously disturbed, inadequate, and troublesome man had called the F.B.I. to tell (accurately) the train he was taking to Washington to assassinate the President. Seemingly "competent" legally despite his imprudence, he pled guilty to a charge carrying a maximum possible prison sentence of up to five years. The report I had requested confirmed that he was disturbed and troublesome, told other things I already knew, and concluded that, "giving serious weight to the nature of the offense and primarily for this reason," the defendant should be given the maximum sentence under the statute. Of course, if there was anything for which the sentencing judge would not be looking to psychologists and other experts outside the law, it was guidance as to "the nature of the offense." Undoubtedly, the vagueness of my inquiry merited no more than this useless response. I have tried since to do better. Sometimes, but rarely, the reports are more helpful.[22]

Judges also request psychiatric reports with some frequency, apparently, when they are confronted with defendants who, though not legally insane, seemingly committed their offense under the pressure of some acute and extreme stress. For example, one prominent judge told me of a case before him in which a man, who had never before had any difficulties with the law, had attempted a robbery—in a manner that suggested he *hoped* to be shot in the attempt—to get some money to pay for his son's upcoming bar mitzvah. A psychiatric presentence report was requested in that case to confirm the judge's suspicion—already formed from the facts presented by the nonpsychiatric probation report—that the defendant was, indeed, not a "bad" man, deeply inclined to crime, but a basically law-abiding citizen who had succumbed to unusual pressures and, given help at least, was unlikely to similarly misbehave again. Following receipt of the report—which, of course, confirmed the judge's perceptions—the judge did mete out an unusually lenient sentence. But again we may ask, Under such circumstances, was such a report really necessary? That is, when a man with a history of well-socialized behavior commits a crime for the first time in his life, and his criminal behavior was apparently triggered by extraordinary pressures, do we really need the opinion of professionals to conclude that such an individual is more amenable to rehabilitative efforts and less dangerous to the community than most offenders who commit superficially similar crimes? Unless such circumstances or similar circumstances exist, is there any basis for assuming that psychiatrists or psychologists can accurately predict which offenders are especially "good risks"?

In sum, let me suggest that there are likely to be few cases in which psychiatric examinations, as such, will produce either data or conclusions that can and will uniquely and validly justify judicial departures from sentencing guidelines. Such departures—whatever their direction—will usually be justified, if at all, by the objective facts of the defendant's crime and history (and by the "common sense" assumptions about human behavior that most judges and mental health professionals share). That does not mean that psychiatric presentence reports are meaningless or valueless. If such reports do no more than ease a judge's mind about acting in other than a rote fashion in certain (unusual) cases, or if they encourage a hesitant judge to take an unorthodox step, that may well justify the expense of such reports. And even if the data and conclusions derived from presentence psychological examinations do no more than confirm a judge's own judgment that unusual or out-of-guideline treatment is called for by the case at hand, such reports will have furthered the goals of sentencing guidelines by helping to ensure that when superficially similar defendants are treated differently from one another, it is not because of the whims of the sentencing judges, but because of the real and meaningful differences among the defendants that lay behind their similarities.

REFERENCES

1. Department of Mental Hygiene. 1978. The Insanity Defense in New York: A Report to Governor Hugh L. Carey. Albany, N.Y.
2. Regina v. Prince, 2 C.C.R. 154, 163 (Brett, J.; dissenting opinion).
3. 1978. Wharton's Criminal Law. 14th edit. C. E. Torcia, Ed.: 134.
4. Powell v. Texas, 392 U.S. 514, 535 (1968).
5. United States v. Brawner, 471 F. 2d 969, 985 (D.C. Cir. 1972).
6. N.Y. Penal Law, section 15.05-1.
7. N.Y. Penal Law, section 15.02-2.
8. See, e.g., United States v. Park, 421 U.S. 658 (1975).
9. Lambert v. California, 355 U.S. 255 (1957).
10. STEPHEN. 1883. A History of the Criminal Law of England: 95.
11. Matter of Torsney, 420 N.Y.S. 2d 192 (1979).
12. Rhodes v. United States, 282 F. 2d 59, 62 (4th Cir. 1960).
13. United States v. Weiser, 428 F. 2d 932, 936 (2d Cir. 1969).

14. See, e.g., Lee v. County Court of Erie County, 27 N.Y. 2d 432, 318 N.Y.S. 2d 705, 267 N. E. 2d 542, cert. denied, 404 U.S. 823 (1971).

15. See Murphy v. Waterfront Commission of New York, 378 U.S. 52, 55 (1964).

16. See, e.g., Lee v. County Court of Erie County, 318 N.Y.S. 2d 710, 713 (1971).

17. People v. Finn, 406 N.Y.S. 2d 800, 801 (1978).

18. See, e.g., PUGH, D. 1973. The insanity defense in operation. Wash. Univ. Law Quarterly 87.

19. SHAPIRO & CLEMENT. 1975. Presentence information in felony cases in the Massachusetts Supreme Court. Univ. Suffolk Law Rev. 49: 66.

20. BOHMER, C. 1973. Judicial use of psychiatric reports in the sentencing of sex offenders. J. Psychiatry Law 1: 223.

21. BOHMER, C. 1976. Bad or mad: the psychiatrist in the sentencing process. J. Psychiatry Law 4: 23.

22. FRANKEL, M. 1973. Law without Order: 45.

WHEN TREATMENT BECOMES COERCION:
A LEGAL PERSPECTIVE

Alan H. Einhorn

Chayet and Sonnenreich, P.C.
Boston, Massachusetts 02110

INTRODUCTION

The struggle to enforce the rights of the institutionalized mentally ill has focused, in recent years, upon the emergence of the right of the patient to determine whether and when to assent to prescribed medical treatment and particularly upon the patient's "right" to refuse unwanted treatment. Efforts to enforce this "right" to refuse have highlighted the critical need to strike an appropriate balance between the rights and needs of the institutionalized mentally ill and the responsibilities of the state to provide for their care. Available judicial mechanisms have thus far proven incapable of providing that balance. This paper will explore the emerging "right" to refuse treatment in light of judicial efforts to adapt that right to the day-to-day realities of institutional psychiatric care. A mechanism will then be proposed that is designed to balance the rights of the patient and the interests of the state in treatment-refusal situations and to render prompt and responsive treatment decisions when such resolution is necessary.

AN HISTORICAL PERSPECTIVE

The American judiciary has long applied traditional notions of assault and battery to protect the individual against unwanted intrusions upon his physical and emotional integrity. The cloak of security that derives from the common law is extensive. Not only is the intentional touching of another's person without authorization defined as a legal wrong, but the "mere apprehension of a harmful or offensive contact" is also actionable.[1] The protection thus afforded "extends to any part of the body and to anything which is attached to it and practically identified with it."[1]

Applied to the relationship between physician and patient, these same notions of physical and emotional integrity are embodied in the doctrine of "informed consent." According to this doctrine, except in an emergency, a physician must inform his patient of the nature, benefits, and risks of a proposed course of treatment and must obtain the patient's consent to that treatment prior to its administration.[2] The premise of the doctrine is

the concept, fundamental to American jurisprudence, that "every human being of adult years and sound mind, has a right to determine what shall be done to his own body."[3]

While the doctrine of informed consent has been applied with some consistency in cases involving the treatment of physical injury or disability, courts have been considerably more reticent to invoke the doctrine in cases involving the institutionalized mentally ill. This reluctance is the result of several factors, all of which reflect the difficulties inherent in applying rote legal principles to the uncertainties of institutional psychiatric care.

One of these factors is directly related to the competency requirement of the informed consent doctrine. As its foundation, the doctrine of informed consent presupposes that the party consenting to treatment can rationally and meaningfully assess the benefits and risks of a suggested procedure, along with those of alternatives, before choosing to proceed with treatment. Persons suffering from acute mental illness are often incapable of this type of rational assessment, however. According to one commentator:

> . . . in psychiatry the problem [of obtaining informed consent] is not acute, but chronic; not sporadic, but endemic. It is the nature of psychiatry to work with patients who suffer from impaired perceptions of themselves and the world. It is an impairment of the "consenting organ" itself which is being treated.[4]

As a result of this impairment that impedes "informed" consent, a physician responsible for the care of a psychiatric patient is often faced with either foregoing treatment he deems essential to the patient's care; treating the patient without consent; or seeking a declaration of incompetence and appointment of a guardian—a procedure that, as described below, is often unresponsive to the patient's immediate needs. Because strict application of the competency requirement of the doctrine of informed consent would thus create formidable barriers to psychiatric treatment, the courts have generally been unwilling to question the medical judgments of physicians confronted with this dilemma. The usual presumption that an adult is competent until proven otherwise—and that he is therefore entitled, unless adjudicated incompetent, to refuse prescribed treatment—has accordingly often been ignored.[5]

Judicial reticence in applying common-law notions to the institutional setting can also be attributed to the judiciary's reluctance to second-guess medical judgments that a "psychiatric emergency" exists. The concept of psychiatric emergency is critical to the formulation of a right to refuse treatment, because the existence of an emergency relieves the physician of the requirement that he obtain a patient's consent before administering treatment.[2,6] Inasmuch as the patient in effect only retains his "right" to refuse treatment in nonemergent circumstances, the definition of "emergency" establishes the parameters of this right.

Attempts to define "emergency" in the institutional setting have provided little guidance to those seeking to ascertain the parameters of a right to refuse treatment. Part of the problem lies in the nature of the psychiatric emergency itself. Unlike many medical emergencies, a psychiatric emergency often has no clearly identifiable onset or duration.

> In fact it can be said that certain [psychiatric] patients are in a chronic emergency state, either in that violent or dangerous behavior is just barely being kept under control, or that they are so sensitive to stimuli that one must be constantly alert for developing signs of a violent outburst.[7]

Institutionalization only complicates the dilemma. The so-called chronic emergency patient may pose an imminent and continuous threat of serious harm not only to himself, but to those around him by virtue of his confinement with others. Under these conditions, and given the special needs of the seriously mentally ill, the courts have been loathe to restrict the treatment prerogatives of institutional medical personnel.

Still another rationale for the reluctance of the judiciary to enforce the doctrine of informed consent within the institutional setting is the changing character of the inpatient population of state psychiatric facilities. State statutes and court rulings,[8,9] increasingly sensitive to the psychological aspects of criminal behavior, have resulted in hospitalization for many persons who would previously have been incarcerated for antisocial conduct. In addition, virtually every state now requires that a person be considered "dangerous" either to himself or others before he can be committed involuntarily for institutional psychiatric care.* As these developments increased the influx of more seriously ill and dangerous patients into state psychiatric facilities, the introduction and widespread use of psychopharmacological agents, as well as a growing acceptance of the concept of community mental health care, began to reduce the number of treatable and less seriously ill patients in state facilities. The net effect of these changes has been an increasingly volatile and disturbed inpatient population, which has laid added stress on an already overburdened, underfinanced, and understaffed state hospital system. The multiplicity of needs of this patient population, added to the burdens already placed on institutional personnel, have further encouraged judicial restraint vis-à-vis those charged with treatment responsibility.

EMERGENCE OF THE "RIGHT" TO REFUSE

Largely as a result of judicial reluctance to apply common-law principles within the institutional milieu, the scales of justice until recently have tipped decidedly against the interests of the patient. Developments over the last several years, however, have begun to readjust that balance.

The courts have finally begun to reverse the disturbing trend of equating the principles of "commitability" and "incompetency" for purposes of authorizing treatment without consent.† And recent state statutes have specifically distinguished those terms[11] so as to eradicate the presumption that incompetency necessarily flows from commitment.[5]

At the same time, judicial rulings in related areas have evidenced a growing sensitivity to the concepts of human dignity and human choice vis-à-vis the administration of unwanted medical treatment.[12,13] Commentators,

---

* In Massachusetts, for example, no person may be committed to a state mental health facility absent a finding that (1) the person is mentally ill, and (2) the discharge of such person from a facility would create a likelihood of serious harm (Mass. G.L.A. c. 123, §8).

† See, e.g., *Winters* v. *Miller*.[10] In that case, the court ruled that a finding of mental illness and commitment to a hospital do not raise even a presumption that the patient is incompetent or unable to manage adequately his own affairs.

including the American Psychiatric Society, have begun to endorse the notion that the involuntary administration of medical treatment is often detrimental to the rehabilitation of the patient and, consequently, to the very purpose of commitment.‡

In conjunction with this increasing sensitivity to the rights and needs of institutionalized psychiatric patients, a growing body of judicial precedent has emerged, reflecting a trend toward the widespread recognition of a "right" to refuse treatment. In *Knecht* v. *Gillman*, for example, the court sustained allegations that the use of an emetic drug on nonconsenting inmates for violations of behavior protocols constituted cruel and unusual punishment.[15] The drug apomorphine had been administered intramuscularly by a nurse as a means to punish undesired behavior. It induced vomiting for periods of 15 minutes to an hour and temporary cardiovascular difficulties. The court enjoined the use of the drug at the facility unless (1) written consent were obtained describing the nature of the treatment proposed, along with its purposes, risks, and effects, and specifically informing the inmate of his right to withdraw his consent at any time; and (2) each treatment administered were authorized by a physician, based upon personal observation, and administered by a physician or nurse.

In *Mackey* v. *Procunier*, the ninth circuit reversed the dismissal of an action brought by an inmate who had been administered succinylcholine as part of a medical experiment.[16] The experiment was designed to ascertain whether behavior could be modified by instilling fear, by inflicting pain, and by psychological suggestion. The court wrote, "Proof of such matters could, in our judgment, raise serious constitutional questions respecting cruel and unusual punishment or impermissible tinkering with the mental processes."[16]

In *Kaimowitz* v. *Michigan Department of Mental Health*, decided the same year as *Mackey*, a Michigan state court enjoined an ongoing experimental psychosurgery program on common-law and constitutional grounds.[17] Although the patient in that instance had actually consented to the surgery, and although the technique had been approved by two hospital committees, the court found that the coercive institutional setting, coupled with the speculative yet irreversible effects of psychosurgery, required the termination of the program. In rendering its decision, the court noted that

psychosurgery is clearly experimental, poses substantial danger to research subjects, and carries substantial unknown risks.[17]

Similar concerns were noted by the court in the landmark case of *Wyatt* v. *Stickney*,[18] in which the Federal District Court for the District of Alabama ruled that institutionalized mental patients have a right to be free

‡ The American Psychiatric Association takes the following position on informed consent: "The American Psychiatric Association is aware of the possibility that the right to adequate care and treatment may be understood and even be used in some cases in a coercive manner. We therefore wish to clearly indicate that our concern is that adequate care and treatment be available. As is the practice generally in medicine, the patient's informed consent for treatment is required except for emergency situations."[14]

from unusual and hazardous treatment procedures, such as lobotomy, electroconvulsive therapy (ECT), and aversive reinforcement conditioning, done without their consent.

While many of the early so-called right-to-refuse cases have recognized such a right only in circumstances involving the use of aversive and intrusive treatment modalities—e.g., psychosurgery, ECT, aversive reinforcement conditioning—or in circumstances where modalities otherwise customarily employed had been used for experimentation or punishment, recent decisions have extended the "right" to refuse to include customary and accepted forms of treatment. Thus, in the case of *In re Boyd*,[19] the lower court dismissed an action brought by an incompetent patient who had refused certain nonessential psychotropic medication on religious grounds. The Court of Appeals for the District of Columbia reversed, indicating that the trial court had failed to give sufficient weight to the patient's religious beliefs. In so ruling, the court acknowledged the principle that medical treatment may not be imposed on a competent person who rejects it, absent a compelling state interest.

Similarly, in *Rennie* v. *Klein*, a federal district court in New Jersey held that involuntary psychiatric patients possess a qualified right to refuse psychotropic medication.[20] And in *Rogers* v. *Okin*, the Federal District Court for the District of Massachusetts ruled that patients confined to psychiatric institutions have the right to be free from forced medication and seclusion in nonemergent circumstances.[21]

The "right" to refuse thus recognized, though perhaps derived from common-law notions of physical and emotional integrity, is based upon a variety of constitutional predicates, including First Amendment freedom of expression, thought,[17] and religion;[6,10,19] the right to privacy under the penumbra of the Bill of Rights;[6,20] the right to be free from cruel and unusual punishment under the Eighth Amendment;[15,16] and the Fifth and Fourteenth Amendment rights to due process protection against invasion of personal liberty.[10]

ENFORCING THE NEWFOUND RIGHT

Although constitutionally based, the "right" to refuse, like other constitutional rights, is not absolute. If the state can establish compelling reasons for imposing treatment against a person's will, courts will allow treatment to proceed.[5,20] In order to conscientiously enforce the "right" to refuse treatment, therefore, there must exist a mechanism whereby both the rights of the patient and the interests of the state are weighed. Such a mechanism must be capable of promptly and sensitively responding to day-to-day treatment dilemmas, protecting patients' rights, assessing the interests of the state, and authorizing the administration of necessary treatment.

Traditionally, psychiatric treatment decisions were made by the attending physician. In theory, the physician was best suited to advise the patient of treatment choices based upon his firsthand knowledge of the patient's illness, history, and needs and the rapport that he had developed with the patient over time. In addition, the physician had presumably been trained to diagnose the patient's illness, assess the various treatment options available, and choose the most appropriate mode. However, at least with respect to physicians in state psychiatric institutions, irregular staffing patterns and insufficient manpower, along with deteriorating facilities, often preclude any one physician from obtaining firsthand knowledge of a patient's illness or history, or from developing a physician-patient relationship. Indeed, treatment regimens are often administered by inadequately educated or trained nonphysician employees and are used for control rather than treatment. As courts have become increasingly aware of these facts, they have grown reluctant to delegate decision-making authority for a patient's well-being to his treating physician.

Presently available judicial mechanisms for the enforcement of the "right" to refuse treatment have similarly proven to be unworkable. One such mechanism is the statutory guardianship procedure existing under state law. The rationale underlying this procedure is that a patient is competent—and thus has the right to make his own treatment choices—unless he is adjudicated incompetent by a court of law, and a guardian appointed to render decisions for him. The guardianship procedure is an expensive, time-consuming process that is unresponsive to the immediate and changing needs of the institutionalized patient. Moreover, the relief afforded by such a procedure is often unnecessarily broad, given the reasons for its invocation. The procedure provides for a finding of general incompetency and the appointment of a guardian over both the patient's person and estate for an indefinite period of time, when all that may be required is a decision with respect to a particular treatment. In addition, a legal determination of "incompetence" deprives the patient of his basic rights as a citizen, e.g., he may no longer enter into legal relationships. Finally, an adjudication of "incompetence" carries with it a social stigma that may be difficult, if not impossible, to overcome.

The procedure originally employed by the court in Rennie v. Klein (Rennie I)§ to evaluate the plaintiff's refusal to accept psychotropic medication typified the impracticality and inappropriateness of traditional judicial mechanisms for everyday treatment decisions regarding the mentally ill. While the Rennie court did not convene a competency/guardianship proceeding, it did provide for a full-scale hearing before a court. In fact, as of November 9, 1978, some 11 months after the case was brought, the Rennie court had conducted two full hearings, resulting in two written opinions, regarding treatment decisions involving but one individual and only two specific treatment episodes.

What becomes clear, based on Rennie I, is that traditional judicial process—encompassing delays, protracted hearings, expert testimony, and written opinions—does not respond to the need for immediate attention and

§ Rennie I refers to the proceedings up to and including the decision reported at 462 F. Supp. 1131 (D.N.J. 1979) (Reference 20.)

continuity of care of patients in psychiatric facilities, where tens or even hundreds of refusals of treatment may occur daily. The enormous burden of time, energy, and expense that will befall courts, institutions, and physicians alike if day-to-day treatment decisions are undertaken by the courts, and the potential for harm to patients resulting from unavoidable and interminable delays, hardly justifies the perpetuation of a *Rennie I*-type scenario, as the *Rennie* court later tacitly acknowledged.

An independent, interdisciplinary review board is another mechanism that has been suggested as a means of deciding issues arising from refusals of treatment. Although such mechanisms are presently used in many psychiatric hospitals for review of protocols for experimentation with human subjects, the process has yet to receive judicial sanction for the purpose of monitoring daily treatment decisions. A specific model for such a mechanism was suggested by the Massachusetts Psychiatric Society in its amicus brief filed in the case of *Rogers* v. *Okin*.[7] This model would provide for a three-member review board, independent of the institution, composed of an attorney and two psychiatrists. The attorney, as chairman, would ensure that patients' rights were considered. The psychiatric members of the board would provide the expertise required to evaluate the correctness of the patient's diagnosis, the appropriateness of the suggested treatment, and the availability of less restrictive alternatives to that treatment.

The function of the board would be to review all refusals of treatment that the attending physician deems essential. In the case of such a refusal, the board would hold an informal hearing at which the patient and his attorney could be present. All relevant testimony and evidence would be received. The board would authorize the treatment only if it determined that the patient's refusal resulted from diminished mental capacity attributable to mental illness and that the patient's overall best interests would be served by the treatment, even if it were administered forcibly. Decisions of the review board would be appealable to the courts.

The review board, like its predecessors, has several flaws that render it unfit for its intended purpose. The first is its hearing procedure, which, much like its judicial counterpart, is unsuited to prompt review and immediate decision making. The second is its size; it is unlikely that a board composed of three professionals will be quick enough to respond to the urgency of many refusal situations. In addition, the mere fact that the board would not be located in the facility ensures delay. Finally, there is the inevitable expense attributable to a system that envisions the employment of three professionals, representation by attorneys, preparation of documents, conducting of hearings, etc. Clearly a less cumbersome, more responsive mechanism is necessary.

The most encouraging development vis-à-vis the creation of a mechanism to enforce the "right" to refuse is the recent order of the Federal District Court for the District of New Jersey in the case of *Rennie* v. *Klein* (*Rennie II*).¶

¶ CA No. 77-2624, Sept. 14, 1979 (Reference 20).

Plaintiff-patients in that action petitioned the court for a preliminary injunction to restrain physicians and institutions from administering psychoactive drugs without the patients' freely given consent obtained under procedural safeguards. In rendering its decision, the court reaffirmed its prior finding that the plaintiffs enjoyed a qualified "right" to refuse treatment; ruled that patients are entitled to some due process protection before psychoactive drugs may be administered to them; held that the "right" to refuse can be enforced only if informed consent is obtained prior to treatment; and held that a patient's refusal of treatment can be overriden only if countervailing state interests so required.‖ At the same time, the court issued an order establishing a mechanism for the enforcement of the patient's rights. That order provided for (1) the obtaining of informed consent on written consent forms prior to the administration of medication; (2) a system of patient advocates to analyze instances in which the treating physician certifies that a patient is incapable of providing informed consent (in which case the advocate would be authorized to seek independent review of the physician's treatment decision) and to serve as informal counsel before an informal reviewer; (3) informal review by an independent psychiatrist before an involuntary patient may be forcibly medicated; (4) enforcement of voluntary patients' right to refuse treatment; and (5) forced medication only in emergency circumstances. The court ruled finally that independent lawsuits alleging violations of patients' civil rights would not be barred by its order.

ANOTHER ALTERNATIVE

The *Rennie II* approach is a constructive step in the search for a mechanism that would responsively and responsibly monitor both the rights of the patient and the interests of the state as they relate to treatment decisions in state psychiatric facilities. The *Rennie II* approach does have several shortcomings, however; perhaps the most important is its failure to impose a different standard of review for patients who are deemed by the independent review to be "functionally competent," as opposed to "incompetent," to make treatment decisions. In addition, the court neglected to indicate whether the mechanism would be available in close proximity to the facility on a continuous basis.

In seeking to improve upon the mechanism established by the court in *Rennie II*, any alternative mechanism should satisfy at least the following criteria: (1) it must be capable of providing a prompt resolution of dilemmas regarding consent to treatment; (2) it must be available on a round-the-

---

‖ Factors to be considered when assessing the countervailing state interests involved were stated to be (1) the nature of the physical threat posed by the patient to other patients and staff; (2) the patient's capacity to make a decision relative to his own treatment; (3) the existence of less restrictive treatment alternatives; and (4) the risk of permanent side effects from the proposed treatment.

clock basis; (3) it must be independent of the institution served, the treating physicians, and the patient; (4) its implementers must have appropriate training to assess the patient's condition and the treatment offered; and (5) the resulting decision must have the force of law. Such a mechanism is described below.

The mechanism proposed is similar to that in *Rennie II*. It shall be referred to as the "civil rights officer" (CRO). CROs would be selected from a panel of qualified psychiatrists appointed by the superior court for the jurisdiction in which the facility is located. They would be selected by the superior court judge and assigned to an individual inpatient treatment facility for 8-hour shifts. One CRO would be assigned to each such facility on a 24-hour-a-day, 7-day-a-week basis. The CRO would be a magistrate of the court, employed and salaried by the court, and would have experience and training in the civil rights area.

The sole function of the CRO would be to review and evaluate treatment decisions either when the patient's ability to render such a decision is alleged to be impaired or when the patient has refused treatment that is considered essential to his well-being. Upon being so notified, the CRO would immediately interview the treating physician and the patient refusing treatment. As in *Rennie II*, the patient would be entitled to informal counsel from a patient advocate, also available on a 24-hour-per-day basis and appointed by the state department of mental health. The CRO could seek information from any person who has knowledge pertinent to the patient's case.

Upon completion of this fact-finding function, the CRO would consider the circumstances and the necessity for providing substitute consent and would, to the extent possible, render an immediate decision which would be entered into the patient record. The following factors would be considered by the CRO for purposes of his decision: the apparent capability of the patient to render a reasoned decision regarding treatment; the degree and intrusiveness of the treatment mode suggested; the permanence and severity of the procedure's effects; the existence of less drastic means of accomplishing the same purpose; the reasons for the patient's refusal; the nature of the symptoms for which the treatment is offered; and the effects on the patient and those around him if treatment were not administered. If the CRO determined that the patient did not have the capability to render a rational decision regarding treatment and that his "best interests," on the basis of the factors noted above, would be served by administration of the treatment, such treatment would be administered. If the CRO determined that the patient did have the capability to render a rational decision regarding treatment, the treatment would be withheld unless there were a compelling reason to override the patient's refusal and no acceptable alternative treatment existed. All decisions of the CRO would be subject to appeal to the local court of general jurisdiction. The CRO would be protected from liability for any injury that might result from a good faith decision rendered by him.

Conclusion

The recent struggle to enforce the rights of the mentally ill has finally awakened our society and its legal system to the needs of those confined to psychiatric facilities. The response of that system, though cautious at first, has grown increasingly sensitive to patients' rights. The challenge now is to design a process that can balance those rights with the critical need for timely and appropriate treatment in the patients' best interests.

References

1. Prosser, W. 1971. Law of Torts. 4th edit.: 37, 34.
2. Watson v. Clutts, 262 N.C. 153 (1962).
3. Canterbury v. Spence, 464 F. 2d 772, 780 (D.C. Cir., 1972), cert. denied, 409 U.S. 1064 (1974).
4. Jonsen, A. R. & B. Eichelman. 1978. Ethical issues in pharmacological treatment. *In* Legal and Ethical Issues in Research and Treatment. D. M. Gallant & R. Force, Eds.: 145. S.P. Medical and Scientific Books. New York, N.Y.
5. Plotkin, R. 1977. Limiting the therapeutic orgy; mental patients' right to refuse treatment. N. L. Rev. **72:** 461, 488.
6. Scott v. Plante, 532 F.2d 939 (3d Cir. 1976).
7. Brief of the Massachusetts Psychiatric Society as Amicus Curiae, Rogers v. Okin, CA 75-1610T, U.S. Dist. Ct., Mass., p. 9.
8. Mass. G.L.A. c. 123, § 16.
9. Durham v. United States, 214 F.2d 862 (D.C. Cir. 1954).
10. Winters v. Miller, 446 F.2d 65, 74 (2d Cir.) cert. denied, 404 U.S. 985 (1971).
11. Brakel, S. & R. Rock, Eds. 1971. The Mentally Disabled and the Law. revised edit.: 49-59. American Bar Foundation. Washington, D.C. (From Reference 5.)
12. In re Quinlan, 70 N.J. 10, 355 A.2d 647, cert. denied, 429 U.S. 922 (1976.)
13. Superintendent of Belchertown State School v. Saikewicz, 1977 Mass. Adv. Sh. 2461, 370 N.E. 2d 417 (1977).
14. American Psychiatric Association Task Force on the Right to Treatment. 1977. Am. J. Psychiatry **134:** 3, note 37.
15. Knecht v. Gillman, 488 F. 2d 1136 (8th Cir. 1975).
16. Mackey v. Procunier, 477 F.2d 877 (9th Cir. 1973).
17. Kaimowitz v. Michigan Department of Mental Health, N. 73-19434 AW-(Cir. Ct. Wayne Cty., Mich., July 10, 1973), excerpted in 2 Prison L. Rpts. 433 (1973).
18. Wyatt v. Stickney, 344 F. Supp. 387 (M.D. Ala. 1972), aff'd. sub nom, Wyatt v. Aderholt, 503 F. 2d 1305 (5th Cir. 1974).
19. In re Boyd, 403 A.2d 744 (D.C. App. 1979).
20. Rennie v. Klein, 462 F. Supp. 1131 (D.N.J. 1979) (individual action); Opinion on Plaintiffs' Motion for a Preliminary Injunction (CA No. 77-2624, Sept. 14, 1979) (class action).
21. Rogers v. Okin, D. Mass., CA 75-1610T, Order and Judgment, October 29, 1979.

THE PATIENT AS OFFENDER: PANEL DISCUSSION

Moderator: Donal E. J. Mac Namara
Panel Members: Albert Axelrod, Alan H. Einhorn,
Maurice R. Green, Thomas R. Litwack, and
Alexander B. Smith

D. E. J. MAC NAMARA *(John Jay College of Criminal Justice, New York, N.Y.)*: I'd like Mr. Einhorn to say a word about society's rights of protection or right to use unattractive alternatives as deterrents against the refusal of treatment.

A. H. EINHORN *(Chayet and Sonnenreich, P.C., Boston, Mass.)*: As a practical matter, when you're dealing with issues that involve police power or issues that are controversial in nature, courts will agree that there's a balancing of interests and that society's interest is clearly one that has to be taken into consideration.

In one such case—involving a ward of the state who was absolutely incompetent to understand the fact that he had leukemia and was dying—the question was whether this individual was going to be subjected to chemotherapy, which would have enormous effects on him and which he would not understand. In that case, the court recognized and laid out one mechanism that would weigh and balance the interests of society against the interests of the individual and decided for the individual that treatment could be refused. In the case of venereal disease, tuberculosis, and various other diseases, it's pretty clear by state statute that there is a balancing of interests that would be applied to those circumstances requiring treatment on society's behalf.

UNIDENTIFIED SPEAKER: I would like to ask my question of Dr. Smith, and it's primarily about the role of confidentiality when working along with the criminal justice system as a psychotherapist. It seems to me that when a parole officer acts in the role of therapist, there is an issue of double jeopardy involved.

Usually, a client assumes confidentiality in a therapist, i.e., that the therapist is not going to reveal the things that are discussed in the session. This engenders trust and helps the therapeutic relationship along. I'm not sure that this kind of relationship can be developed with a parole officer.

Also, when a therapist in a mental health center is asked by the court to act as a therapist, the therapist is subject (at least in New Jersey) to be subpoenaed by the court, and the records are also subject to subpoena. That also raises the question of confidentiality in the case—whether or not the client can trust in the therapist when he is acting, at least in part, as an arm of the court.

A. B. SMITH *(John Jay College of Criminal Justice, New York, N.Y.)*: That's a good question. Supposing we take the outside agency first. That's easier because the point is that if the outside agency will tell the court in advance that they will not handle the case unless they can maintain confidentiality (as they have this right), then the court may decide whether or not to make the referral. I'm not making this up on the spur of the moment—for a number of years I was attached to the BARO Clinic, which was a psychiatric clinic that was established in Brooklyn in the middle 1950s. The moving force was the then District Attorney Edward Silver, because a clinic of that kind was needed in Brooklyn. There were no agencies that could handle the prepsychotic, the postpsychotic, and the highly disturbed offenders who were placed on probation or parole. These offenders came to the clinic knowing that the ground rules were that confidentiality had to be maintained, that otherwise the clinic wouldn't take the referral.

Now as far as the other situation is concerned, by the very nature of the relationship of a probation officer to the court, or a parole officer to the parole commission, there are certain things that happen between the patient and the officer that must transcend the bounds of confidentiality. Whatever an offender tells a probation officer or a parole officer is not confidential, especially if it has anything to do with the possibility of his committing another crime or the disclosure that he has already committed a crime.

UNIDENTIFIED SPEAKER: I'd like to ask Professor Mac Namara to give us a list of those things that work. Wouldn't it be in the public interest to try to get those things applied?

D. E. J. MAC NAMARA: I would be very hesitant to state dogmatically that any single approach works in a generality of cases. There are some techniques that have been shown in one or more experiments to work with a larger number of offenders than do other techniques that are presently being used, or that have been shown to work better than no technique at all. However, in the opinion of many persons who are concerned with prison reform, inmate's rights, political rights, etc., most of these techniques are considered to be assaultive, aggressive, invasions of privacy, mandatory or coercive treatment when no treatment is wanted, or a hurtful or punitive treatment even though punishment might not be its objective. Those persons have been strong enough in their pressures to disclose these techniques and get further public, shall we say, condemnation of them. They have been strong enough in their pressures to influence a major agency of the United States government to change the entire five-year development plan for a penal institution. They have been strong enough to influence courts to sabotage the Maryland program that was working at least somewhat better than any of the others.

Now my colleague who has just passed away, Robert Martinson—in his book *The Effectiveness of Correctional Treatment,* a very massive study—came pretty much to the conclusion that nothing works very well. But also in the process of doing that study, Martinson made it very clear that nothing much was being attempted and even those things that *were* attempted were done in such a slipshod way, with such poor methodology and such poor controls, that we don't have the documentation that you asked for.

I would like to have an experimental institution in the United States, where we could try out even wild ideas over a period of time until we could discover something that works. Perhaps a United States version of Hersted-vester or something of that sort. So, I must admit that I cannot give you a direct answer, but those are some things I'll throw out at you.

UNIDENTIFIED SPEAKER: I'd like to direct my question to Mr. Axelrod. I was wondering whether guided group interaction is given concomitantly with other kinds of treatment.

A. AXELROD* (*Highfields Residential Group Center, Hopewell, N.J.*): To the best of my knowledge, programs utilizing guided group interaction use it solely as a treatment approach. That's generally true in New Jersey and in other programs that I'm aware of.

UNIDENTIFIED SPEAKER: I have a second question for Mr. Axelrod. You state that a basic assumption of the program is that antisocial behavior is learned by association and, conversely, that unlearning of antisocial behavior can be accomplished by association with peers who exhibit social behavior. Now if that were true, then would not the best peer group consist of those adolescents who have persistently exhibited prosocial behavior rather than those who are antisocial?

A. AXELROD: Actually, I think that all juveniles are both social and an-tisocial, that is, I think that everyone's behavior is prosocial in most aspects. It's only in limited areas that people act antisocially. So if you have a group made up of juvenile delinquents, for the most part they are oriented socially. In terms of making identification with each other, which is an im-portant factor in developing an effective group, I think it's better if the peo-ple have something in common, such as identifying themselves as people who have gotten into trouble.

In sum, even though they are delinquent, they have prosocial values and can be effective in helping each other to improve their adjustment to the institutional setting and to the broader society.

D. E. J. MAC NAMARA: I'm going to allot Dr. Litwack 30 seconds to respond to the remark I made about his presentation.

T. R. LITWACK: (*John Jay College of Criminal Justice, New York, N.Y.*): Actually, I'd rather make another comment about something else you said. I'm not so sure that Dr. Mac Namara is correct in saying that the courts, as a result of suits brought by civil liberties lawyers, have significant-ly constrained the ability of correctional personnel to rehabilitate offenders. For example, Patuxent Institution in Maryland is still functioning—much to the displeasure of civil libertarians—and I'd like Dr. Mac Namara to be more specific about how these suits have forestalled adequate treatment.

As long as I have the microphone, I'd also like to add a few other, very quick points. One is that the Supreme Court ruled just last spring that before individuals can be committed to mental hospitals, there must be clear and convincing evidence that they meet the standards for commitment; so

* Mr. Axelrod presented the paper by A. Elias, as the author could not attend the sym-posium.

presumably it should now be the law that before someone can be forced to undergo treatment, there must be clear and convincing evidence that they need the treatment.

The other point I want to make, in response to Dr. Mac Namara's comments to my paper, was that while it seems to me that we need to reduce sentencing discretion (because some offenders are now incarcerated for too long a period of time and others for too short a period of time), and while the major goal of sentencing should be to protect the community, if you do get rid of sentencing discretion, you will still be left with a problem. Some people—who have really been entirely law abiding all of their lives—will suddenly, as the result of some very acute environmental pressure, go and commit a crime. And if there is no sentencing discretion, those people will be subject to long prison terms despite the fact that (without a finger lifted to rehabilitate them) chances are they would never commit a crime again.

For example, one told to me by a judge, a fellow who had a history of purely prosocial behavior, but who was very strapped for money to pay for his son's bar mitzvah, stuck up a store to get money to pay for the bar mitzvah—and did so under circumstances that suggested that he really hoped he would be killed in the attempt. Do we really want to treat that person like any other offender? And if we have the discretion to treat him otherwise, how do you limit discretion in other cases?

"SCARED STRAIGHT" AND THE PANACEA PHENOMENON: DISCUSSION

Discussant: James O. Finckenauer

School of Criminal Justice
Rutgers University
Newark, New Jersey 07102

Juvenile delinquency is one of the most difficult and intractable social problems facing America today. For example, one of only four priorities for action set by the National Advisory Commission on Criminal Justice Standards and Goals in 1973 was that of preventing juvenile delinquency. "Street crime is a young man's game," the Commission said in support of this priority. Our efforts to prevent and control juvenile delinquency over the past two decades might be described as a search for an elusive panacea. In the words of David Rothenberg of the Fortune Society, "We always seem to seek simple solutions for complex situations." If nothing else, the causes of delinquency are incredibly complex. Delinquency generally results from some combination of the following factors: perceptions of limited opportunities, peer group pressures, normlessness, poor early socialization experiences, social disorganization at home and/or in the community, and negative labeling. Because of the multiple paths to delinquency, it follows that there can be no easy or simple answers. But that doesn't seem to keep us from trying.

Webster defines panacea as a remedy for all diseases; a cure-all. One of the causes *and* effects of our failures and frustrations in dealing with juvenile crime has been a search for a cure-all. This search has been conducted not only by the general public, but by politicians, lawmakers, juvenile-justice officials, and social scientists as well. In this article, I will examine the panacea phenomenon in some detail; look at some of the reasons for our sense of frustration; discuss the "Scared Straight" program as a classic case in point; and suggest some possible implications.

The 1960s and 1970s have been replete with failures in the war on juvenile crime—and these failures were in no small part a result of programs being oversold at the outset. One early example was the massive ($12.5 million) Mobilization for Youth (MFY) project launched on New York's Lower East Side in 1962. This project was designed to combat juvenile delinquency by opening the neighborhood opportunity structure to deviant or potentially deviant youths. It failed largely because it did not account for other causes of delinquency; but responsible persons acted as if it were a surefire answer.

The War on Poverty begun by President Johnson in 1964 was built on the Mobilization for Youth model. Specific aspects such as the Job Corps and Neighborhood Youth Corps were further attempts to combat juvenile

213

delinquency by enhancing legitimate opportunities for youths. These skirmishes against youth crime can be characterized as oversell and underperform. The first is an example of the panacea phenomenon, while the second has certainly contributed to our sense of frustration arising from failure.

The Omnibus Crime Control Act which created the Law Enforcement Assistance Administration (LEAA) in the U.S. Department of Justice has spent millions on crime control and criminal justice since 1968 without reducing juvenile delinquency. The same can be said of the Juvenile Justice and Delinquency Prevention Act of 1974. This is not to say that individual successes have not been achieved through both of these efforts, but rather that the oversell/underperform problem has plagued each of them. In each instance, dramatic breakthroughs were forecast but not realized.

On a more specific level, the diversionary programs and youth service bureaus that were advocated by the National Advisory Commission have, in the words of Bullington and his colleagues, been "widely advertised as a panacea not only for delinquency but also for the inequities and imperfections of the juvenile justice system."[1] Thus, whether it is on the massive scale of MFY, the antipoverty program, or LEAA, or whether it's on the individual program level, the vicious cycle continues. Legislation and programs or projects of various kinds are posed as cure-alls; they fail to live up to expectations which are frequently unrealistic; frustration sets in; and the search for the next panacea begins anew.

Social scientists and researchers also do not seem to be immune to this phenomenon. Here examples can be found when the issue is approached from the opposite direction—namely that of evaluation of treatment efforts. An excellent example is the work of Lipton, Martinson, and Wilks who reviewed 231 treatment studies in corrections—including juvenile corrections—published between 1945 and 1967. This review resulted in Martinson's assessment that "with few and isolated exceptions, the rehabilitative efforts that have been reported so far have had no appreciable effect on recidivism."[2] This became translated into a "nothing works" doctrine with Martinson's statement on a CBS "Sixty Minutes" broadcast that "there is no evidence that correctional rehabilitation reduced recidivism."

Martinson has been criticized for seeking universals in his evaluation, which is another way of saying he was looking for cure-alls. In a recent article, Michael Gottfredson points out that seeking universals is a widely known treatment-destruction technique.[3] He indicates that in seeking universals, an evaluator simply shows that although the treatment method has been found to work with some offenders, it is not effective with others; or that it has not been tried with all offenders. These are simply different versions of the panacea phenomenon.

One of the most recent answers to the juvenile delinquency problem seems to be to scare delinquents or suspected delinquents straight. "Scared Straight" has become the label for the Juvenile Awareness Project at New Jersey's Rahway State Prison. This label derives from the title of an Oscar award–winning film about the project which has been repeatedly aired across the country.

The film was first shown on November 2, 1978 by KTLA, Channel 5 in

Los Angeles. *TV Guide* for that evening carried the following blurb: "SCARED STRAIGHT! Special: Inside a maximum security prison. This hour-long program follows 17 juvenile offenders as they learn, at first hand, about the realities of prison life. Using brutally frank and frequently obscene language, 'Lifers' at Rahway (N.J.) State Prison tell the young people about the ultimate pay-off for their criminality." The film points out that some 8,000 juveniles had visited Rahway and that 80% of them had been "scared straight." Actor Peter Falk narrates the documentary, a factor that seems to enhance the authenticity and drama of the film.

In the time since the first showing of this film, there has been a clamor in some 38 states and foreign countries to create, mandate, and legislate similar programs in everything from local jails to state prisons. This new approach has been touted as the way to stop juvenile delinquency once and for all. Why?

Its appeal seems to stem partly from the fear of crime—juvenile crime—and particularly of the violent young hoodlums who are presumed to stalk the streets. It comes too from a sense of frustration that nothing else works. The ingredients for such a program—convicts, delinquents, and prisons—are readily available everywhere, and it costs little or nothing. Best of all, its success rate is claimed to be close to 90%. It is this unbeatable combination that seems to be responsible for a "Scared Straight" bandwagon, read panacea.

The core of this combination is the success rate. First, what about the 17 youths portrayed in the film? All but one of the 17 are claimed to have been scared straight based on a three-month follow-up. A field survey by the Washington-based National Center on Institutions and Alternatives resulted in a report that for 10 juveniles identified from the film, no involvement in the serious crimes alluded to in the film could be found. Some youngsters reported having committed some minor offenses, but were certainly not hard-core delinquents. Offenses included setting off firecrackers, smoking marijuana, and stealing cookies and candy bars. Some youngsters appearing in the film "Scared Straight" had previously attended the program, contrary to the impression given in the film.

What about the famed overall success rate? Almost from its beginnings, great claims of success for the project have been made by sponsors and supporters and by the lifers themselves. The figures used, however, are so subject to error and inaccuracies as to render them totally invalid. Among the problems with the figures are the following:

a. More than half of the juveniles attending have no record of delinquency. The fact that nondelinquents remain nondelinquent is no great achievement. These are not successes.

b. Some data are collected by means of letters sent to parents/guardians and sponsors within a short time after the juveniles visit the project. These letters ask for information on the subject youngsters' conduct after their visit. This method of collecting data is of the "to your knowledge" variety, and is thus too subjective and haphazard to be valid.

c. Replies to the aforementioned letters are frequently based upon

follow-up periods of only days or a few weeks. The most hard-core delinquent may remain crime free over such a short period under any circumstances. Again, these are not successes.

    d. Self-selection dictates responses to the letters. Because only some
parents and agencies respond, they cannot be considered a representative
sample of the whole. It is possible that only some who have good things
to say, do so.

    e. Recidivism is not defined or uniform for all those reporting.
Does it mean rearrest or reconviction? Does it mean further problems in
school? Does it mean further incorrigibility? Or, What does it mean?
"Recidivism" for a nondelinquent is clearly a misnomer.

    Results from a 16-month evaluation of the project, which is the only
controlled study to date, show a success rate (no recorded arrests during a
six-month follow-up) of 59% for an experimental group of 46 juveniles. A
similar group of 35 youngsters who were used for comparison purposes
showed a success rate of 89%. This study showed that more of the 46 at-
tenders committed subsequent offenses, and also that they committed more
offenses and more serious offenses than did their counterparts in the comparison group. Overall, the project was not successful with any subgroup in
the attending sample when outcomes were compared to those of the comparison sample.[4]

    Since this study was released in April 1979, an official survey of the
records of 67 youths from Mercer County, New Jersey, sent to the project,
disclosed that 51 (76%) were subsequently rearrested. Two other surveys
reportedly undertaken in New Jersey counties resulted in failure rates of
about 40% and 60% respectively.

    A recent study by the Michigan Department of Corrections of a project
called JOLT (Juvenile Offenders Learn Truth) resulted in its suspension.
The project at the State Prison of Southern Michigan was determined to be
of "no measurable benefit for those juveniles who toured the prison."[5] It is
becoming more and more obvious that it is not possible to simply scare kids
straight, at least to those who ever thought that there was a possibility.

    The film "Scared Straight" seems to have misled the American public
and some officials into thinking this is a miracle cure for juvenile crime. It
has misrepresented the lifers' Juvenile Awareness Project by overemphasiz-
ing the scare tactics and by giving little or no attention to other aspects of
the lifers' approach. It could result in the brutalizing, terrorizing, and
traumatizing of youngsters across the country. For example, a report from
Pennsylvania about a "scared straight"-type program disclosed that
youngsters had been burned and otherwise physically abused by inmates. It
may cause the exploitation of inmates and, at the same time, the demise of
existing inmate efforts to help youngsters. In the long run, "Scared
Straight," the film, could be the worst thing that ever happened to the
Juvenile Awareness Project.

    Beyond the seemingly inevitable conclusion that it is not possible to
simply scare kids straight, we once again face the folly of searching for

simplistic solutions—for panaceas. That road seems destined to lead only to further failure and frustration.

References

1. BULLINGTON, B., J. SPROWLS, D. KATKIN & M. PHILLIPS. 1978. A critique of diversionary juvenile justice. Crime and Delinquency **24**(1): 59–71.
2. MARTINSON, R. 1974. What works?—questions and answers about prison reform. The Public Interest (Spring): 22–54.
3. GOTTFREDSON, M. R. 1979. Treatment destruction techniques. J. Res. Crime Delinquency **16**(1): 39–54.
4. FINCKENAUER, J. 1979. Juvenile Awareness Project: Evaluation Report No. 2. New Jersey Department of Corrections. Newark, N.J. (Unpublished.)
5. YARBOROUGH, J. 1979. Evaluation of JOLT as a Deterrence Program. Michigan Department of Corrections. (Unpublished.)

A THEORETICAL PERSPECTIVE ON JUVENILE INTERVENTION PROGRAMS: DISCUSSION

Discussant: Leendert P. Mos

Center for Advanced Study in Theoretical Psychology
The University of Alberta
Edmonton, Alberta, Canada T6G 2E9

It is my intent to sketch a theoretical perspective to evaluate intervention programs aimed at delinquency prevention and/or control, and the results obtained by James Finckenauer and colleagues in their study of Juvenile Awareness Project Help (JAPH).[1,2] Briefly, Finckenauer found that Juvenile Awareness Project Help did not influence juveniles' attitudes towards "justice," "law," "policeman," "prison," "punishment," and "self," or towards "punishment" and "obedience"; however, the project did result in more negative attitudes toward "crime." More importantly, the project did not prevent or control subsequent delinquency. In fact there was some evidence of an increase in delinquency and severity of delinquency following JAPH intervention. While these results may be disturbing to some, they should hardly come as a surprise considering the complexity of human conduct.

Traditionally, human conduct is viewed as normatively regulated. The basic assumption being that in the course of development, individuals internalize norms and values of their culture, community, or primary group and that these come to guide behavior. All education and socialization are based upon this assumption, namely that (prescriptive) beliefs are causally efficacious in conduct. Similarly, from this perspective, deviant behavior is viewed as failure to internalize norms and values or as internalization of deviant norms and values. Several ancillary assumptions are usually invoked to complete this story. The acquisition or internalization of norm and value beliefs and changes in these beliefs frequently require an affective context or relationship; and behavior following from these beliefs must have positive consequences for the individual holding such norm and value beliefs. These qualifications are important because they point out that the internalization of prescriptive beliefs must be supplemented by an account of the acquisition and role of beliefs about the anticipations and behavior of others. Indeed the nature of such beliefs, derived from the perceived anticipations of others, takes on a categorical character for the individual not unlike the prescriptive beliefs internalized during the course of socialization. It is the interactive process concerning prescriptions and anticipations that constitutes the basis for self-definition (self-concept). Presumably, prescriptive beliefs come to influence conduct only after the individual has acquired some beliefs about the anticipations of others, and the latter are probably best understood in terms of felt gratification relative to perceived opportunity. In any case, the claim that human behavior is normatively regulated must be qualified by a recognition that beliefs based on the anticipations and behavior of others might well result in suspension of or change in one's prescriptive beliefs, with a view to rationalizing behavior inconsistent with these beliefs but in some sense appropriate to the perceived anticipations of others.

The conceptual distinction between prescriptive beliefs and beliefs about the anticipations of others—one that is honored in one form or another in psychodynamic, behavioristic, and cognitive theories of personality—is made here for the purpose of evaluating intervention programs only. Thus, programs that are solely designed to change individual or group prescriptive beliefs—attitudes, values, and norms—with the assumption that these changes will result in the modification of behavior consistent with these changed prescriptive beliefs, deal with only one-half of the story. Conforming behavior is not merely a function of acquiring community prescriptions; it is also a function of beliefs acquired about the anticipations of others that may or may not have its basis in, or be consistent with, prescription-guided conduct. In fact, others' anticipations are more likely based on categorical attributions of inadequacy as the result of stereotype, prejudice, or ideology—and always on the basis of felt gratification and perceived opportunity experienced in concrete interpersonal relationships.

The distinction between prescriptive beliefs and beliefs based on others' anticipations can be brought out more forcefully if we consider a two-by-two matrix of beliefs about prescriptions and beliefs about others' anticipations. When prescriptive beliefs and beliefs about others' anticipations coincide, we have a situation where community standards are reflected in the anticipations of significant others and representatives of community institutions. Hence, a situation exists where individuals are "insulated against delinquency." In other words the individual in such a community has maximal opportunity for behaving in a prescribed manner and finds his conformity recognized and gratifying. Instrumental behavior is both appropriate to the anticipations and behavior of others and consistent with internalized norms and values. However, if within a particular community prescriptions are uniform but others' anticipations, for whatever reasons, are quite variable and at variance with prescriptions, we might expect behavior that is deviant from prescribed norms but appropriate to conditions of restricted opportunity and limited gratification. Similarly, if prescriptions are variable for members of the same community but the anticipations of others are uniform (a conflict of prescriptions is characteristic of a pluralistic society), we might expect deviant behavior that is nevertheless appropriate to perceived loss of opportunity and gratification. Finally, when both prescriptions and anticipations are variable, even when these coincide for particular subgroups within a larger socially mobile community, we essentially have a situation where individuals are "sensitized to delinquency."

Of course, an analysis in terms of prescriptions, anticipations, and self-identity is not novel, but the perspective does serve to bring out the complex and interdisciplinary nature of studying human conduct. Thus we might theorize about the psychological mechanisms that mediate prescriptions and anticipations (e.g., dissonance); point to self-identity as the pivotal process (rather than the mere information-processing flow from norms to behavior) for understanding (deviant) conduct; and suggest the relevance of biological considerations in the interaction of cognitive (beliefs) and emotional (gratification) factors in socialization and, hence, the development of self-identity. Furthermore the analysis has the virtue of being primarily social in nature. Self-identity has its roots in the perceived anticipations of others—which in turn are based on the self-identity of significant others and representatives of institutions—and the more formal processes of education, instruction, and nurture of prescriptions. Finally, the relative standing of prescription to anticipation beliefs avoids defining deviant behavior as necessarily against something, and instead views it in terms of self-identity validation. Therefore we might better appreciate the tenacity of the deviant behavior of those juveniles who have little to gain by conformity or much to lose by nonconformity.

Many intervention programs rely on the assumption that deviant behavior is either the result of ineffective internalization of prescriptive norms or effective internalization of deviant norms. Within this context, programs may attempt to change the values and attitudes of individuals or groups through some process of modeling or identification using credible or likable models. Alternatively, individual or group programs may attempt to normalize deviant values and attitudes by demonstrating that behavior following from these restricts individual opportunity and gratification—at least in the long run. It is not my intention to be critical of such programs, only to point out that they fail to recognize the importance of the anticipations (and consequent behavior) of others that constitute the basis of beliefs about opportunity and gratification and, hence, a self-identity that may well be at variance with wider community prescriptions. Conduct that is always selective with regard to self-identity can be most effectively modified by changing conditions of opportunity and gratification, that is, by changing the anticipations of significant others and representatives of community institutions. It is probably not too daring to suggest that programs aimed at delinquency control should probably have as their target representatives of community institutions, while prevention programs are best aimed at those who stand in a primary relationship to juveniles. In terms of the preceding matrix of prescriptions and anticipations, prevention programs are most effective when prescriptions are uniform and anticipations vary and when prescriptions vary and anticipations are uniform, while control programs are best restricted to situations where prescriptions and anticipations are at variance resulting in a sensitization to delinquency.

With respect to the Juvenile Awareness Project Help (JAPH), which is based on the deterrence conception of prevention, my preceding sketch suggests certain criticisms. The intent of the JAPH program is to prevent or control delinquency by impressing upon juveniles certain possible consequences of incarceration—consequences primarily of an aggressive and sexual nature committed by inmates against newly incarcerated juveniles. The impact of the program is presumably heightened by the fact that it was initiated and is conducted by inmates ("lifers") in a prison setting. No attempt will be made here to evaluate the proper application of the conception of deterrence; but it should be noted that the evaluation of potential risk (incarceration and assault) of unintended events (deviant behavior) might affect attitudes towards such events (e.g., Finckenauer did find increased negative attitudes toward "crime"), but they are unlikely to affect behavior that may or may not eventually lead to involvement in crime (*certainty,* not severity of punishment, is the most effective aspect of the deterrence notion). This is not to deny the relevance of the rationality of weighing consequences, but to deny the relevance of these consequences when they are far removed from, or irrelevant to, self-identity-validating (deviant) behavior. Another way of making the same point is to note that beliefs acquired on the basis of the lifers' anticipations are unlikely to affect self-identity because lifers are neither significant others nor representatives of community institutions, and they are themselves unsuccessful in maximizing their opportunities and gratification. It is not surprising then that there were no attitudinal effects relating to "law," "justice," "self," etc., since beliefs about these are acquired either as prescriptions or anticipations. According to the preceding analysis, if the juveniles' attitudes towards the "*self*" had in fact changed, we might then have some basis for expecting attitudes towards "policeman," "prison" and "punishment," etc., to have changed. Also, it is not surprising to find some change in attitudes toward the punishment of criminals if we consider that, despite all the verbal threats expressed by the lifers, they remain what they are, namely, lifers, who are losers and perhaps deserving of some consideration (syntony). In summary, with respect to attitude change as a result of JAPH intervention, we might do better to evaluate attitude changes of the interveners (lifers) than of their juvenile victims.

Without effecting changes in self-identity we would not expect changes in behavior. Nevertheless, exposure to JAPH intervention did appear to increase delinquency ("boomerang effect"). This is a puzzling result that deserves continued investigation. It is perhaps not irrelevant to point out, however, that the *content* of this community-sanctioned program is at variance with community prescriptions! This axiological oddity, which deserves study in its own right, might well serve to reinforce the difficulties juveniles face in attempting to forge culturally normative self-identities on the basis of varying prescriptions and anticipations resulting at best in self-deception and at worst in the deception of others. (The fact that JAPH intervention was more successful with nondelinquents than with delinquents supports this notion insofar as the former might well have better established self-identities and, therefore, are better able to consider distant consequences of their behavior.) Finally, while it is no doubt tempting to expose thousands of juveniles to a project that is economically and politically appealing, the time is past when such intervention programs can be implemented without a firm theoretical basis and a quality evaluation component.

REFERENCES

1. FINCKENAUER, J. O. & J. R. STORTI. 1979. Juvenile Awareness Project Help: Evaluation Report No. 1. Rutgers School of Criminal Justice. Newark, N.J.
2. FINCKENAUER, J. O. 1979. Juvenile Awareness Project Help: Evaluation Report No. 2. Rutgers School of Criminal Justice. Newark, N.J.

A SOCIAL PSYCHOLOGIST VIEWS "SCARED STRAIGHT": DISCUSSION

Discussant: Alfred Cohn

New College
Hofstra University
Hempstead, New York 11550

I have chosen to react to the film and to the lifers' program not in terms of whether the latter "works," a matter which I believe will be amply covered in this discussion, but as an academic social psychologist whose interests include persuasion, propaganda, attitude change, youth and identity, the criminal justice system, and ethics. I wish to raise some general questions from this complex frame of reference.

It is well known that the key to the successful solution of a problem in human behavior is often the definition of the problem. If we define our difficulty in cooperating with a coworker as: "He is an arrogant, self-centered, greedy individual," our action is likely to be very different from what it would be if we defined the problem as: "He is a shy and needful individual." The success of our attempts to alter our relationship hinges on the accuracy of our definition.

The lifers are seeking to deter youngsters from running afoul of the law. Their particular target, at least according to the film, is that group of boys and girls who have been, or appear likely to be, "in trouble." Their method of deterrence includes threats, intimidation, emotional shock, loud and angry bullying, and persuasion. They attempt to persuade their youthful targets, primarily with fear-arousing appeals, to eschew antisocial acts.

Let us speculate for a moment about this. Erik Erikson has suggested that young people are sometimes drawn to delinquency as a means of establishing a sense of self, an identity, albeit a "negative" identity. He writes that a "turn towards a negative identity prevails in the delinquent . . . youth of our larger cities, where conditions of economic, ethnic, and religious marginality provide poor bases for any kind of positive identity. If such 'negative identities' are accepted as a youth's 'natural' and final identity by teachers, judges, and psychiatrists, he not infrequently invests his pride as well as his need for total orientation in becoming exactly what the . . . community expects him to become."[1] A negative identity is described as "an identity perversely based on all those identifications and rules which, at critical stages of development, had been presented . . . as most undesirable or dangerous and yet also as most real."[1]

While the effects of fear-arousing appeals are not fully understood, it does seem that they are more influential if an alternative path is clearly mapped so that the target knows what must be done in order to avoid the dreadful fate depicted for him. It has also been suggested that persons who feel vulnerable to the threat may be so frightened as to feel compelled to deny, derogate, or otherwise reject the persuasive appeal altogether. A person who feels incapable of complying with the fear-arousing persuasion is also likely to reject it. Finally, persons who feel competent will be less influenced by such appeals.[2]

Now to the first point. Those young people who establish the "negative identity" of delinquent (a subgroup of youngsters in trouble) would be placed in a frightening conflict situation to the extent that they find the visit to Rahway pertinent and convincing. The conflict is between maintaining the (negative) identity and facing incarceration, on the one hand, and renouncing the (probably hard-won) identity and minimizing the threat of incarceration, on the other.

It is conceivable that, in response to the threat, one might even seek to strengthen the fragile identity by undertaking more delinquent behavior than one might otherwise have done.

A second point has to do with the desirability of exposing young people to this form of "The Treatment" at all. No psychologist could ethically subject research participants to such an experience. Number Seven of the *Ethical Principles in the Conduct of Research with Human Subjects* states that "the ethical investigator protects participants from physical and mental discomfort, harm and danger. If the risk of such consequences exists, the investigator is required to inform the participant of that fact, secure consent before proceeding, and take all possible measures to minimize distress. . . ."[3]

To be sure, dissuading a young person from criminal activity is a worthy goal. Similarly, involving offenders in humane public service is a worthy goal. However, one cannot but wonder whether these goals justify the procedures used and the stress generated. It is a terrible commentary on our country that we have men and women locked up, often for decades, and subject to the dehumanizing experiences and tensions of prison life. One wishes that our fabled ingenuity had yielded less destructive ways of protecting society and punishing malefactors, and it is gratifying to note recent changes in this direction. To me, it is desirable that the American public be made more aware of the conditions of incarceration so that people can be encouraged to develop viable alternatives. The lifers' program, as depicted in the film, is consistent with the latter goal but seems to encourage the very abuses that prisoners and the public ought to be challenging. The risk, as I see it, of viewers saying, "Look how effective our prison system is," is not to be denied.

To the extent that a macho young man feels humiliated in this frightening situation, and to the extent that his identity is threatened by the humiliation, he may attempt to strengthen his sense of self by reasserting his machismo in some antisocial manner.

To the extent that he feels frightened by the experience and lacks a means of coping with it, he may attempt to discredit what the lifers struggled to impart.

To the extent that he is present involuntarily, he may question the values and ethics of those who subject him to this scary program in order to brutalize him into conformity with society's requirements.

There is no denying that crime among young people is a major problem for all of us. Probably half of the people in this room have been victimized in recent years by offenders of tender years and tough exteriors. But the magnitude of the problem does not justify the reflexlike adoption of such a program as this. The very fact that it is appealing to a public that is fed up with young thugs, the very fact that it provides satisfaction and purpose to persons doomed to spend years in cages, makes it attractive at first glance. It seems useful and, if the film is to be believed, effective. It is inexpensive and, if effective in persuasion, probably cost effective as far as the public is concerned. But it appears to treat heterogeneous young people as being "all alike." It fails to take account of the individual differences among the youths exposed to it. Society seems unwilling to provide sufficient personnel and services to aid young people in trouble. Presentation of the lifers' program as a panacea, as is done in this film, allows us all to breathe a sigh of relief. We can "let the cons do it" and feel virtuous and vindicated.

In other words, we, as a society, are encouraged to "cop out." Perhaps some would-be offenders are deterred by this process of emotional flagellation. But where are the *different* strokes for other folks?

REFERENCES

1. ERIKSON, E. H. 1968. Identity: Youth and Crisis: 88, 174. W. W. Norton & Company. New York, N.Y.
2. MIDDLEBROOK, P. N. 1974. Social Psychology and Modern Life: 168–170. Alfred A. Knopf, Inc. New York, N.Y.
3. American Psychological Association. 1973. Ethical Principles in the Conduct of Research with Human Subjects: 61. American Psychological Association. Washington, D.C.

"SCARED STRAIGHT": DISCUSSION

Discussant: William J. Maguire

Rahway Prison
Rahway, New Jersey 07065

It has been said that the whole concept of the Rahway State Prison lifers' program, their Juvenile Awareness Program, can't possibly work. That it simply isn't possible to scare anybody into or out of anything. It's especially not possible to scare people straight.

It's been said that the hard-core criminals, the real dregs of our society who have been indicted, convicted, and incarcerated for the worst kinds of crimes against our society, are the last people on earth to properly impress any youngster and especially a youngster flirting with a life of crime.

Most pointedly, it has been said that the "Scared Straight" Program is self-defeating, that it possibly could have a romanticizing effect on impressionable young people, and that attempts to scare them straight from a life of crime are doomed to failure. This part of the debate surrounding the lifer's program has had the greatest impact on me. This lofty principle that it simply isn't possible and is indeed dangerous to scare anybody in or out of anything has struck me as the worst sort of argument.

Isn't it true that one of the first object lessons we learn as children is that if you play with fire, you're going to get burned? Isn't it true that we, as adults and parents of impressionable young people, have used the phrase for years? Isn't it true that our alcohol and drug-abuse programs, many funded by agencies of our federal government, at least in part try to scare young people straight by emphasizing the ways alcohol and drugs can adversely affect their lives, much the same as crime can affect their lives?

Isn't it true that our bicycle safety programs try to scare young people into realizing the dangers of two on a bike? Isn't it true that the national defensive-driving program, already attended by fifteen million Americans and compulsory if you have been convicted of moving violations, shows a fatal head-on crash in the first segment of its film? Isn't this an attempt to scare us into driving safely?

In so many ways and in so many areas of our young people's lives, in their impressionable years, we try to scare them straight about drugs, alcohol, bicycles, fire, auto safety, venereal disease, and crime. That's what the lifers' program is about. If we added crime to the above list, which the professionals don't want to do, the lifers' program could be viewed as an adult attempt and an innovation to help and influence young people.

There is nothing so very unique about the program. It's people who are there telling young people they don't want them there. Think about this one too: "Life or breath." How many times a night do you see that on TV? I must assume that most of you work during the day, but you must see it at night. "Life or breath." Scaring us away from smoking. I'm a two-pack-a-day guy, and I'll probably not see 90 years of age.

It's really not the scaring straight, but who is doing the scaring, that boggles the mind of the experts. The experts who have been trying for 200 years and have failed. They cannot accept the fact that the scum of society has come up with a program that works. Fifteen thousand children have gone through the program. Don't tell me it doesn't work. I've talked to too many parents. I've talked to too many children. I've talked to too many other experts. Judge Nicola from Middlesex County, one of the originators of the program, monitored 210 of the kids he sent to Rahway Prison personally, and followed them for one year.

He's an expert. I don't challenge him. I don't challenge Judge Kleiner from Burlington County who has sent approximately 300 children through the program and monitored 100 for a period of six months. He is now working on the second six-month period. I don't challenge his credentials. I don't challenge the credentials of Congressman Ike Williams. After the film was shown, it created such a controversy that people from all over the world were writing to the Rahway State Prison asking penal people, judicial people, and probation people: How do we start it in our own state? How do we start it in our own country?

And lo and behold, 69, 90, 120 days prior to that, the Finckenauer report becomes public. I don't challenge the credentials of Professor Finckenauer. He has the academic credentials to do this kind of work. But I do question both the academic background and the work experience of some of his analysts. That is subject to question. His was the only adverse opinion, from a professional, to come forth. But I have already listed half a dozen others. And I can give you a dozen others if you ask for them, I have their names, whose credentials cannot be criticized. They are professionals.

I'm not a professional. I'm a former mayor, one who had the powers of appointment from my juvenile commission. I'm a former county executive, responsible for the operation of our county jail. I'm now in the New Jersey Assembly on appropriations. So before me every year comes an endless line of money seekers. Every year they are looking for more money, more people, and more space—including my commissioner, William Fowler.

So I have a little bit of experience, but I'm not an expert. I have letters with me from parents, and I have letters with me from children. I tell you the program does work. The bottom line is, Who is doing the scaring? It's our convicted felons. That's why the experts are challenging it. I urge you to support the program. We've had over 15,000 children in this program.

The lifers are booked for the next 90 days, 5 days a week, 9:30 in the morning, and 1:30 in the afternoon. The children keep coming. Penal experts send them, mothers send them, school teachers send them, judges send them, psychiatrists send them, and psychologists send them. Are all of these people wrong? Hell, no! And the nice part about it is that—as a taxpayer you will appreciate this—not one penny of the New Jersey taxpayer's money is used to fund this program. Think of your tax dollars that have been spent on our alcoholic problem and look at the success that even the experts agree is marginal.

Look at the tax dollars that have been spent on the drug-abuse programs. Even the experts admit their success has been marginal. Here we have a program that doesn't cost the taxpayers of the State of New Jersey one lousy copper, and the alleged experts are shooting it down. They'll do it over my dead body.

SOCIAL STRESS AND MARITAL VIOLENCE IN A NATIONAL SAMPLE OF AMERICAN FAMILIES*

Murray A. Straus

Department of Sociology
University of New Hampshire
Durham, New Hampshire 03824

The work of the Family Violence Research Program over the past eight years has accumulated evidence that the family is the most violent institution, group, or setting that a typical citizen is likely to encounter.[27,28,29,33] There are of course exceptions, such as the police or the army in time of war. But the typical citizen has a high probability of being violently assaulted only in his or her own home.

This can be made clear (without, at this point, giving detailed statistics) by pointing out that the Uniform Crime Reports give data on violent crimes in rates per hundred thousand. By contrast, we found it more appropriate to report rates per *hundred,* rather than per hundred thousand or even per thousand.[33]

THE PARADOX OF FAMILY VIOLENCE AND FAMILY STRESS

Family Violence

These data point to the first of many ironies or paradoxes about the family. In this case, the paradox is that the family is also the group to which people look for love, support, and gentleness. The hallmark of family life is *both* love and violence.

Much of the work of the Family Violence Research Program at the University of New Hampshire has been designed to unravel this paradox. We are a long way from a complete explanation. However, some progress has been made. This paper examines one of the several factors that contribute to the explanation: the link between stress and violence.

Stress in Families

Another irony of family life is that, although the family is often seen as a place where one can find respite from the tensions of the world, the family tends to be a group with an inherently high level of conflict and stress.

* This paper is one of a series of publications of the Family Violence Research Program at the University of New Hampshire. The program is supported by the University of New Hampshire and by National Institute of Mental Health Grants MH27557 and T32–MH15161.

The theoretical case for this view is presented in detail elsewhere.[6,10] In this paper, there is space to illustrate only two of the stress-producing factors of the family.

First, in addition to the normal differences and conflicts between two or more people, the family has built into its basic structure the "battle of the sexes" and the so-called generation gap.

A second source of stress is inherent in what is expected of families. For example, families are expected to provide adequate food, clothing, and shelter in a society that does not always provide the necessary resources to do this. Another example is the expectation that families bring up healthy, well-adjusted, law-abiding, and intelligent children who can get ahead in the world. The stress occurs because these traits and the opportunity to get ahead are factors beyond the control of any given family to a greater or lesser extent.

The basic argument of the paper is that the second of these stress-producing factors is part of the explanation for the first. Specifically, a major cause of the high rate of violence in families is the high level of stress and conflict characteristic of families. Of course, this is only a plausible argument. Brenner, for example, has shown a clear relationship between stress as indexed by unemployment rate and the rate of assault and homicide in the United States, Canada, and Great Britain.[3] But is it other members of their own families who are assaulted or murdered by the unemployed? This needs to be demonstrated with empirical data. Consequently, a major part of this paper is devoted to such an empirical study.

THE THEORETICAL MODEL

Although the empirical findings will start with the relationship between the levels of stress and violence in families, it is not argued that stress *directly* causes violence. Violence is only one of many possible responses to stress. Among the alternatives are passivity, resignation, or just leaving. University departments, for example, are also stressful environments, but the rate of physical violence within such departments is close to zero.

The absence of a *necessary* link between stress and violence is shown in Brenner's data on the correlates of unemployment.[3] Unemployment is highly correlated with assault and homicide. But it is also correlated with hypertension, deaths from heart attacks, mental hospital admissions, and alcoholism. Similarly, Brown and Harris[4] studied a random sample of women in London, using highly reliable and valid data on life stresses. They demonstrated a clear tendency for these women to respond to stress by *depression* rather than violence.

Mediating Variables

FIGURE 1 suggests that other factors must be present for stress to result in violence. The center box of FIGURE 1 illustrates some of the other variables that must also be present to produce a correlation between stress and violence. For example, people are unlikely to respond to stress by violence unless this is part of the socially scripted method of dealing with stress and frustration—as it is in our society. Therefore, an important part of the model is the existence of norms or images of behavior that depict striking out at others when under stress as part of human nature.

However, these are very general behavioral scripts. They cannot explain *family* violence because they are part of the society's image of basic nature in *all* types of situations. These general scripts may be part of the explanation, but they are not sufficient. To find the additional variables that will lead to a sufficient explanation, one has to look at the nature of the family itself.

Normative Legitimacy of Family Violence

One very simple, but nonetheless important, factor is that the family has different rules about violence than do other groups. In an academic department, an office, or a factory, the basic rule is that no one can hit anyone else, no matter what they do wrong. A person can be a pest, an intolerable bore, negligent, incompetent, selfish, or unwilling to listen to reason. But that still does not give anyone the right to hit such a person. In

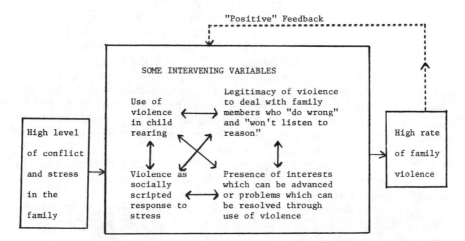

FIGURE 1. Partial model of relationship between stress and family violence. This diagram is labeled as a partial model for two main reasons: The most obvious reason is that it includes only a sampling of the intervening variables that could be included in the center box. Second, the model omits negative feedback loops (i.e., deviation dampening processes) which must be present. Without them the violence would escalate to the point where the system would self-destruct—as it sometimes, but not typically, does. See Reference 27 for a systems model of family violence which includes negative feedback processes and other elements of a cybernetic system.

the family the situation is different. There, the basic rule is that if someone does wrong and won't listen to reason, violence is permissible and sometimes even required.

This is clearly the case in respect to the rights and obligations of parents; but it also applies to spouses. As one husband said about an incident in which his wife threw a coffee pot at him: "I was running around with other women—I deserved it." Statements like that are made by many husbands and wives. In fact, the evidence suggests that a marriage license is also a hitting license.[28,31] Still, that does not explain why or how such a norm arose or why it persists. Here again, there are a number of factors, one of which is the use of violence in child rearing, that is, physical punishment (FIGURE 1).

Family Socialization in Violence

Physical punishment provides the society's basic training in violence but, of course, training that applies most directly to behavior in the family. At least some use of physical punishment is just about universal in American society, typically beginning in infancy.[24] What are the reasons for saying that learning about violence starts with physical punishment?

When physical punishment is used, several things can be expected to occur. Most obviously, the infant or child learns to do or not to do whatever the punishment is intended to teach; for example, to not pick up things from the ground and put them in his or her mouth. Less obvious, but equally or more important, are four other lessons, which are so deeply learned that they become an integral part of one's personality and world view.

The first of these unintended consequences is the association of love with violence. Parents are the first and usually the only ones to hit an infant. For most children this continues throughout childhood.[26] The child therefore learns that his or her primary love objects are also those who hit.

Second, since physical punishment is used to train the child or to teach about which dangerous things are to be avoided, it establishes the moral rightness of hitting other family members.

The third unintended consequence is the "Johnny I've told you ten times" principle—that when something is really important, it justifies the use of physical force.

Fourth is the idea that when one is under stress, tense, or angry, hitting—although wrong—is "understandable," i.e., to a certain extent legitimate.

Involuntary Nature of Family Membership

The last of the mediating variables for which there is space to discuss is the simple fact that the family is only a semivoluntary institution. This is most obvious in the case of children. They cannot leave, nor can parents throw them out, until a legally set age. So leaving—which is probably the most widely used and effective method of avoiding violence—is not available as an alternative in the parent-child aspect of the family.

To a considerable extent the same is true for the marital relationship. Ninety-four percent of the population marries, and anything done by this large percent of the population is not likely to be voluntary. No system of socialization is that effective. In fact, we all know the tremendous informal social pressures that are put on people to get married and stay married. Although divorces are now easier to get, the economic, social, and emotional barriers to breaking up a marital relationship are still extremely strong. Even couples who are living together without a formal marriage find it difficult to end the relationship. In cities like Boston and New York, there is a booming business in marriage counseling for the unmarried.

There are a number of other factors that should be included in FIGURE 1 and in this discussion. Those that have been discussed, however, should be sufficient to illustrate the theory that guided the analysis reported in this paper.†

By way of summary, the theory underlying this paper rejects the idea that people have an innate drive toward aggression, or an innate tendency to respond to stress by aggression. Rather, a link between stress and aggression occurs only if (a) the individual has learned an "aggressive" response to stress; (b) if such a response is a culturally recognized script for behavior under stress; and (c) if the situation seems to be one that will produce rewards for aggression.

SAMPLE

The data used to examine this theory were obtained in January and February of 1976. Interviews were conducted with a national area-probability sample of 2,143 adults. To be eligible for inclusion in the sample, each respondent had to be between 18 and 70 years of age and living with a member of the opposite sex as a couple. However, the couple did not have to be formally married. A random half of the respondents were female and half were male. Interviews lasted approximately one hour and were completely anonymous. Furthermore, interviewers were of the language or racial group that was predominant in the sampling area for which they were responsible. Further details on the sample are given in Straus, Gelles, and Steinmetz.[33]

---

† FIGURE 1 illustrates the general nature of the theory, without listing all of the variables that need to be taken into account. There are two aspects of the model that are included simply to alert readers to their importance, but that are not analyzed. First, this paper will not deal with feedback processes. Second, in the center box the arrows show that each intervening variable is related to the others. They are a mutually supporting system, and interaction effects are no doubt also present. However, in this paper, these and other intervening variables will be dealt with singly.

DEFINITIONS AND MEASURES OF STRESS

There has been a vast debate on the concept of stress.[15,16,18,19,22,23] For example, one issue is whether stress is a property of the situation (such as illness, unemployment, family conflict, getting married, or getting promoted to a new job) or whether it is a subjective experience. For some people a new set of job responsibilities is experienced as stress, whereas for others, *lack* of such new responsibility is a stress.

The definition of stress used here treats stress as a function of the interaction of the subjectively defined demands of a situation and the capabilities of an individual or group to respond to these demands. Stress exists when the subjectively experienced demands are inconsistent with response capabilities. This inconsistency can be demands in excess of capabilities or a low level of demand relative to response capabilities.‡

In fact, there is a gap between the definition of stress given above and data I will actually report. This is because the methodology of this paper *assumes* (a) that some life event, such as moving or the illness of a child, produces a certain but unknown degree of demand on parents; (b) that on the average this is subjectively experienced as a demand; (c) that the capabilities of parents to respond to these demands will not always be sufficient; and (d) that the result is a certain level of stress. On the basis of these assumptions, it is then possible to investigate the relationship between such stressful life events and the level of violence in the family. Obviously, that leaves a large agenda for other investigators to develop a more adequate measure of stress.

As indicated in TABLES 1 and 2, the aspect of stress that is measured in this study is limited to what are called "stressor stimuli." The data were obtained by a modified version of the Holmes and Rahe stressful life events scale.[13] Because of limited interview time, the scale was restricted to the 18 items listed in TABLE 1. (See APPENDIX, Section I.) The scores on this scale ranged from 0 to 18, with a mean of 2.4 and a standard deviation of 2.1. In addition to the overall stress score, we also considered different subgroupings of items. The subscores and their means are given in TABLE 2.

Sex Differences

The first thing to notice in TABLE 1 is that the experiences reported by the men and women respondents are quite similar. The exceptions are events for which men and women have different exposure. Thus, fewer women have paid employment, so it is not surprising that two to three times as many men as women experienced an occupationally related stress, such

‡ A more adequate formulation of stress includes a number of other elements. Farrington[6] has identified six components used in research on stress: the stressor stimulus, objective demands, subjective demands, response capabilities, choice of response, and stress level. Important as these six components are, there is no way to investigate them with the data from the sample.

TABLE 1

PERCENT EXPERIENCING 18 LIFE STRESSES DURING PREVIOUS YEAR

Life Event	Male (N = 960)	Female (N = 1,183)	Total (N = 2,143)
1. Troubles with the boss	25.8	9.9	17.0
2. Troubles with other people at work	31.4	11.2	20.3
3. Got laid off or fired from work	10.0	5.9	7.7
4. Got arrested or convicted of something serious	1.9	0.9	1.3
5. Death of someone close	41.5	38.8	40.0
6. Foreclosure of a mortgage or loan	1.5	1.6	1.6
7. Being pregnant or having a child born	8.1	15.8	12.4
8. Serious sickness or injury	18.9	16.7	17.6
9. Serious problem with health or behavior of a family member	23.0	29.0	26.3
10. Sexual difficulties	9.0	13.1	11.6
11. In-law troubles	10.9	12.0	11.5
12. A lot worse off financially	15.8	12.1	13.7
13. Separated or divorced	3.6	2.6	3.0
14. Big increase in arguments with spouse/partner	8.1	9.4	8.8
15. Big increase in hours worked or job responsibilities	28.9	16.3	21.9
16. Moved to different neighborhood or town	17.2	16.4	16.8
17. Child kicked out of school or suspended	1.6	1.6	1.6
18. Child got caught doing something illegal	2.7	3.0	2.8

as troubles with a boss or losing a job.§ There are a few other interesting sex differences.

Item 4 shows that twice as many men were arrested or convicted of a serious crime. An interesting sidelight is that to a noncriminologist, an annual arrest or conviction rate of 2 per 100 men seems quite high.

The only other item with a nontrivial difference is item 10, having had some type of sexual problem in the previous year. The rate for women is half again higher than the rate for men (13.1 versus 9.0).

Frequency of Different Stressors

The most frequently occurring stress among the 18 items is the death of someone close to the respondent (item 5). This happened to 40% of our respondents during the year we asked about. The next most frequent stress is closely related—a serious problem with the health or behavior of someone in the family (item 9). This occurred in the lives of about one out of four. For men, however, occupational stresses occurred more frequently. Item 2 shows that about 30% had a difficulty with their boss, and at the positive end about the same percentage had a large increase in their work responsibilities (item 15).

§ The sex difference in item 7 (being pregnant or having a child) is probably due to men misunderstanding the question. It was meant to apply to the men as well as the women in the sample, in the sense of whether the wife was pregnant or had a child in the last year.

TABLE 2

MEAN SCORES ON STRESS INDEXES

Index	Items	Mean Score*		
		Male (N = 960)	Female (N = 1,183)	Total (N = 2,143)
Overall stress index	1 to 18	14.9	12.4	13.5
Occupational stress	1, 2, 15	28.7	12.4	19.7
Economic stress	3, 6, 12	9.0	6.5	7.6
Occupational and economic stress	Occ. + Econ.			27.3
Interpersonal stress	5, 9, 11, 16	23.1	24.1	23.6
Health stress	7, 8	13.3	16.2	14.9
Spousal stress	10, 13, 14	7.1	8.2	7.7
Parental stress	17, 18	2.7	3.1	2.9
Nuclear family stress	Spousal + Parental	14.3	14.2	14.2

* The scores are in percentage form in order to make the scores on each index somewhat comparable. Each is a percentage of the maximum possible raw score. Thus, a mean of 14.9 on the overall stress index means that this group averaged 14.9% of the 18 points that are possible; a mean of 28.7 on the occupational stress index means that this group averaged 28.7% of the three points that are possible on this index. See Reference 35, Chapter 2 for further explanation of percentage standardization.

DEFINITION AND MEASURES OF VIOLENCE

I can deal more adequately—both conceptually and operationally—with violence. This is because violence has been the focus of my research on families for the past seven years, and is the main focus of this study.

The definition of violence that underlies this research treats violence as one type of aggressive act. Therefore, I will first define aggression. *Aggression* is an act carried out with the intention of, or perceived as having the intention of, hurting another person. *Violence* is an act carried out with the intention or perceived intention to cause physical hurt, pain, or injury to another person. Violence, as I am using that term, is therefore synonymous with physical aggression.

Although this is the basic definition of violence used in studies undertaken as part of the Family Violence Research Program at the University of New Hampshire, it is usually necessary to take into account a number of other characteristics of the violent act. These include (a) the severity of the act, ranging from a slap to torture and murder; (b) whether it is instrumental to some other purpose, such as forcing another to do or not to do something, or expressive, i.e., an end in itself; (c) whether it is a culturally permitted or required act, or one that runs counter to cultural norms (legitimate versus illegitimate, or criminal, violence).

To illustrate these three dimensions in relation to violence within the family—a child may be slapped mildly for some misdeed or beaten so severely that medical treatment is necessary; the spanking or beating may be instrumental to teaching the child not to run into a busy street, or it may be done out of exasperation and anger—and the child may be of an age when the legitimacy of parents hitting a child is virtually unquestioned, as compared to the general illegitimacy in our society of hitting an 18-year-old child.

As in the case of the measurement of stress, there is a gap between what this set of definitions demands and what is available for analysis. The technique used is known as the Conflict Tactics Scales.[30] It consists of a check list of acts of physical violence. Respondents were asked about conflicts and difficulties with other family members. They were then asked whether, in the course of such conflicts in the past year, any of the items on the list had occurred. The list starts with nonviolent tactics, such as talking things over, and then proceeds on to verbally aggressive tactics, and finally to physical aggression, that is, violent acts.

The descriptions of violent acts in turn were designed to permit a measure of the severity as well as the frequency of family violence. The list starts out with pushing, slapping, shoving, and throwing things. These are what can be called the "ordinary" or "normal" violence of family life. It then goes on to kicking, biting, punching, hitting with an object, beating up, and using a knife or gun. This latter group of items was used to compute a measure of "severe violence," which is comparable to what social workers call child abuse, feminists would call wife beating, and criminologists would call assaults.

TABLE 3

INCIDENCE RATES FOR SEVERE VIOLENCE INDEX, OVERALL VIOLENCE INDEX, AND ITEMS MAKING UP THESE INDEXES

Conflict Tactics Scale Violence Indexes and Items	Rate Per 100 for Violence By:		Frequency*			
			Mean		Median	
	H	W	H	W	H	W
Wife Beating and Husband Beating (N to R)	3.8	4.6	8.0	8.9	2.4	3.0
Overall Violence Index (K to R)	12.1	11.6	8.8	10.1	2.5	3.0
K. Threw something at spouse	2.8	5.2	5.5	4.5	2.2	2.0
L. Pushed, grabbed, shoved spouse	10.7	8.3	4.2	4.6	2.0	2.1
M. Slapped spouse	5.1	4.6	4.2	3.5	1.6	1.9
N. Kicked, bit, or hit with fist	2.4	3.1	4.8	4.6	1.9	2.3
O. Hit or tried to hit with something	2.2	3.0	4.5	7.4	2.0	3.8
P. Beat up spouse	1.1	0.6	5.5	3.9	1.7	1.4
Q. Threatened with a knife or gun	0.4	0.6	4.6	3.1	1.8	2.0
R. Used a knife or gun	0.3	0.2	5.3	1.8	1.5	1.5

* For those who engaged in each act, i.e., omits those with scores of zero.

It can be seen from this description of the violence indexes of the Conflict Tactics Scales that they take into account the dimensions of intent and severity. However, we do not have data on whether the act was primarily instrumental versus expressive, or on whether the act was one that the members of that family believed to be illegitimate or, in the circumstances, legitimate.

Spouse Violence Rates

The first row of TABLE 3 shows that violence by a husband against his wife that was serious enough to be classified as wife beating occurred as a rate of 3.8 per 100 couples. Violence by a wife serious enough to be classified as husband beating occurred at an even higher rate—4.6 per 100 couples. However, it is important to remember that these data are based on attacks, rather than on injuries produced. If one uses injuries as the criterion, then wife beating would far outdistance husband beating. (See APPENDIX, II.)

What proportion of these attacks were isolated incidents? Our data suggest that this was rarely the case. For those who experienced an assault, the medians in the last column of TABLE 3 show that assaults happened about three times during the year. If the means are used as the measure of the frequency of occurrence, the figure is much higher—about eight or nine times. But this is because of a relatively few couples at the extreme for whom such violence was just about a weekly event.

STRESSFUL LIFE EVENTS AND ASSAULT BETWEEN SPOUSES

For purposes of this analysis, the Stress Index was transferred to Z scores and grouped into categories of half a Z score. Therefore, in FIGURE 2, each horizontal axis category indicates the families who fall within a band that is half a standard deviation wide.

The data plotted in FIGURE 2 clearly show that the higher the stress score, the higher the rate of assault between husband and wife. For the wives, the curve approximately fits a power function. For the husbands the relationship shows a general upward trend, but is irregular.¶

Both the smooth shape of the curve and the fact that the line plotted for the women is above the line for the men at the high stress end of the graph suggest that stress has more effect on violence by wives than on violence by husbands. At the low end of the scale, women in the −1.0 to −1.4 stress group have an assault rate about half that of the men in this group (1.1 per 100 versus 2.2 for the men). But at the high stress end of the

¶ The numbers of husbands and wives, on which each of the rates in FIGURE 2 is based, are: −1.0 = 361 and 365; −0.5 = 459 and 460; 0.0 = 414 and 415; +0.1 = 304 and 303; +0.6 = 224 and 218; +1.1 = 128 and 129; +1.6 = 45 and 45; +2.1 = 103 and 105.

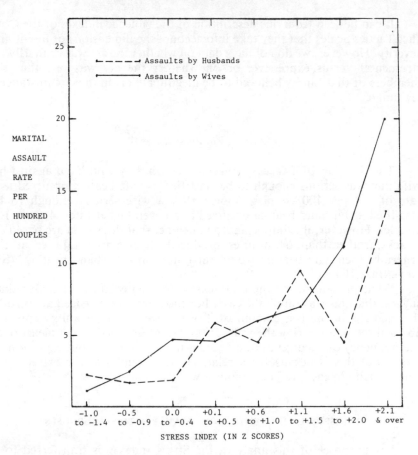

FIGURE 2. Marital assault rate by stress index score.

scale, women in the +1.6 to +2.0 and +2.1 and over categories have assault rates that are, respectively, 150% and 50% greater than the rates for the husbands who experienced this much stress. It seems that in the absence of stress, women are less violent to their spouse than are men, but under stressful conditions women are more violent.

An analysis identical to that in FIGURE 2 was done, except that the dependent variable was not limited to the types of severely violent acts used in FIGURE 2. That is, the measure included pushing, slapping, shoving, and throwing things. Except for the fact that the rates are much higher—they start at 5 per 100 and range up to 48 per 100—the results are very similar.

The importance of this similarity is that it helps establish a connection that is extremely important for understanding serious assaults. Again and again in our research, we find a clear connection between the "ordinary" violence of family life, such as spanking children or pushing or slapping a spouse, and serious violence, such as child abuse and wife beating. Actually, the connection goes further. *Verbal* aggression is also part of this pattern

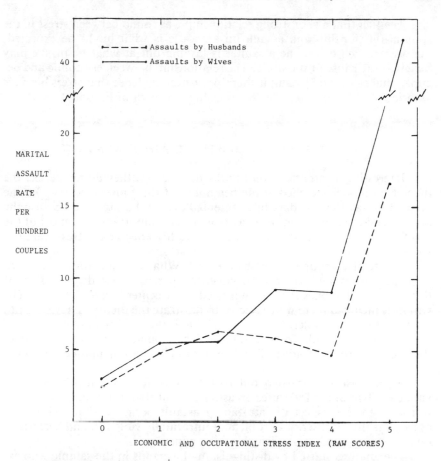

FIGURE 3. Marital assault rate by economic plus occupational stress index.

of relationships. People who hurt another family member verbally are also the ones most likely to hurt them physically.[29] Moreover, the same set of causal factors applies to both the milder forms of violence and acts of violence that are serious enough to be considered child abuse or an assault on a spouse. The similarity of the relationship between stress and the overall violence index and the relationship between stress and serious assaults is but one of many such examples found for this sample.[33]

TYPES OF STRESSORS AND ASSAULTS

The analyses just reported were also carried out using each of the stress subscores listed in TABLE 2 as the independent variable. In each case, as the amount of stress increased, so did the assault rate. These relationships were strongest for the "spousal stress" and the "economic plus occupational stress" subscores.

The fact that a very strong relationship was found between stress in the spousal relationship and assault on a spouse is what might be expected, because in such cases, the assaulter is lashing out at what he or she may believe is the cause of the stress. The relationship between economic and occupational stress and assault is therefore better evidence that stress per se is associated with violence. This relationship is shown in FIGURE 3.‖

FACTORS LINKING STRESS AND WIFE BEATING

Interesting as are the findings presented so far, they do not reflect the theoretical model sketched at the beginning of this paper (FIGURE 1). One might even say that the data just presented distort the situation because the graphs tend to draw attention away from a very important fact: most of the couples in this sample who were subject to a high degree of stress were not violent.

A critical question is raised by this fact. What accounts for the fact that some people respond to stress by violence whereas others do not? Part of the answer to that question was suggested in the center box of FIGURE 1. The variables included there were selected to illustrate the theory. They were not intended to be a complete list, either of what is theoretically important or of the variables available for this sample. The available data actually cover three of the four variables listed in FIGURE 1 plus a number of other variables.

An analysis was carried out to take into account these intervening variables. This analysis focuses on assaults by husbands on their wives. It is restricted to this aspect of intrafamily assault because, along with child abuse, it is the most serious problem of intrafamily violence, and because of limitations imposed by the length of the paper.

The analysis started by distinguishing husbands in the sample who experienced none of the stressful events in the past year ($N = 139$) from those in the high quartile of the index ($N = 258$). Each of these groups was further divided into those who were in the high quartile of each mediating variable versus those in the low quartile. This enables us to see if the presumed mediating variable was, as specified in the theoretical model, necessary for life stresses to result in violence.

If the theory outlined in FIGURE 1 is correct, the men who had the combination of high stress and the presence of a mediating variable will have a high rate of violence, whereas the men who experienced a similar high amount of stress but without the presence of mediating variable will *not* be more violent than the sample as a whole, despite the fact that they were under as much stress during the year as the others.

‖ The numbers of husbands and wives, on which each of the rates in FIGURE 3 is based, are: 0 = 1,053 and 1,058; 1 = 544 and 548; 2 = 258 and 256; 3 = 135 and 130; 4 = 43 and 44; 5 = 12 and 12.

TABLE 4

EFFECT OF INTERVENING VARIABLES ON THE INCIDENCE OF ASSAULT BY HUSBANDS
EXPERIENCING HIGH STRESS

Intervening Variable	Assault Rate per 100 Husbands when Intervening Variable Was:		N*	
	Low	High	Low	High
A. Childhood Experience With Violence				
Physical punishment after age 12 by mother (0 vs. 4+ per yr)	7.1	6.7	85	89
Physical punishment after age 12 by father (0 vs. 4+ per yr)	7.4	8.4	81	83
Husband's father hit his mother (0 vs. 1+ per yr)	5.4	17.1	167	41
Husband's mother hit his father (0 vs. 1+ per yr)	4.6	23.5	176	34
B. Legitimacy of Family Violence				
Approval of parents slapping a 12-year-old (0 vs. high ¼)	5.9	9.9	34	71
Approval of slapping a spouse (0 vs. any approval)	2.7	15.0	150	100
C. Marital Satisfaction and Importance				
Marital satisfaction index (low vs. high quartile)	12.3	4.9	73	61
Marriage less important to husband than to wife = high	5.9	11.7	17	34
D. Socioeconomic Status				
Education (high vs. low quartile)	6.1	5.4	49	56
Husband a blue collar worker = low	9.2	5.4	284	202*
Income (low ≤ $9,000, high ≥ $22,500)	16.4	3.5	122	113*
E. Marital Power				
Power norm index (high = husband should have final say)	4.2	16.3	71	55
Decision power index (high = husband has final say)	5.2	16.1	58	62
F. Social Integration				
Organizational participation index (0 vs. 11+)	10.5	1.7	86	60
Religious service attendance (0–1/yr vs. weekly)	8.9	5.4	79	56
Relatives living near (0–2 vs. 13+)	5.7	11.9	124	118*

* The Ns vary because, even though the intent was for the high and low groups to be the
upper and lower quartiles, this was not always possible. In the case of occupational class, for
example, the comparison is between a dichotomous nominal variable. In the case of continuous variables, we sometimes wanted to preserve the intrinsic meaning of a score category, such
as those with a score of zero, even though this might be more or less than 25% of the sample.
Another factor causing the Ns to vary is that the division into quartiles was based on the distribution for the entire sample of 2,143 rather than just the high stress subgroup analyzed in this
table. Finally, there are three variables for which the data were obtained from the wife as well
as the husband (husband's occupation, family income, and relatives living nearby). The Ns for
these variables are roughly double those for the other variables because they are based on the
entire sample, rather than only on those families where the husband was the respondent.

Socialization for Violence

The first row of TABLE 4 runs directly contrary to the theory being examined. It shows that the men who were physically punished the most by
their mother when they were teenagers were slightly *less* violent under stress
than the men who were not or only rarely hit at this age by their mother. On
the other hand, having been physically punished on more than just a rare

occasion by a *father* does relate to assaulting a wife. Husbands whose father hit them the most have an assault rate against their wives that is slightly higher than do husbands who were under equally high stress that year but who did not experience this much violence directed against them as a teenager. The difference between the effect of having been hit by one's mother versus by one's father suggests that violence by the father against a teenage boy is a more influential role model for violent behavior that the son will later display under stress.

The next two rows of TABLE 4 refer to violence *between the parents* of the husbands in this sample. These two rows show large differences between husbands who are the sons of parents who engaged in physical fights and those who are sons of parents who did not. The assault rate by husbands whose own father had hit their mother was 216% higher than the rate for the men whose father never hit their mother (17.1 per 100 vs. 5.4). Surprisingly, the largest difference of all is in the much greater assault rate by husbands who had grown up in families where their *mother* had hit their father. This contradicts the idea of the same sex parent being a more influential role model. Whatever the intervening process, however, Section A of TABLE 4 shows that the men who assaulted their wives were exposed to more family violence as teenagers than were the men who were not violent despite an equally high level of stress.

Legitimacy of Family Violence

Section B of TABLE 4 reports "semantic differential" scores[20] in response to questions about slapping a child and slapping one's husband or wife. Each score is made up by combining the ratings for how "necessary," "normal," and "good" the respondent rated slapping.

The first row of Section B shows that husbands who approved of slapping a child had a 68% greater rate of assaulting their wives than did the husbands with a score of zero on this index. When it comes to approval of slapping *a spouse,* there is a 456% difference in the predicted direction. These findings are consistent with the theoretical model asserting that the relation between stress and violence is a process that is mediated by social norms, rather than a direct biologically determined relationship. However, since these are cross-sectional data, the findings do not prove the correctness of the model. It is also quite plausible to interpret the greater assault rate by men who approve of violence as an after-the-fact justification. Except for a few variables that clearly occurred at a previous time, such as violence experienced as a child, this caution applies to most of the findings to be reported.

Marital Satisfaction and Importance

The first row of Section C compares men who were low in marital satisfaction with men in the high quartile. The low quartile men had a 151%

higher assault rate. A similar difference is shown by comparing men who rated their marriages as a less important part of their lives than the marriage played in the lives of their wives. Of course, these differences, like a number of others reported in this paper, could reflect the effect of marital violence rather than the cause. Only a longitudinal study can adequately sort out this critical issue. The findings of this study are not inconsistent with the idea that men under stress are more likely to be violent if they do not find the marriage a rewarding and important part of their lives.

Socioeconomic Status

Three aspects of socioeconomic status are examined in Section D of TABLE 4. The first of these, the educational level of the couple, shows findings that many will find surprising. The husbands in the high quartile of education were only slightly less violent than those in the low quartile. This is inconsistent with the widely held view that less educated people are more violent. Actually, a careful review of the available studies fails to support this widespread idea.[31] A number of studies (including an analysis of this sample[7]) suggest there is little or no difference in aggression and violence according to education.

On the other hand, when it comes to indicators of present socioeconomic position, the low groups are, as expected, more violent. The second row of Section D, for example, shows that the assault rate of blue collar husbands is 70% greater than the assault rate of the white collar employed husbands. If the combined income of the couple was $9,000 or less, the rate of assault by husbands on their wives was 368% higher than in families with a more adequate income (16.4 per 100 versus 3.5 per 100).

What could account for the sharply different findings for education as compared to occupation and income? One fairly straightforward possibility is that low income and low status occupations are indirect indicators of even more stress than is measured by the stress index. Low or high education, on the other hand, does not necessarily mean that the couple is currently in an economically bad position, such as is indicated by a total family income of $9,000 and under.

Marital Power

One of the most important factors accounting for the high rate of marital violence is the use of force by men as the "ultimate resource" to back up their position as "head" of the family.[1,12,28,29] Section E provides evidence that this may be part of the explanation for why some men assault their wives when under stress and others do not.

The first row of Section E shows that the assault rate of husbands who feel that husbands *should have* the final say in most family decisions is 288% higher than it is for husbands who are not committed to such male dominance norms. The second row suggests that when this is translated into actual decision power, the differences are almost as great. The husbands who actually did have the final say in most family decisions had an assault rate of 16.1 per 100 as compared 5.2 for the husbands who were also under high stress but shared decisions with their wives.

Social Integration and Isolation

The last set of mediating factors included in this paper explores the theory that violence will be higher in the absence of a network of personal ties. Such ties can provide help in dealing with the stresses of life, and perhaps intervene when disputes within the family become violent.

The first row of Section F shows that men who belonged to no organizations (such as clubs, lodges, business or professional organizations, or unions) had a higher rate of assault than did the men who participated in many such organizations. The same applies to men who attended religious services as compared to men who rarely or never attended services.

The third row of Section F, however, shows opposite results. Couples who had many relatives living within an hour's travel time had a *higher* rate of assault than did couples with few relatives nearby. This finding is not necessarily inconsistent with social network theory. The usual formulation of that theory *assumes* that the network will be prosocial.That is usually a reasonable assumption. However, a social network can also support antisocial behavior. This is the essence of the differential association theory of criminal behavior. A juvenile gang is an example.

In respect to the family, Bott[2] and others have shown that involvement in a closed network helps maintain sexually segregated family roles, whereas couples not tied into such networks tend to have a more equal and shared-task type of family organization and to be less traditional.[25] In the present case, the assumption that the kin network will be opposed to violence is not necessarily correct. For example, a number of women indicated that when they left their husband because of a violent attack, their mothers responded with urgings for the wife to deal with the situation by being a better housekeeper, by being a better sex partner, or by just avoiding him, etc. In some cases, the advice was "you just have to put up with it for the sake of the kids—that's what I did."

SUMMARY AND CONCLUSIONS

This study was designed to determine the extent to which stressful life experiences are associated with assault between husbands and wives, and to explore the reasons for such an associaton. The data used to answer these questions come from a nationally representative sample of 2,143 American couples. Stress was measured by an instrument patterned after the Holmes and Rahe scale. It consisted of a list of 18 stressful events that could have occurred during the year covered by the survey. Assault was measured by the severe violence index of the family Conflict Tactics Scales. This consists of whether any of the following violent acts had occurred in the course of a family dispute during the past year: punching, kicking, biting, hitting with an object, beating up, and using a knife or gun.

The findings show that respondents who experienced none of the 18 stresses in the index had the lowest rate of assault. The assault rate increased as the number of stresses experienced during the year increased. This applies to assaults by wives as well as by husbands but is most clear in the case of the wives. Wives with a stress score of zero had a lower rate of assault as compared to the assaults by husbands with a stress score of zero. But the assault rate of wives climbed steadily with each increment of stress, and gradually became greater than the assault rate of the husbands. Thus, although wives were less assaultive under normal conditions, under stress they were more assaultive than the husbands.

The second part of the analysis was based on the theory that stress by itself does not necessarily lead to violence. Rather, it was assumed that other factors must be present. Several such factors were examined by focusing on men who were in the top quartile in stresses experienced during the year. These men were divided into low and high groups on the basis of variables that might account for the correlation between stress and violence. If the theory is correct, the men who were in the high group of the presumed intervening or mediating variable should have a high assault rate, whereas the men in the low group on these variables should not be more assaultive than the sample as a whole, despite the fact that they were under as much stress during the year as were the other high-stress subgroup of men.

The results were generally consistent with this theory. They suggest the following conclusions:

1. Physical punishment by fathers and parents who hit each other train men to respond to stress by violence.

2. Men who assault their wives believe that physical punishment of children and slapping a spouse are appropriate behavior. Their early experience with violence therefore seems to have carried over into their present normative stance. However, a longitudinal study is needed to establish whether this is actually the causal direction.

3. Men under stress are more likely to assault their wives if the marriage is not an important and rewarding part of their life.

4. Education does not affect the link between stress and violence. However, low income and a low status occupation do, perhaps because these are indicators of additional stresses.

5. Men who believe that husbands should be the dominant person in a marriage, and especially husbands who have actually achieved such a power position, had assault rates from one and a half to three times higher than the men in more equalitarian marriages who were also under stress.

6. Men who were socially isolated (in the sense of not participating in unions, clubs, or other organizations) had higher rates of assault on their wives, whereas men who were involved in supportive networks only rarely assaulted their wives despite being under extremely high stress.

Of course, these conclusions, although consistent with the findings reported in this paper, are not proved by the findings. Many of the findings are open to other equally plausible interpretations, particularly as to causal direction. The question of causal direction can only be adequately dealt with by a longitudinal study. In the absence of such prospective data, the following conclusions must be regarded as only what the study suggests about the etiology of intrafamily violence.

We assume that human beings have an inherent capacity for violence, just as they have an inherent capacity for doing algebra. This capacity is translated into actually solving an equation, or actually assaulting a spouse, *if* one has learned to respond to scientific or technical problems by using mathematics, or if one has learned to respond to stress and family problems by using violence. Even with such training, violence is not an automatic response to stress, nor algebra to a scientific problem. One also has to believe that the problem is amenable to a mathematical solution or to a violent solution. The findings presented in this paper show that violence tends to be high when certain conditions are present; for example, where people are taught the use of violence through childhood experiences and where the need of an individual to dominate a marriage provides a situation that is likely to yield to violence. If conditions such as these are present, stress is related to violence. If these conditions are not present, the relation between stress and violence is absent or minimal.

ACKNOWLEDGMENTS

It is a pleasure to acknowledge the many helpful criticisms and suggestions by the members of the Family Violence Research Program seminar: Joanne Benn, Diane Coleman, Ursula Dibble, David Finkelhor, Jean Giles-Sims, Cathy Greenblatt, Suzanne Smart, and Kersti Yllo; the computer analysis of Shari Hagar; and the typing of this paper by Sieglinde Fizz.

REFERENCES

1. ALLEN, C. & M. A. STRAUS. 1980. Resources, power, and husband-wife violence. *In* The Social Causes of Husband-Wife Violence. M. A. Straus & G. T. Hotaling, Eds.: Chapter 12. University of Minnesota Press.
2. BOTT, E. 1957. Family and Social Network. Tavistock Publications. London, England.
3. BRENNER, M. 1976. Estimating the social costs of national economic policy: implications for mental and physical health, and criminal aggression. Paper presented to the Joint Economic Committee, U.S. Congress, 1976; Revised version to be published as The impact of social and industrial changes on psychopathology, a view of stress from the standpoint of macrosocietal trends. *In* Society, Stress, and Disease. 1979. L. Levi, Ed. Oxford University Press.
4. BROWN, G. W. & T. HARRIS. 1978. Social Origins of Depression: A Study of Psychiatric Disorder in Women. Tavistock Publications. London, England.
5. BULCROFT, R. A. & M. A. STRAUS. 1975. Validity of husband, wife, and child reports of conjugal violence and power. (Mimeographed paper.)
6. FARRINGTON, K. 1980. Stress and family violence. *In* The Social Causes of Husband-Wife Violence. M.A. Straus & G. T. Hotaling, Eds.: Chapter 7. University of Minnesota Press.

7. FINKELHOR, D. 1977. Education and marital violence. (Mimeographed paper.)
8. GELLES, R. J. 1975. Violence and pregnancy: note on the extent of the problem and needed services. Family Coordinator 24: 81–86.
9. GELLES, R. J. 1976. Abused wives: Why do they stay? Journal of Marriage and the Family 38: 659–668.
10. GELLES, R. J. & M. A. STRAUS. 1979. Determinants of violence in the family: toward a theoretical integration. In Contemporary Theories About the Family. W. R. Burr, R. Hill, I. Nye & I. L. Reiss, Eds. Chapter 21. The Free Press. New York, N.Y.
11. GERSTEN, J. C., T. S. LANGNER, J. G. EISENBERG & L. ORZEK. 1974. Child behavior and life events: undesirable change or change per se. In Stressful Life Events: Their Nature and Effects. B. S. Dohrenwend & B. P. Dohrenwend, Eds.: 159–170. John Wiley & Sons, Inc. New York, N.Y.
12. GOODE, W. J. 1971. Force and violence in the family. Journal of Marriage and the Family 33: 624–636. (Also reprinted in Reference 24.)
13. HOLMES, T. H. & R. H. RAHE. 1967. The social readjustment rating scale. Journal of Psychosomatic Research 11: 213–218.
14. HOTALING, G. T., S. G. ATWELL & A. S. LINSKY. 1979. Adolescent life changes and illness: a comparison of three models. Journal of Youth and Adolescence 7(4): 393–403.
15. LAZARUS, R. S. 1966. Psychological Stress and the Coping Process. McGraw-Hill Book Co. New York, N.Y.
16. LEVINE, S. & N. A. SCOTCH. 1967. Toward the development of theoretical models. II. Milbank Memorial Fund Quarterly 45(2): 163–174.
17. MARTIN, D. 1976. Battered Wives. Glide Publications. San Francisco, Calif.
18. MCGRATH, J. E. 1970. A conceptual formulation for research on stress. In Social and Psychological Factors in Stress. J. E. McGrath, Ed.: 10–21. Holt, Rinehart, & Winston, Inc. New York, N.Y.
19. MECHANIC, D. 1962. Students Under Stress: A Study in the Social Psychology of Adaptation. The Free Press. New York, N.Y.
20. OSGOOD, C., G. SUCI & P. TANNENBAUM. 1957. The Measurement of Meaning. University of Illinois Press. Urbana, Ill.
21. PAYKEL, E. S. 1974. Life stress and psychiatric disorder: applications of the clinical approach. In Stressful Life Events: Their Nature and Effects. B. S. Dohrenwend & B. P. Dohrenwend, Eds.: 135–149. John Wiley & Sons, Inc. New York, N.Y.
22. SCOTT, R. & A. HOWARD. 1970. Models of Stress. In Social Stress. S. Levine & N. A. Scotch, Eds.: 259–278. Aldine Publishing Co. Chicago, Ill.
23. SELYE, H. 1966. The Stress of Life. McGraw-Hill Book Co. New York, N.Y.
24. STEINMETZ, S. K. & M. A. STRAUS, Eds. 1974. Violence in the Family. Harper & Row Publishers. New York, N.Y.
25. STRAUS, M. A. 1969. Social class and farm–city differences in interaction with kin in relation to societal modernization. Rural Sociology 34: 476–495.
26. STRAUS, M. A. 1971. Some social antecedents of physical punishment: a linkage theory interpretation. Journal of Marriage and the Family 33: 658–663.
27. STRAUS, M. A. 1973. A general systems theory approach to a theory of violence between family members. Social Science Information 12: 105–125.
28. STRAUS, M. A. 1976. Sexual inequality, cultural norms, and wife-beating. Victimology 1: 54–76; reprinted in Victims and Society. 1976 E. C. Viano, Ed. Visage Press. Washington, D. C. and in Women into Wives: The Legal and Economic Impact on Marriage. J. R. Chapman & M. Gates, Eds. 2. Sage Publications. Beverly Hills, Calif.
29. STRAUS, M. A. 1977. Wife-beating: How common and why? Victimology 2: 443–458. Reprinted in Reference 34.
30. STRAUS, M. A. 1979. Measuring intrafamily conflict and violence: the Conflict Tactics (CT) scales. Journal of Marriage and the Family 41: 75–88.
31. STRAUS, M. A. 1979. Socioeconomic status, aggression, and violence. (Paper in preparation.)
32. STRAUS, M. A. 1980. The marriage license as a hitting license: evidence from popular culture, law, and social science. In The Social Causes of Husband-Wife Violence. M.A. Straus & G. T. Hotaling, Eds.: Chapter 3. University of Minnesota Press.
33. STRAUS, M. A., R. J. GELLES & S. K. STEINMETZ. 1980. Behind Closed Doors: Violence in the American Family. Anchor/Doubleday. New York, N.Y.

34. STRAUS, M. A. & G. T. HOTALING, Eds. 1980. The Social Causes of Husband-Wife Violence. University of Minnesota Press.
35. STRAUS, M. A. & F. KUMAGAI. 1979. An empirical comparison of eleven methods of index construction. *In* Indexing and Scaling for the Social Sciences with SPSS. M. A. Straus, Ed.: Chapter 2. (Book in preparation. A mimeographed copy of this chapter is available upon request).
36. WOLFGANG, M. E. 1956. Husband-wife homicides. Corrective Psychiatry and Journal of Social Therapy **2**: 263–271. Reprinted *In* Deviancy and the Family. C.D. Bryand, Ed. F.A. Davis. Philadelphia, Penn.

APPENDIX

I. STRESS INDEX MODIFICATIONS

The stress index used in this study departs from the Holmes and Rahe scale in ways other than length. One of the criteria used to select items from the larger original set was the elimination of stresses that have a positive cathexis. Methodological studies show that the negative items account for most of the relationship between scores on the stress index and other variables.[11,21] We modified some items and added some that are not in the Holmes and Rahe scale to secure a set of stressors best suited for this research. The Holmes and Rahe weights were not used in computing the index score for each respondent. This decision was based on research that found the weighting makes little difference in the validity of scales of this type[35] and of the Holmes and Rahe scale specifically.[14]

An important limitation that this stress index shares with the Holmes and Rahe index is that one does not know the time distribution of the stressful events. At one extreme, a person who experienced four of the stressors during the year could have had them spread out over the year, or at the other extreme, all four could have occurred at roughly the same time.

II. WIVES AS VICTIMS

Although these findings show high rates of violence *by wives*, this should not divert attention from the need to give primary attention to wives *as victims* as the immediate focus of social policy. There are a number of reasons for this:

a. A validity study carried out in preparation for this research[5] shows that underreporting of violence is greater for violence by husbands than it is for violence by wives. This is probably because an act of violence, so much a part of the male way of life, is typically not the dramatic and often traumatic event that it is for a woman. Physical violence is not unmasculine. But it *is* unfeminine according to contemporary American standards. Consequently, if it was possible to allow for this difference in reporting rates, even in simple numerical terms, wife beating would probably be the more severe problem.

b. Even if one does not take into account this difference in underreporting, the data in TABLE 3 show that husbands have higher rates in the most dangerous and injurious forms of violence (beating up and using a knife or gun).

c. TABLE 1 also shows that when violent acts are committed by a husband, they are repeated more often than is the case for wives.

d. These data do not tell us what proportion of the violent acts by wives were in response to blows initiated by husbands. Wolfgang's data on husband-wife homicides[36] suggest that this is an important factor.

e. The greater physical strength of men makes it more likely that a woman will be seriously injured when beaten up by her husband than the reverse.

f. A disproportionately large number of attacks by husbands seem to occur when the wife is pregnant,[8] thus posing a danger to the unborn child.

g. Women are locked into marriage to a much greater extent than are men. Because of a variety of economic and social constraints, they often have no alternative but to endure beatings by their husbands.[9,17,28,29]

VIOLENCE-PRONE FAMILIES

Suzanne K. Steinmetz

Individual and Family Studies
University of Delaware
Newark, Delaware 19711

Introduction

The intent of this paper is to present an overview of the characteristics of violence-prone families. Given the recent attention paid to family violence, one might believe that this topic has a long, rich research tradition. However, it has only been since the late 1960s that family violence has been identified as a legitimate topic for academic research. Yet, an examination of some of the first written laws suggests that not only did violence between family members exist, but it was an institutionalized, very acceptable way for those in a dominant, superior position to control those in a weaker, subordinate position. Perhaps it is only when that position is questioned, when we become cognizant of the amount and destructiveness of violence within families, that attempts to study the phenomena are undertaken.

The concept of children as property of their parents is illustrated in the Hammurabi Code of 2100 B.C. and the Hebrew Code of 800 B.C., which considered infanticide to be an acceptable practice. The Bible gives us the earliest and best known account of sibling violence, the story of Cain killing his brother Abel.

> and Cain talked with Abel his brother: and it came to pass, when they were in the field, that Cain rose up against Abel, his brother, and slew him (Genesis 4:8)

The Bible also provides us with the dictum "spare the rod and spoil the child," perhaps one of the earliest written accounts of child-rearing philosophy.

A 1646 colonial law attempted to help parents control their rebellious children, noting that unless parents "had been very unchristianly negligent in the education of such children or so provoked them by extreme cruel correction," any child over 16 years of age of sufficient understanding who cursed, smited, and would not obey his natural mother or father "would be put to death."[1]

Colonial custom also demanded that couples cohabit peacefully. However, evidence from court records and diaries suggests that not all spouses were loving. Joan Miller was charged with "beating and reviling her husband and egging her children to healp her, bidding them to knock him in the head and wishing his victuals might choke him."[2] One man in Plymouth Colony was punished for abusing his wife and "kiking her off from a stolle into the fier"; and another man for "drawing his wife in a uncivil manner on the snow."[2]

Concern for protecting children from abuse erupted in 1874 when the story of 9-year-old Mary Ellen who was physically abused by her parents was reported. While protection of animals was available through the Society for the Prevention of Cruelty to Animals (SPCA), there were no laws to protect children. Social workers, by defining Mary Ellen as a member of the animal kingdom, were able to provide help and protection.[2] In 1885, the Pennsylvania legislature considered enacting a bill that would publicly whip wife beaters, as a tax-saving alternative to imprisonment. While the use of violence to control violence is questionable (and not likely to influence the husband to return home as a warm and loving mate), it was an improvement over the 1824 law permitting husbands to chastise their wives with a twig no bigger than their thumb.[2]

The level of violence found within the contemporary family has suggested to some researchers that every role relationship in the American family is characterized by rates of violence that make the problem of violence in the streets pale by comparison.[3] These researchers, summarizing their data from a national sample of 2,143 families, noted that whereas the uniform crime reports for assaults are reported in rates per 100,000, their data were reported in rates per 100. Statistics also indicate that you are at greater risk of injury in your home among family, friends, and neighbors than you are in the crime-ridden streets, and that family members make up the single largest category of homicide victims. Furthermore, domestic disturbance calls are reported to be the most dangerous calls for the police to answer, and more police are injured and killed answering domestic disturbance calls than any other single category of calls.[4]

Frequency of Domestic Violence

One of the more recent studies on child abuse reported 300,000 incidents of abuse; 40,000 cases requiring protective service intervention and 2,000 deaths during 1975.[5] A national sample survey of 2,143 intact families found that 20% hit a child with an object, 4.2% "beat up" a child, 2.8% threatened a child with a knife or gun, and 2.9% used a knife or gun on a child.[6] Furthermore, they predicted that between 1.5 and 2 million children are severely abused each year. These figures are even more disturbing when one realizes that the sample surveyed only intact families (single parents are at higher risk of abuse) and only the parent-child interaction for children age 3–18 (toddlers are at higher risk).

Sibling Violence

Probably the form of family violence considered to be most normal is violence between sibs. One study of college freshmen found that 62% reported that they had used physical violence on a sibling during the last year.[7] Other studies, based on a broad-based nonrandom sample[8] and a random sample,[9] found rates ranging from 63–78%. Straus, Gelles, and

Steinmetz[6] found that during the past year, 75% reported using physical violence and averaged 21 acts per year. Thirty-eight percent of siblings kicked or hit, 14% "beat up," 0.8% threatened to use a gun or knife, and 0.3% used a gun or knife. When we extrapolate these percentages to the 36.3 million children between 3–17 who have siblings, we find that 6.5 million children have been "beaten-up" by a sibling and that nearly 2 million children at sometime during their childhood have faced a gun or knife.

Marital Abuse

The data for marital abuse suggest that violence is unfortunately prevalent in many families. Gelles found that 55% of 80 families experienced marital violence and 21% beat their spouses regularly.[10] Straus reported that 16% of a sample of college freshmen saw their parents engage in marital violence during the past year.[7] Based on a random sample of New Castle County, Delaware, Steinmetz found that 60% of 57 families experienced marital violence.[9] For 10% of the couples, physical violence was a regular occurrence. When these data were combined with police statistics, it was revealed that severe physical abuse was experienced by 7% of wives and 0.6% of husbands.[11] The national survey of family violence[6] reported that during a one-year period, one out of six couples had a violent episode, 5% experienced severe physical abuse, and 4% used a gun or knife.

THE SOCIAL AND PSYCHOLOGICAL CHARACTERISTICS OF VIOLENCE

Psychiatric Conditions

The reporting of statistics on family violence points up the incongruence between the view of the family as the unit that provides love, comfort, protection, and support, and data that indicate the prevalence of violence between family members.

As a result we look for a scapegoat to help us understand the use of extreme violence. It is easy to comprehend why child abusers or wife batterers are labeled as mentally ill—obviously normal people would not behave this way. Likewise, a battered wife is described as having psychiatric defects—Why else would she allow herself to become a victim?

An examination of early studies of child abuse attributed numerous psychiatric defects, such as depression, immaturity, impulsiveness, and dependency, to abusing parents.[12,13,14] Forty-eight percent of the mothers in one British study were described as being neurotic, and a high percentage of fathers in this study were diagnosed as psychopaths.[15] Although the above finding suggests that psychiatric disorders produce child abuse, the evidence to the contrary is overwhelming. Steel and Pollock[14] noted that abusive parents did not exhibit excessive aggressive behavior in other areas of their lives and were not much different from a cross section of the general populations. Kempe and Helfer[15] state that less than 10% of parents who abuse children are seriously mentally ill. Furthermore, electro-encephalographic examination of abusive parents found no evidence of a relationship between child abuse and organic dysfunction.[16]

Based on empirical evidence[17] as well as a critical examination of the literature,[18] it appears that, as a group, child abusers are no more or less mentally ill or emotionally disturbed than any randomly selected group of parents. Being identified and labeled as a child abuser appears to be the major distinguishing feature. While there is some evidence of pathology in the profiles of offenders and victims in studies of spouse abuse,[19] the question of cause and effect needs to be raised.

Hilberman and Munson,[20] in their study of 60 battered women, found that almost the entire sample of 60 women had sought medical help for stress-related complaints and many evidenced symptoms commonly associated with the rape-trauma syndrome. Furthermore, more than half had evidence of prior psychological dysfunction, including classic depressive illness, schizophrenia, manic-depression, alcoholism, and severe character disorders. Thirteen of the group had been hospitalized with violent psychotic behavior. There has been an assertion that since certain types of women are more prone to be a victim and since these women often appear to avoid taking steps to resolve their problems, they are at fault for being abused. The assumption is made that all women can control their lives if they choose to. Research describing the personality characteristics of a battered wife often leaves an impression that these victims, by their own weaknesses, had enabled this type of interaction to occur. A woman is likely to become a victim of spouse abuse when she displays the characteristics of a weak, vulnerable woman: she is isolated,[10,20] helpless, and depressed;[25] she has fewer resources;[21-25] she is overcome by anxiety;[21,25,26] and full of guilt and shame.[20,27]

Often it is suggested that by changing the woman's social and economic resources; increasing her education and job skills; teaching her to be less submissive; helping her to have a better self-concept; or teaching her to interpret her husband's moods, the violence can be reduced. While these are valid mechanisms for helping a victim escape from the battering environment, they tend to emphasize the ability of a woman to control her environment, an ability many battered women are lacking. Thus, a profile emerges of a woman who displays a learned helplessness that enables her to be further victimized.[28]

It is suggested that contrary to the notion that these psychiatric conditions cause women to be at risk of being beaten, it is the dynamics of the beating itself that produce these manifestations.[29] This phenomenon is closely related to the processes involved in brainwashing. Isolation from family, friends, and social support systems reinforces the victim's dependency on the abuser for confirmation of her worth. Unfortunately, the confirmation supports the woman's negative self-image, filling her with shame and guilt.

Social Class

While possibly more prevalent among lower classes, family violence is by no means limited to lower-class families. The disproportionate representation of working and lower classes noted by Blumberg,[30] Gil,[17] Holter and Friedman,[13] and Elmer[12] might have resulted from the practice, in earlier research, of utilizing medical facilities to obtain study populations. An underrepresentation of reported violence in middle-class families may be a consequence of the privacy surrounding middle-class acts and the services utilized by middle-class families. Lower-class families usually rely on social control agencies, such as the police, social service or family court workers, and clinics; agencies that keep "public" records. Middle- and upper-class families have access to private social support systems, such as family counselors, private doctors, ministers, and lawyers, that maintain the privacy of the professional relationship.

Blue Collar/White Collar

While the various dimensions of social status show inconsistencies when we use the broad categorization of blue collar/white collar (working class/middle class) classification, the relationship is quite clear. Blue collar status predicts greater levels of family violence for both males and females.[6,9] It may be that the blue collar/white collar category is too broad to clearly discern patterns. However, it may also reflect a broad class-based difference. Middle-class families may have been socialized to sharpen their communication skills because of the desirability of mediation and compromise rather than overt aggression.[31] Since the inability to communicate is highly related to physical violence between spouses,[9,25] this may also contribute to the differences in levels of family violence with respect to social class.

Income

Income is another aspect of social class. Because of the purchasing power associated with it, income provides families with resources useful for mediating many stress-producing and potentially violent situations. Greater financial resources enable parents to procure stress-reducing mechanisms, such as baby sitters, vacations, nursery schools, and camps, which provide them with "time-out" from childrearing/homemaking responsibilities. An examination of the interaction between stress and income and the effect on family violence is provided by the data from the national survey.[6] Increased stress, as rated by 18 items, had no effect on the very poor (family income below $6,000) or on those with family incomes above $20,000 (where income provides a cushion) but did increase the likelihood of child abuse for the middle income group. However, only those families with incomes over $20,000 were immune from the effects of stress-related spousal violence.

When physical or medical problems arise, possessing a higher income enables one to secure medical and psychological help from a private physician. Prescott and Letko[25] found that wives of professional men were four times more likely to have contacted a therapist than wives of men in low-status jobs.

Finally, mothers in higher income families have had greater access to contraception and abortion, thus enabling them to have greater control over family size and spacing, a factor related to family conflict and violence.[31-34] Among Gil's[17] abused families, 40% had 4 or more children, while in Johnson and Morse's[31] sample of 101 abused children, 35% were from families with 4 or more children.

In general there is a consistent decrease in violence as income levels go up. For families with incomes of under $6,000, 53% of families reported abuse between siblings, 22% reported child abuse, and 11% reported for both wife and husband abuse. In contrast, for those families with incomes of $20,000 and over, 41% reported sibling violence, 11% reported child abuse, and 2% each reported husband and wife abuse.

Education

Education is usually considered one of the major components of social class. It defines the range of occupations one is eligible to fulfill and thus is closely linked to income (from the job) and prestige (obtained by working in a given job). Steinmetz[9] found that a husband's education showed a strong negative correlation with spousal violence and father-child violence; a wife's education showed a similar relationship for spousal violence but virtually no relationship (0.04) for the mother-child violence. Gelles'[10] finding of an inverse relationship between husband's educational levels and violence was consistent with that noted by Steinmetz. However, while Gelles noted rather high levels of violence for women college graduates, in the national data there were fewer college graduates who were offenders or victims of spousal violence and college graduates were the least violent parents.

While other studies tended to find a negative relationship between education and violence, the national data[6]—which categorized education into four levels: eighth grade or below; some high school; high school graduate; and college—did not support this finding. For both men and women there was a positive relationship between the first three levels of education and child abuse (11%, 15%, and 18% for men; 12%, 14%, and 17% for women). It was only among those parents who had been exposed to college that a decrease in child-abuse rates occurred (11% for both men and women).

A curvilinear relationship also appeared for spouse abuse, with high school drop-outs having the highest abuse rates (6% each) as well as the highest victimization rates (7% each). The effect of college education on the probability of victimization is noteworthy. While a college education reduces the likelihood of a woman being victimized (2%), it increases the likelihood of victimization for men (5%).

Employment Status

The employment status of the husband/father and satisfaction with occupational/homemaking roles are also predictors of family violence. Unemployment is often perceived by males as incompetency in fulfilling their provider roles. This has been linked to child abuse and wife beating. Gil[17] reported that nearly half (48%) of the fathers in his sample of abusers experienced unemployment during the year preceding the abuse. McKinley[35] found that the lower the job satisfaction, the higher the percentage of fathers who used severe corporal punishment—a relationship that was not affected by social class.

The national survey[6] revealed a consistently lower level of child and spouse abuse among families where the husband was employed full time. Furthermore, part-time employment was more likely to predict family violence than was unemployment. A study of battered women who replied to a request for information in *Ms. Magazine* reported that husbands who were unemployed or employed part-time were extremely violent compared with husbands who were employed full time.[25]

Also related to the use of violence is job satisfaction and perceived inability to fulfill the breadwinner/head-of-household role.[25,36,37] Since middle- and upper-class parents are usually better educated, they are more likely to have fulfilling jobs and have the flexibility to change jobs. They are also likely to reside in larger, more comfortable homes, and have adequate resources for carrying out the homemaker/childbearing role. As a result, parents in the middle and upper classes are less likely to be locked into unfulfilling jobs in the marketplace and in the home.

Occupational Environment

Occupational environment, a concept that focuses on the tasks and ideology inherent in specific occupations, was found to predict, with more accuracy than social class, the parents' use of violence on children.[38,39] This same idea was upheld in studies of the police. These studies found that police showed no evidence of abnormal aggressiveness or rebellious tendencies,[40] sadistic or authoritarian attitudes or behavior,[41] and scored lower on a measure of punitiveness.[42] It appears that it is not the individual who selects law enforcement as a career, but the training and job itself that produce punitive, authoritarian, violent behavior. A recent study found similar results for military personnel in which the ideology and goals of the unit (not just the tasks the individuals actually perform) predicted the levels of violence used.[43]

Isolation

Families who lack close personal friendships and are poorly integrated into the community are likely to experience family violence for several reasons. First, they are lacking the friendship network which could provide support during times of extreme stress, and second, they are not likely to be influenced by the community's expectations of normal social behavior. Merrill[44] reported that 50% of abusive families belonged to no formal group association and 28% had only one such membership. Lenoski[45] found that 89% had unlisted phones. Elmer and Gregg[46] reported that abusive mothers were also found to score higher on an anomie scale.

Gil[17] and Schlosser[47] found that in some instances this isolation results from high mobility, which cuts these families off from kinship and friendship groups. In other instances the isolation results because the abusive families are not fully accepted by their community[44] or are actually rebuffed.[47] There appears to be a certain circularity to this process. The parent who batters the child, or the wife who experiences batterings from her husband, is likely to avoid becoming friendly with neighbors because of embarrassment and fear of discovery. This isolation, however, increases the likelihood of the problems continuing, since the family has no one to discuss problems with or to seek advice and help from. Of course, it is possible that once the aberrant behavior is discovered (most likely when the police are called), the isolation becomes enforced by the community rather than voluntary on the part of the family.

Age and Length of Marriage

O'Brien[37] found that violence was spontaneously mentioned in 64% of longer duration marriages and in 36% of shorter duration marriages. Roy's[24] examination of 150 cases of battered women found that the violence first peaked between 2.5 and 5 years.

In their national study, Straus and his colleagues[6] found that over 80% of those under 30 years of age were more likely to consider the slapping and spanking of 12-year-olds to be necessary, normal, and good. Less than 66% of the group 50 years and older supported this view. Although there is this decrease in the percentage who view the use of physical force on adolescent-aged children as necessary and good, approximately two-thirds of the population over 50 years of age still held a view that is contrary to a large body of research on child rearing, as well as popular advice on child rearing.

This survey reported that the use of violence on children decreased as both the children and parents matured. Eighty-six percent of children 5–9 years old; 54% of children 10–14 years old; and about 33% of children 15–17 years old were hit by their parents during the survey year.

Furthermore, 21% of parents under 30 years of age, 13% of the parents 31–50 years, and 4% of those 51 through 65 used abusive violence on a child. No parent 65 or older used abusive violence on a child, but this may reflect the age of their "child" (a middle-aged adult) rather than a change in child-rearing philosophy. Age appears to be a major influence on spousal violence. While 15% of the couples under 30 years of age used abusive violence on each other, only 4% of those 31 to 50 years and 1% of the group 51 through 65 years of age used abusive violence.

Sex Differences

Lansky, Crandall, Kagan, and Baker,[48] Toby,[49] and Whitehurst[50] found males' behavior to be more violent than females'. This difference has been observed in infants[51] and among Western and non-Western societies.[52] However, when marital and parental roles are examined, the data are not as clear-cut. Women, for example, outnumber men as child abusers.[53] While this is understandable, since women have the major caretaking responsibility, it does suggest that women are not immune from perpetrating violence.

In the national survey[6] men were more likely than women to express the belief that slapping is necessary, normal, and good, but mothers (68%) were more likely to have used violence on the child than were fathers (58%) during the survey year. Furthermore, with the exception of using or threatening to use a gun or knife (admitted only by fathers), mothers used each type of violence more frequently. About 4.4% of mothers kicked, hit, punched, or beat up a child compared with 2.7% of the fathers.

While mothers were more likely to abuse children, it was sons who were at greater risk of abuse: 4.5% for sons versus 2.8% for daughters.

Although media presentations have focused on wife beating as a major problem, husband beating must also be considered. Straus'[7] study of 385 couples showed little difference in the frequency with which husbands and wives committed physically violent acts against each other. Steinmetz,[54] in a comparison of data from five other studies, found that virtually identical percentages of husbands and wives resorted to throwing things, hitting with the hand, and hitting with an object. The only modes that husbands used more frequently than wives were pushing and grabbing—modes requiring superior physical strength—and these differences disappeared in the "high users" group. Furthermore, an examination of husbands and wives who used violence revealed that wives resorted to violence more frequently. Secondary analysis of previously published data revealed that the average violence scores of wives as compared with husbands were all slightly higher in the three studies (4.04 vs. 3.52;[9] 7.82 vs. 6.00;[55] and 7.00 vs. 6.60[8]). The national study[6] found that wives committed an average of 10.1 acts of violence against their husbands during 1975, while husbands averaged only 8.8 acts against their wives. Only Gelles[10] found husbands to exceed their wives in use of physically violent modes. He found that 11% of the husbands and 5% of the wives engaged in marital violence between 2 and 6 times a year, and 14% of the husbands and 6% of the wives used violence between once a month and daily. Wives exceeded husbands in one category, however; 11% of the husbands and 14% of the wives noted that they "seldom" (defined as between two and five times during the marriage) used physical violence against their spouses. Gelles[10] found that husbands exceeded wives in the frequency with which they used violence, but noted that wives tended to slap, throw things, and hit with an object, modes that deemphasize physical strength. The importance of physical strength must not be overlooked; while women and men are nearly equal in their use of violence, women because of smaller size and less strength receive a greater degree of injury. Severe abuse rates, based on a random sample of families and compared to police statistics, suggest that 7% of the women as compared with 0.6% of the men are likely to be severely abused in any given year.[11] Furthermore, battered women, even those with occupational, financial, and family resources, are psychologically trapped—a phenomenon not experienced by men.[29]

Curtis[56] reported that while violence by men against women was responsible for about 27% of the assaults and 17.5% of the homicides, violence by women against men accounted for only 9% of the assaults and 16.4% of homicides. Thus, while women commit only one-third as many assaults against men as men commit against women, the number of cross-sex homicides committed by the two groups is nearly identical. Wilt and Bannon warn that caution should be applied when interpreting the above findings. They note that "non-fatal violence committed by women against men is more likely to be reported to the police than is violence by men against women; thus, women assaulters who come to the attention of the police are likely to be those who have produced a fatal result."[57]

Residence

Like other areas of violence the highest rates of family violence tended to be found in urban (large city) areas. However, data from the national survey[6] did not show a consistent relationship between size of the residential area and family violence. In fact, the family violence rates for wife and child abuse were as high or higher among rural families as among urban families. Furthermore, the rates among rural families for child abuse were higher than rates found in small cities and suburbs. However, urban families and rural families share several things in common: isolation, lower educational levels, and lower incomes all were found to contribute heavily to child abuse and wife beating.

Race

Race was found to predict levels of family violence.[6] While blacks tended to be more violent than whites for child, wife, and husband abuse, they reported lower rates of sibling violence. Those families categorized racially as "other" were consistently highest in all categories except wife abuse (blacks were higher). These groups tend to have more unemployment, lower levels of education and income, larger families producing overcrowding, and to be confined to urban areas that experience higher levels of violent crime.

Pregnancy

Pregnancy is closely related to family violence in several ways. Premarital pregnancy or unplanned pregnancies, which strain limited resources, often result in the child's being resented; this is a precursor to abuse.[13,15,16,58] The financial and emotional stress that accompanies pregnancy has been linked to husbands' frequent and severe physical attacks on their wives.[10,34,27,57] Although many wives reported being the victim of beatings before and after the birth of the child, those that occurred during the pregnancy were described as being considerably more brutal and often included being kicked or punched in the stomach, a phenomenon that Gelles[56] has labeled intrauterine child abuse.

Alcohol

Wertham[59], Gil,[17] and Young[33] found a relationship between the use of alcohol and child abuse. The use of alcohol was also found to be closely linked to wife beating.[10,25,27] MacAndrew and Edgerton[60] suggest that the effects of alcohol on a social behavior are influenced by cultural expectations and socialization. Thus, in some societies the use of alcohol is associated with considerable violence, while in others no relationship exists, or exists only under certain circumstances. Several researchers[2,10,6] have noted that difficulty in ascertaining the actual sequence: Do men drink, lose control, and then beat their wives?; or Do men wish to vent their anger on their wives and drink in order to gain the courage to do so and to provide an excuse for their action?[7] Gelles[10] suggests that the association between alcohol and violence reflects the process of deviance disavowal—men get drunk to give them an excuse for their abusive behavior toward their wives.

Violent Histories

Probably the most important predictor of family violence is a pattern of a history of violence. The axiom, "an abusing parent was often an abused child," has been well documented.[12,14,15,61] Roy[24] found that 81% of husbands who beat their wives were beaten as children or saw their mothers being beaten. However, only 33% of the beaten women reported being beaten or seeing their mother beaten. Being beaten as a child also predicts other types of violence. Owens and Straus,[62] in a secondary analysis of a survey conducted for the Commission on the Causes and Prevention of Violence, found a relationship between experiencing violence as an observer or a victim during childhood and violent behavior as an adult. This finding was supported by Sedgely[63] in a secondary analysis of National Opinion Research Center data. Gayford,[64] in a study of battered wives, discovered that both the batterer and victim had a violent childhood. These patterns were found to continue over several generations in studies of child abuse—a cycle in which the battering parents had experienced abuse from their own parents.[62,65,66,67] Wilt and Bannon[57] note that over one-fourth of the individuals who committed assault or murder reported having had frequent arguments with their parents. Furthermore, their analysis of 90 intrafamilial homicides revealed that 62% had been preceded by previous assaults on the same family member. Even in less violent forms, the use of physical force is passed on from generation to generation.[6,8,9] Perhaps one of the more intriguing findings of the national survey[6] is that while the probability of nonviolent parents being violently attacked by their children is about 1 out of 400, the probability of parents who use severe violence on their children being attacked by their children is 200 out of 400.

Based on a study of 34 boys and 39 girls in a family treatment program, Gladston expressed belief that "children who have received significant exposure to violent behavior before the age of two are likely to have identified with this pattern of response in a fashion that proves to be essentially irreversible, although a great deal can be done subsequently to contain it."[68] He notes that intervention before the age of 18 months greatly enhances the possibility of modifying the child's violent behavior.

CONCLUSION

Much of the literature presented has shown the effect of violence in one generation on the behavior of the next generation. However, violence witnessed and experienced by children often is the precursor to violence against society. Experiencing violence during childhood was found to be characteristic in the backgrounds of murderers, assault and batterers, rapists, political assassins, and individuals who commit suicide. Thus none of us are immune from the effects of violence in the family. We experience violence directly within our family or indirectly by having to reside in a violent society caused, in part, by violent socialization practices.

While considerable data have been amassed during the last decade on family violence, we really have only begun to scratch the surface. The evolution of research and theory in this field has produced a questioning of biological-based, instinctual theories or Freudian psychoanalytic theories to explain violence. They have been replaced with theories emphasizing the social/cultural context. The data presented in this article support this theoretical perspective—violence as a learned behavior transmitted from one generation to the next. Obviously this explains only part of the family violence phenomenon.

On the frontier of knowledge, research is focusing on the intricate body processes as a key to violent behavior. Investigation of chromosomal and hormonal influence on violence must not be discounted, especially since trends have appeared across generations.

Research being conducted at the Universities of Maryland and Pennsylvania on organic brain dysfunction is especially exciting. The distinctive brain scan patterns have been found to exist over several generations. This suggests one alternative to social-learning theories as an explanation for family violence existing over several generations.

Personality changes caused by chronic or deteriorating diseases such as diabetes and arteriosclerosis are being examined as a possible link in understanding family violence in certain circumstances.

While social/cultural linkages to family violence will probably predominate at this time, these new areas of exploration will provide additional insights necessary for a more complete understanding of this complex, destructive behavior.

ACKNOWLEDGMENTS

I wish to acknowledge Clella Bay Murray who prepared the references and provided technical editing of this paper. I also want to thank Sarah Roberts Foulke who offered suggestions for improving the manuscript. Finally, I want to express my gratitude to Marge Murvine for her patient typing of numerous drafts (always with my promise that this would be the last).

REFERENCES

1. BRENMER, R. H. 1970. Children and Youth in America: A Documentary History 1: 37. Harvard University Press. Boston, Mass.
2. STEINMETZ, S. K. 1978. Violence between family members. Marriage and Family Rev. 1(3): 1–16.
3. STRAUS, M. A., R. J. GELLES & S. K. STEINMETZ. 1978. Physical violence in a nationally representative sample of American families. Presented at the 9th World Congress of Sociology, Uppsala, Sweden, August 14–19.
4. PARNAS, R. I. 1967. The police response to domestic disturbances. Wisc. Law Rev. 914: 914–960.
5. BESHAROV, D. J. 1975. Building a community response to child abuse and maltreatment. Children Today 4(5): 2–4.
6. STRAUS, M. A., R. J. GELLES & S. K. STEINMETZ. 1980. Behind Closed Doors: Violence in the American Family. Doubleday & Co., Inc. New York, N.Y.
7. STRAUS, M. A. 1974. Leveling civility and violence in the family. J. of Marriage and the Family 36: 13–19.
8. STEINMETZ, S. K. 1977. The use of force for resolving family conflict: the training ground for abuse. The Family Coordinator 26: 19–26.
9. STEINMETZ, S. K. 1977. The Cycle of Violence: Assertive, Aggressive and Abusive Family Interaction. Praeger Publishers. New York, N.Y.
10. GELLES, R. J. 1974. The Violent Home: A Study of Physical Aggression between Husbands and Wives. Sage Publications. Beverly Hills, Calif.
11. STEINMETZ, S. K. 1977. Wifebeating—husband beating—a comparison of the use of physical violence between spouses to resolve marital fights. In Battered Women: A Psychosociological Study of Domestic Violence. M. Roy, Ed.: 63–72. Van Nostrand Reinhold Co. New York, N.Y.

12. ELMER, E. 1971. Studies of child abuse and infant accidents. *In* The Mental Health of the Child. U.S. National Institute of Mental Health. U. S. Government Printing Office. Washington, D.C.
13. HALTER, J. C. & S. B. FRIEDMAN. 1968. Principals of management in child abuse cases. Am. Orthopsychiatry 38(1): 127–138.
14. STEEL, B. F. & D. A. POLLOCK. 1974. A psychiatric study of parents who abuse infants and small children. *In* The Battered Child. R. E. Helper & C. H. Kempe, Eds.: 89–134. University of Chicago Press. Chicago, Ill.
15. KEMPE, C. H. & R. E. HELPER, Eds. 1972. Helping the Battered Child and His Family. J. P. Lippincott Co. Philadelphia, Penn.
16. SMITH, S. M., L. HONIGSBERGER & C. A. SMITH. 1973. EEG and personality factors in baby beaters. Br. Med. J. 3: 20–22.
17. GIL, D. G. 1970. Violence Against Children: Physical Child Abuse in the United States. Harvard University Press. Cambridge, Mass.
18. GELLES, R. J. 1973. Child abuse as psychopathology: a sociological critique and reformation. Am. J. Orthopsychiatry 43: 611–621.
19. SNELL, J., R. ROSENWALD & A. ROBEY. 1964. The wifebeater's wife. A study of family interaction. Arch. Gen. Psychiatry 11: 107–112.
20. HILBERMAN, E. & I. MUNSON. 1977–78. Sixty battered women. Victimology 2: 460–470.
21. GELLES, R. J. 1967. Abused wives: Why do they stay? J. Marriage and the Family 38: 659–668.
22. STRAUS, M. A. 1973. A general systems theory approach to a theory of violence between family members. Social Science Info. 12: 105–125.
23. STRAUS, M. A. 1977–78. Wifebeating: How common and why? Victimology 2: 443–457.
24. ROY, M. 1977. Battered Women: A Psychosociological Study of Domestic Violence. Van Nostrand Reinhold Co. New York, N.Y.
25. PRESCOTT, S. & C. LETKO. 1977. Battered: a social psychological perspective. *In* Battered Women: A Psychosociological Study of Domestic Violence. M. Roy, Ed.: 72–96. Van Nostrand Reinhold Co. New York, N.Y.
26. RIDINGTON, J. 1977–78. The transition process: a feminist environment as reconstitutive milieu. Victimology 2: 563–575.
27. RESNICK, M. 1976. Wife Beating. Counselor Training Manual #1. NOW—Wife Assault Task Force. Ann Arbor, Mich.
28. WALKER, I. E. 1977–78. Battered women and learned helplessness. Victimology 2: 525–534.
29. STEINMETZ, S. K. 1978. Wife beating: a critique and reformation of existing theory. Bull. Am. Acad. Psychiatry and Law 4(3): 322–334.
30. BLUMBERG, M. 1964–65. When parents hit out. Twentieth Century 173: 39–44.
31. JOHNSON, B. & H. A. MORSE. 1968. Injured children and their parents. Children 15: 147–152.
32. STRAUS, M. A. 1976. Sexual unequality, cultural norms and wifebeating. Victimology 1: 54–76.
33. YOUNG, L. R. 1964. Wednesday's Children: A Study of Child Neglect and Abuse. McGraw-Hill Book Co. New York, N.Y.
34. FARRINGTON, K. 1977. Family violence and household density; Does the crowded home breed aggression? Paper presented at the Annual Meeting of the Society for the Study of Social Problems, Chicago, Ill., September 5–9.
35. McKINLEY, D. G. 1964. Social Class and Family Life. The Free Press. New York, N.Y.
36. LEVINGER, G. 1966. Sources of marital dissatisfaction among applicants for divorce. Am. J. Orthopsychiatry 36 (5): 803–807.
37. O'BRIEN, J. E. 1971. Violence in divorce-prone families. J. Marriage and the Family 33: 692–698.
38. STEINMETZ, S. K. 1971. Occupation and physical punishment: a response to Straus. J. Marriage and the Family 33: 664–666.
39. STEINMETZ, S. K. 1974. Occupational environment in relation to physical punishment and dogmatism. *In* Violence in the Family. S. K. Steinmetz & M. A. Straus, Eds. Harper and Row, Publishers. New York, N.Y.

40. SKOLNICK, J. H. 1969. Justice Without Trial: Law Enforcement in Democratic Society. John Wiley & Sons, Inc. New York, N.Y.
41. NIEDERHOFFER, A. 1967. Behind the Shield, The Police in Urban Society. Doubleday & Co., Inc. Garden City, N.Y.
42. MACNAMARA, D. E. & E. SAGARIN. 1971. Perspectives on Correction. Thomas Y. Crowell. New York, N.Y.
43. SHWED, J. A. 1979. The military environment and physical child abuse. M. A. Thesis. University of New Hampshire. Durham, N.H.
44. MERRIL, E. J. 1962. Protecting the Battered Child. Children's Division, American Human Association. Denver, Colo.
45. LENOSKI, E. F. 1974. Translating injury data into preventative and health care services— physical child abuse. University of Southern California School of Medicine. Los Angeles, Calif. (Unpublished manuscript.)
46. ELMER, E. & G. S. GREGG. 1967. Developmental characteristics of abused children. Pediatrics 40: 596–602.
47. SCHLOSSER, P. 1964. The abused child. Bull. of the Menninger Clinic 28: 260.
48. LANSKY, L. M., V. S. CRANDALL, J. KAGAN & C. T. BAKER. 1961. Sex differences in aggression and its correlates in middle class adolescents. Child Dev. 32: 45–58.
49. TOBY, J. 1966. Violence and the masculine ideal: some qualitative data. Ann. Am. Acad. Political and Social Sci. 364: 19–27.
50. WHITEHURST, R. N. 1974. Violence in husband-wife interaction. In Violence in the Family. S. K. Steinmetz & M. A. Straus, Eds. Harper and Row, Publishers. New York, N.Y.
51. HOFFMAN, L. W. 1978. Changes in family roles, socialization, and sex differences. In Family Factbook: 59–72. Marquis Academic Media. Chicago, Ill.
52. WHITING, B. 1965. Sex identity conflict and physical violence: a comparative study. Am. Anthropol. 67: 123–140.
53. RADBILL, S. X. 1968. A history of child abuse and infanticide. In The Battered Child. R. E. Helper & C. H. Kempe, Eds. University of Chicago Press. Chicago, Ill.
54. STEINMETZ, S. K. 1977–78. The battered husband syndrome. Victimology 2(3–4): 499–509.
55. STEINMETZ, S. K. 1977. Secondary analysis of data from a United States-Canadian comparison of intra-family conflict. Canadian Conferences on Family Violence, Simon Fraser University, Burnaby, Canada, March 12.
56. CURTIS, L. A. 1974. Criminal Violence: National Patterns and Behavior. Lexington Books. Lexington, Mass.
57. WILT, G. M. & J. D. BANNON. 1976. Violence and the Police: Homicides, Assaults and Disturbances. The Police Foundation. Washington, D.C.
58. GELLES, R. J. 1975. Violence and pregnancy: a note on the extent of the problem and needed services. The Family Coordinator 24(1): 81–86.
59. WERTHAM, F. 1972. Battered children and baffled adults. Bull. N.Y. Acad. Med. 48: 887–898.
60. MACANDREW, C. & R. B. EDGERTON. 1969. Drunken Comportment: A Social Explanation. Aldine Press. Chicago, Ill.
61. WASSERMAN, S. 1967. The abused parent of the abused child. Children 14: 175–179.
62. OWENS, D. J. & M. A. STRAUS. 1975. The social structure of violence in childhood and approval of violence as an adult. Aggressive Behavior 1(2): 193–211.
63. SEDGELY, J. & D. LUND. 1979. Self reported beatings and subsequent tolerance for violence. Public Data Use 7(1): 30–38.
64. GAYFORD, J. J. 1975. Wife-beating: a preliminary survey of 100 cases. Br. Med. J. 1: 194–197.
65. OLIVER, J. E. & A. TAYLOR. 1971. Five generations of ill-treated children in one family pedigree. Br. J. Psychiatry 119: 473–480.
66. SILVER, L. B., C. C. DUBLIN & R. S. LOURIE. 1969. Does violence breed violence? Contribution from a study of the child abuse syndrome. Am. J. Psychiatry 126: 404–407.
67. ZALBA, S. R. 1966. The abused child: a survey of the problem. Social Work 11: 3–16.
68. GLADSTON, R. 1975. Preventing the abuse of little children: the parents' center project for the study and prevention of child abuse. Am. J. Orthopsychiatry 45(3): 372–381.

THE CHARISMATIC LEADER AND THE VIOLENT SURROGATE FAMILY

Fred Wright

Department of Psychology
John Jay College of Criminal Justice
New York, New York 10019

Phyllis Wright

The New York Counseling and Guidance Service
New York, New York 10024

In recent times a new kind of violent behavior has emerged that is both shocking and puzzling. A variety of familylike groups, usually religiously oriented and often headed by highly charismatic leaders, have engaged in unusually bizarre and violent behavior. Generally referred to as cults, they have carried out their activities in a fairly methodical and cohesive fashion. The most dramatic example, of course, is the murder of the United States Congressman Leo J. Ryan and members of his investigating party, as well as the subsequent mass suicide of more than 900 members of the People's Temple, that occurred in Guyana on November 18, 1978. Other examples of violent cults abound. There was the Charles Manson group, which functioned in the early 1970s and which murdered a number of people in California in an unusually grim and sadistic manner. Recently, members of Synanon, a well-known California-based group, originally founded to treat drug addiction and lately reported to be taking on the characteristics of a cult, has been accused of the attempted murder of a prosecutor by putting a rattlesnake in his mailbox. In 1977, a self-styled renegade Mormon prophet named Immanuel David—who, like Jim Jones, had been visited by holocaustic visions—killed himself. The next morning, his wife helped their seven children jump from their eleventh floor hotel room and then followed them. Another renegade Mormon prophet, Ervil Le Baron, who heads a sect called the Church of the Lamb of God, has been convicted of inciting some of his followers to murder his own brother, as well as others, apparently to consolidate his leadership position within his group.

Coercion and violence appear to be a common and an accepted characteristic of many other cults as well. According to reports by the news media,[22] investigating governmental agencies,[28] and ex-members of these organizations,[4] psychological pressure, physical punishment, and/or violent threats are used against those who violate group norms or criticize the cult.

It is the purpose of this paper to develop a clearer understanding of these phenomena by reviewing and discussing the research, theories, and explanations of behavioral scientists that are relevant.

Recently, there has been some empirical research directly related to cult phenomena. Three of the studies reviewed are consistent in their findings regarding the needs of individuals who join cults.[13,24,25] These researchers, working independently of each other, all found that members had experienced significant emotional distress before entering the cult, and that they usually experienced, at least for a time, considerable relief from this distress once involved in the cult. Two of the studies account for this relief by concluding that cult members' hunger for ideology was nourished, for a while at any rate, through membership.[13,25] This has been a frequently given explanation for religious conversion.[5,17] However, the data from the Ullman study[24] of conversion to mainstream religious groups, as well as conversion to the newer sorts of groups under discussion here, don't support this conclusion. Her study was the only one that directly compared converts to regular members on the basis of a search for truth or meaning. She found no difference between the two groups in interest for the search for explanations of topics like the scientific notion of truth or problems of social injustice. She did find that, among the converts, there was a strong need for an accepting authority figure to calm emotional turmoil rooted in childhood. Eighty percent of the experimental subjects, compared to 20% of the controls, had negative feelings about their fathers, or their fathers had been absent while they were growing up. Therefore, Ullman concludes that a high percentage of subjects were looking for father figures and believes that this lends support to Freud's theory that religious conversion, in part, represents a search for a father figure.

In light of Ullman's findings and the fact that psychoanalytically oriented writers have spent a great deal of time and effort exploring the nature of relations between authority figures and subjects via the notion of transference, it would be of value to the purpose of this paper to review that notion as it relates to the topic under discussion. As already noted, Freud accounted for religion-seeking behavior partly as a search for a father figure. He repeats this theme in a number of his books, and also introduces the concept of transference to further explain this kind of behavior.[7-11] According to Freud, people defend themselves against the terrors of life by transferring onto a deity feelings that they had, as children, directed towards their father. In effect, they transfer their dependency needs from their real-world father onto an exalted, heavenly father who will then protect and nourish them if they behave properly, i.e., if they are good children.

Erich Fromm, another leading psychoanalytic writer, developed Freud's views on the transference of authority, particularly in his well-known book *Escape from Freedom.*[12] Here he points out that people have a tendency to give up the independence of their own individual self and to strive to fuse or bind themselves up with somebody or something outside of themselves in order to acquire the strength that they feel they lack.

Fromm focuses particularly on the kind of person he refers to as the authoritarian character. This is the individual who seeks a "magic helper," as Fromm describes it. This helper is a person or personification, such as a principle or God, who will protect, help, and develop the individual; be with him or her always; and never leave the individual alone. When real persons assume this role, according to Fromm, they are endowed with magic qualities. Those who endow do so out of an inability to stand alone and to fully express their own individual potentialities. They hope to get everything they want from life through the magic helper, instead of through their own actions. This process is illustrated by the Unification Church's practice of having the church leader, Rev. Moon, select marriage partners as well as arrange the weddings for church members.[2]

This kind of dependency can result in an individual's whole life being focused almost entirely on getting the helper to fulfill his or her wishes. People differ in the means they use to achieve this. Some use obedience, some "goodness," while for others suffering is the main means of manipulating the magic helper. This dependency creates a certain amount of security but also results in a feeling of weakness and bondage. In effect, the individual feels enslaved by the helper.

More recently Ernest Becker, in his Pulitzer Prize winning book *The Denial of Death,*[1] has synthesized the notions of a number of psychoanalysts who have discussed transference to authority figures. One aspect of the authority transference, according to him, is in its use as a control device. Through it we are, or believe we are, capable of opposing reality and keeping it ordered or "fixed" so that we can pursue our own expansion and fulfillment. By allying ourselves with another who seems to be made up of all the qualities we feel we are missing, we reduce ambiguity and achieve clarity and boundedness; in short, we believe we have gained control over the world and our fate rather than their controlling us.

Another aspect of the transference to leaders, according to Becker, is that it enables us to overcome our fear of life, of emerging into the world, and of realizing our own individuality, experiencing, and living. By binding ourselves to one person we believe we will tame this terror. For example, by incorporating another's ideology, we hope to free ourselves from the difficult work of having to develop one of our own.

The third use of transference noted by Becker is that through it people believe immortality will be gained. Via transference, the individual fantasizes she or he will overcome even death. That is, in deifying others by placing them on pedestals or by endowing them with extraordinary powers, the believer becomes more powerful. It is as though the more the idealized other possesses, the more the believer possesses and thus feels more secure. This notion helps us to understand the extraordinary mourning and panic that can occur when a leader dies or gets ill. When a leader with whom we have merged our identity and who has become our bulwark against death goes, we too go. We are abruptly faced with mortality at that point, and, most important, our own end comes into sharp focus. The transference object, endowed with supernatural powers, keeps us from perceiving that as long as she or he remains in good health.

Finally, Becker describes an authority transference as an "urge to higher heroism."[1] People need to infuse their life with value so that they can call it good. Transference, thus, is a talent in that it is a form of "creative fetishism,'' according to Becker. Through it, we take this mystery (our lives and the meaning of our lives) and dispel it by addressing our performance of heroics to another human being who then judges its value. We know if it is bad by the reaction of the idealized other and thus are able to change it. We are now in a position to achieve heroic self-validation, even though it comes through surrender to another's world-view. Thus, the traditional psychoanalytic view of transference as simply unreal projection is rejected. True, it is a distortion of reality but a distortion with two dimensions: distortion due to fears (of loss of control, of life, and of death), but also distortion due to the heroic attempt to assure self-expansion. Thus transference is not necessarily a cowardly maneuver, it can also be seen as a life-enhancing illusion.

Another aspect of transference not discussed by Becker, and yet of relevance to this paper, has to do with the notion of the "transitional object."[26] This is a concept frequently called upon by contemporary psychoanalysts to account for human behavior, and it becomes particularly valuable for this paper in light of the findings[13] of Galanter et al., mentioned earlier. They found that many of their subjects had been in transition at the time of their conversion to the cult. For example, many were ex-college students in the process of moving away from a school setting.

Winnicott was the first to describe transitional objects.[26] He saw them as the "first not-me possession" and referred to such objects as soft dolls, teddy bears, and security blankets. The notion of transitional phenomena grows out of the process of normal infant development. In the beginning , it is thought that children do not distinguish themselves from the mothering one. As development proceeds, however, the mother begins to withdraw her complete support, and the child must adapt to an existence separate from mother. In order to accomplish this separation, a bridge between mother and the outside world must be established. According to Winnicott, a soft object, such as a blanket, becomes the transitional object that enables the growing child to negotiate this separation. This object symbolizes the mother and at the same time is not the mother. It provides an anchor point from which to approach reality and integrate subjective and objective experiences, as well as serving as a defense against anxiety.

Others have indicated that the concept of the transitional object can be broadened to cover a variety of human behaviors other than those of early developmental stages.[16,19,14] For example, Halpern has said "we may define it as applying to any object or habit that a person of any age may use to span the gap between any developmental stage and the one following by carrying the illusion of the previous stage with him until he is ready to stand unaided in the next."[14] These notions enable us then to conceive of the cult leader as a transitional object for certain people who are in a transition. The leader is invested with properties from the member's subjective needs and experiences, as well as retaining part of his or her external identity. The leader-object then enables the person to separate from or leave an earlier developmental stage and move on to something else while at the same time retaining remnants of what was left behind. For example, a young person who joins a cult may separate from the family of origin and simultaneously retain parental and sibling surrogates and, therefore, a family feeling.

Other groups or organizations that may serve the same function are youth gangs, underworld organizations, college fraternities and sororities, encounter groups, psychotherapy groups, or the fan clubs that form around popular entertainers. The gang leader, godfather, housemother, group therapist, or celebrity entertainer serves the same function in fantasy as the cult leader. This may explain, in part, the need of a cult leader like Jim Jones to maintain his heroic, "star" image by, for example, dyeing his hair pitch black and "performing miracles," i.e., faith healing. He could be perceived as doing so, at least in part, in order to retain his position as a glamorous and therefore comforting transitional object for his followers.

Thus far the research reviewed has shown that those who are most susceptible to the appeals of cults are people who are experiencing considerable emotional distress, as well as those who are in a state of transition, or—as Margaret Singer, a psychologist who has also studied modern cults, puts it—who "are between meaningful affiliations."[6]

The Ungerleider et al.[25] study found something else that is of particular relevance to this paper. They assessed hostility and found that those who remained in cults, when compared to those who joined and eventually left, were significantly higher on the variables of "anger at family members" ($P < 0.007$), as measured by the Minnesota multiphasic personality inventory, and "overcontrolled hostility" ($P < 0.05$), as measured on a subscale developed by Megargee.[18] The authors reasoned that the "cults appear to serve as externalized superego substitutes," helping members manage hostile impulses. Thus those who remain in cults appear to be people who are having difficulty managing their aggression. The cult becomes a vehicle through which they can gain control of themselves, and more specifically, it may very well offer them a means to express their anger at family members by rejecting them for another, "better" family and at the same time legitimate their anger. Rev. Moon, for example, describes his church as a "true family" and casts the external world and the family or origin in highly negative terms.[4] These findings suggest that anger at authority figures may be a particular problem for cultists, and yet one that they have not coped with very successfully. Thus another dimension would be added to the cultists' need for the cult leader. That is, the leader helps them in their efforts to govern their own aggression.

It would appear, at least in violent cults, that not only does the leader help members to control their hostility, he also helps members to express it. Wilfred Bion[3] and Fritz Redl[20] have written extensively about this latter phenomenon. As Redl puts it, the leader, or a central person in the group, is unconflicted about matters that the rest of the group members feel inhibited about. Members thus admire this person for being unconflicted about matters they too experience, but feel conflict or shame over. Further, when this unconflicted person initiates an antisocial act, the meaning of that act is changed, freeing others to act because the risk had been taken by the leader. That is, they avoid the guilt or responsibility for acting incurred by the leader and therefore the members can act in a guiltless or nonresponsible fashion. The leader therefore transforms the world for the followers, making it possible for them to do that which they always wanted to do but which was forbidden by internalized norms or repressions, e.g., engage in promiscuous sex or aggression towards others or the self.

Bion extends this notion regarding the "use" people in groups make of leaders.[3] According to him, the leader is as much a creature of the group and its shared emotion, as the group members are his creatures. In fact, he must reflect or mirror their assumptions and feelings in order to qualify for leadership in the first place. Leaders become leaders to particular people because they epitomize or represent in a very concrete way something that is within their followers that the followers are either unable, unwilling, or afraid to acknowledge and express.

The research of Edwin Megargee[18] is also helpful in furthering understanding of this matter. He finds that when comparing offenders who engage in unusually excessive violent behavior (e.g., impulse murderers) to other criminal groups (e.g., moderate aggressors, property offenders, burglars), the violent offenders were assessed as less hostile, less aggressive, and more controlled. In fact, the excessively violent were "overcontrolled." He showed that such people tended to be extremely dependent, submissive, and passive individuals with rigid control over aggressive impulses as long as their dependency was gratified. When the dependency gratification was withdrawn they would become murderously assaultive toward the depriver. The history of these individuals showed that they had had maternal figures who had emphasized conformity to the rules of the social system, and that to gain affection they'd had to deny or repress any hostility. Thus they had never learned how to express hostile feelings. Megargee further hypothesizes that the excessively violent response is not determined by the immediate stimulus but rather that it is a function of the absolute or total amount of instigation to aggression that had been slowly building up over a preceding period of time. This partially accounts for the violent behavior that appears to be all out of proportion to the immediate stimulus (e.g., the response of the People's Temple to Congressman Ryan's investigation).

Megargee suggests as treatment for the overcontrolled a psychotherapy that aims to reduce excessive inhibitions so that the individual can learn to acknowledge and accept his feelings of hostility and learn ways of satisfaction while still not posing too great a threat to society.

Thus far in this paper we have drawn largely on the notions of psychoanalytic thinkers in our efforts to understand abnormal group behavior. However, there are other formulations that can be of use to us as well. For example, susceptibility to suggestion and/or imitation are frequently offered as explanations for hard-to-understand group responses. In fact, those who have analyzed the conversion process in the new religious groups have shown that the recruiters go to great lengths to generate conditions that make it easier for suggestion to take hold. Christopher Edwards, an ex-member of the Unification Church and author of the book on his experiences in this church entitled *Crazy for God,*[4] describes in detail the well-organized technology involved: the chanting, singing, confessions, and group activities that tend to mesmerize and lower the sense of being a separate, independent being; the physical demands and inadequate diet that sap the energy required to thoroughly think issues through; and the constant repetition of the group's ideology coupled with reinforcements contingent upon attitudes and behaviors acceptable to the group.

Stanley Cath, a psychiatrist who had treated ex-cult members, contends, in fact, that there are neurophysiological factors that are being manipulated by technology-wise cult leaders, thereby altering individuals' levels of consciousness and making them far more susceptible to the leader's wishes and influence.[21]

Another explanation for irrational group behavior is presented by Ralph Turner and Lewis Killian in their excellent and comprehensive book *Collective Behavior*.[23] According to them, both psychoanalytic and contagion or suggestion/imitation theories make valuable contributions toward understanding bizarre collective behavior. They qualify their support, however, by indicating that these theories neglect the complexity of people. According to these writers not all members in a group feel and act the same way. They agree with psychoanalytic theory that people have latent or repressed tendencies, but they contend that rather than having only one or a few such tendencies people have several latent tendencies that are relevant to a given situation. If this is the case, then it also becomes important to explain how a group of people with a variety of different urges winds up acting in what, at least to the outside observer, looks like a form of united craziness.

Their explanation lies in what they term "emergent norms."[23] They say that in a particular situation interaction among group members occurs, and that norms then emerge that are specific to the situation. "These 'emergent' norms define those acts that, out of many sorts of behavior that might be possible in the situation, are expected or permitted in this particular crowd. Tendencies to behave in a different fashion are then restrained, and individuals who remain a part of the crowd experience pressure to behave in the manner that has been defined as appropriate."[23] That is, a common or shared understanding as to what sort of behavior is expected in a particular situation develops. This shared understanding encourages behavior consistent with the norm, inhibits behavior contrary to it, and justifies restraining action against individuals who dissent. Since the norm is to some degree specific to the situation, differing in degree or in kind from the norms governing noncrowd situations, it is an "emergent" norm.

They are saying, then, that bizarre group or crowd behavior is similar in many respects to routine crowd or organized behavior. People define their situation, taking into account all the knowledge or information that is available to them at the time, and take on roles or particular functions in their group, for example, becoming leaders and followers. As a result, though the behavior may appear irrational and asocial from outside the crowd, given the fund of information available within the group at that particular time and place and the collective definition of the situation they arrive at as a result of that fund, the behavior members then pursue may seem quite appropriate to them. In effect, an "irrational" group defines the situation differently than the larger group it is part of would define it and, as a result, is governed by norms that are at variance with those of the larger society.

One last point made by Turner and Killian of relevance to this paper has to do with the matter of the significance of anonymity for crowd behavior. They point out that "if crowd behavior is subject to social control under an emergent norm, it is important that the individual in the crowd have an identity so that the control of the crowd can be effective."[23] According to this perspective, the control of the crowd should be greatest among persons who are known to one another rather than among anonymous persons. Therefore, control should be greatest in cults, in comparison to other sorts of crowds or collectives, because people are very well known to each other.

Christopher Edwards confirms this in his account of his life in the Unification Church, where he shows how the proselytizing group went to great lengths to let the initiates know that they were indeed not only well known by the group, but were in fact very highly regarded for their potential to become outstanding supporters of the group's normative system.[4] Where control is great in a group it can be expected that the group as a whole, without dissent or with minimal dissent, will be likely to engage in prescribed behavior regardless of how this behavior appears to people who are not part of that social system.

The last matter to be dealt with in this paper is the cult leaders themselves and their appeal. What information do we have that will enable us to understand these people and the oftentimes enormous influence they have over their followers?

Otto Kernberg,[15] an American psychiatrist and psychoanalyst, describes a personality syndrome that sounds a great deal like that of the various cult leaders who have received public attention in recent times. Specifically, he writes about a subgroup of borderline patients referred to as the narcissistic personality. He describes these patients as presenting excessive self-absorption, usually coinciding with a superficially smooth and effective social adaptation, but with serious distortions in their internal relationships with people. That is, they have serious deficiencies in their capacity to love and to empathize with others. As a consequence, exploitativeness and ruthlessness toward others are also characteristics of these patients.

Further, according to Kernberg, these patients are characterized by various combinations of intense ambitiousness, grandiose fantasies, and overdependence on external admiration and acclaim. They are on a continuous search for gratification of strivings for brilliance, wealth, power, and beauty. Finally, he stresses the presence of chronic, intense envy in these people, and defenses against such envy—particularly devaluation of others, omnipotent control, and narcissistic withdrawal—as major characteristics of their emotional life.

What is the etiology of such a personality type according to Kernberg? First, chronically cold parental figures with covert but intense aggression are a frequent feature in the background of such patients. There is a parental figure, usually the mother or mother surrogate, who functions well on the surface in the home, but with a fair degree of callousness, indifference, and nonverbalized and spiteful aggression. The need for children to defend against the expression of their own envy and hatred in such an environment is obvious, thus leading to the devaluation, control, and withdrawal defenses just mentioned. Another consequence of this childhood environment is the development of a deep conviction of being unworthy, and a view of the world as devoid of nurturance and love.

In addition, the histories of such patients show that they often possessed a quality that could have aroused the envy or admiration of others. For example, unusual physical attractiveness or a special talent became refuge against feelings of being unloved and even hated. Sometimes these patients were used by other family members as a means to garner attention and admiration. Often they were designated the "brilliant" child in the family who was slated to fulfill the family's or a family member's aspiration for greatness. This special position in the family became the source around which the patients' grandiose fantasies became crystallized. Clearly, people with needs and traits like these would be logical candidates for the role of cult leader; such a position or "job" would be highly attractive to them and complement their emotional profile.

Another view of this character type has been explored by Robert Ellwood, a researcher of religious movements. According to him, there are striking parallels between the religious phenomena of primitive shamanism and modern cults. In fact, he says "the cult phenomena could almost be called a modern resurgence of shamanism."[5]

The shaman, in primitive society, provided a variety of valuable services. First, he was usually a person who had gone through a severe emotional disorder of his own, and would probably be defined as mentally ill by ordinary standards. The sickness, however, became the vehicle for explorations of realms beyond the normal perimeters of the human spirit, which put the shaman in a position of healer. That is, through his own personal struggle with, and overcoming of, illness he is in a position to show others the way out of evil or illness. As a result, most shamans are medicine men in their cultures, but not all medicine men are shamans. For shamans usually have special qualities and techniques that enable them to induce mystical, ecstatic experiences. Thus, not only do they heal, they can also provide one with a new spiritual life. Further, Ellwood points out that it is the shaman who, during times of social and spiritual upheaval, breaks free of the traditional bonds and founds new faiths, thereby allowing people to cope with the new experience forced upon them. In summary, the shaman or cult leader's appeal rests in his or her capacity, or apparent capacity, to lead followers out of distress or illness as well as to provide them with a means for survival, even ecstasy, in a difficult and changing world.

Our understanding of the source of the cult leader's power is also furthered by recent research that shows that a person in a position of authority can be highly influential despite consciously striving to be the opposite. Wright, Buirski, and Smith studied graduate-level college students who had formed laboratory groups to study their own group process as well as the nature of group leadership.[27] The authors were surprised to learn the extent to which the group leaders were unknowingly influencing the group members' preferences for, attention to, and attributions about other members. This was measured by responses on a number of research instruments. The leaders themselves strove to conduct themselves in a nondirective and low-disclosing style, and believed they had done so. That is, their conscious intention was to avoid communicating preferences or directing members' attention or attributions. The striking thing about the research is how thoroughly unsuccessful they were in carrying out this intention. Group members sensed the leaders' preferences and interests and followed suit. Apparently, just being assigned the role of leader in a group is enough to profoundly influence the psychological processes of followers.

In sum, a review of the research and literature relevant to cult phenomena was undertaken in this paper in an effort to gain insight into the psychology of cult members, leaders, and the cult itself as an entity. In particular, an attempt was made to understand the sources of the extreme violence engaged in by a number of cults. Results from empirically oriented studies were focused on and related to the theoretical formulations of a number of behavioral scientists for further clarification. Findings indicated that cult members tended to be emotionally distressed people prior to cult membership and that once involved, they obtained considerable relief from this distress at least for a time. Further, research shows that many cult members had been in a state of transition at the time of conversion. People who remain in cults have also been found to be high on the variables of "anger at family members" and "overcontrolled hostility." Cult leaders appear to satisfy a variety of the needs of members as a result of their own personality structure in conjunction with the authority inherent in the role of group leader. Other group-level processes were analyzed in an effort to further account for the phenomena under study.

REFERENCES

1. BECKER, E. 1973. The Denial of Death. The Free Press. New York, N.Y.
2. BERNARD, J. 1979. 700 couples got engaged in the city yesterday . . . and many didn't know each other. New York Post (May 14): 30.
3. BION, W. R. 1959. Experiences in Groups. Basic Books. New York, N.Y.
4. EDWARDS, C. 1979. Crazy for God. Prentice-Hall Inc. Englewood Cliffs, N.J.
5. ELLWOOD, R. S. 1973. Religious and Spiritual Groups in Modern America. Prentice-Hall Inc. Englewood Cliffs, N.J.
6. FREEMAN, M. 1979. Of cults and communication: a conversation with Margaret Singer. A.P.A. Monitor (July/August): 6-7.
7. FREUD, S. 1919. Totem and Taboo. Paul Kegan. London, England.
8. FREUD, S. 1932. Leonardo Da Vinci. Paul Kegan. London, England.
9. FREUD, S. 1934. The Future of an Illusion. Hogarth Press. London, England.
10. FREUD, S. 1934. Civilization and Its Discontents. Hogarth Press. London, England.
11. FREUD, S. 1939. Moses and Monotheism. Hogarth Press. London, England.
12. FROMM, E. 1941. Escape from Freedom. Rhinehart and Winston, Inc. New York, N.Y.
13. GALANTER, M., R. RABKIN, J. RABKIN & A. DEUTSCH. 1979. The "Moonies": a psychological study of conversion and membership in a contemporary religious sect. Am. J. Psychiatry 136: 165-170.

14. HALPERN, H. M. 1968. Transitional phenomena: constructive or pathological. Voices 3: 44.
15. KERNBERG, O. 1975. Borderline Conditions and Pathological Narcissism. Jason Aronson, Inc. New York, N.Y.
16. KOSSEFF, J. W. 1975. The leader using object relations theory. *In* The Leader in the Group. Z. Liff, Ed. Jason Aronson, Inc. New York, N.Y.
17. LIFTON, R. J. 1956. Thought Reform and the Psychology of Totalism. W. W. Norton & Co., Inc. New York, N.Y.
18. MEGARGEE, E. I. 1966. Undercontrolled and overcontrolled personality types in extreme anti-social aggression. Psychological Monographs 80 (611).
19. MURRAY, M. E. 1974. The therapist as a transitional object. Am. J. Psychoanal. 34: 123–127.
20. REDL, F. 1942. Group emotion and leadership. Psychiatry 5: 573–596.
21. SHAPIRO, B., Producer. 1979. Cults: In the Name of God? American Broadcasting Companies, Inc. New York, N.Y. (Television program.)
22. THOMAS, J. & N. SHEPPARD, JR. 1979. Cults in America. New York Times (September 21): 1, 52.
23. TURNER, R. H. & L. M. KILLIAN. 1972. Collective Behavior. Prentice-Hall, Inc. Englewood Cliffs, N.J.
24. ULLMAN, C. 1979. Change of mind or change of heart? Some cognitive and emotional characteristics of religious converts. Ph.D. Thesis. Boston University. Boston, Mass.
25. UNGERLEIDER, T. & D. K. WELLISHCH. 1979. Coercive persuasion (brainwashing), religious cults, and deprogramming. Am. J. Psychiatry 136: 279–282.
26. WINNICOTT, D. W. 1958. Collected Papers: Through Paediatrics to Psycho-analysis. Tavistock Publications. London, England.
27. WRIGHT, F., P. BUIRSKI & N. SMITH. 1978. The implications of leader transparency for the dynamics of short-term process groups. Group 2: 210–219.
28. Attorney General of the State of New York. 1974. Final report on the activities of the Children of God. Charity Frauds Bureau.

PORNOGRAPHY AND VIOLENCE AGAINST WOMEN: EXPERIMENTAL STUDIES*

Edward Donnerstein

*Department of Psychology
University of Wisconsin
Madison, Wisconsin 53706*

Recently, the National Institute of Mental Health designated that an understanding of the conditions that lead to sexual attacks against women is a major problem area and requires an increased focus. While there are many potential avenues of investigation, one that seems to be of current concern is the role of media effects in the possible elicitation of such aggressive acts, particularly in the area of pornography. Although the 1970 Presidential Commission on Obscenity and Pornography concluded that there was no evidence of a relationship between exposure to erotic forms of presentations and subsequent aggression (particularly sexual crimes), recent criticisms of these findings[1-3] have led a number of investigators to reexamine this issue. Specifically, research by a number of individuals in the social-psychological area has indicated that under appropriate conditions exposure to erotic forms of media presentations can facilitate subsequent aggressive behavior.[4-8] While this research has been directed at the effects of erotic media presentations on behavior, the issue of whether such presentations can in some manner be related to increased aggressive attacks against women has been only recently of concern.[8,9] It is generally believed by a large proportion of the population that many sexual materials can precipitate violent sexual crimes, such as rape.[10] Basic research directed at examining this concern, in regard to erotic forms of media and other presentations that depict women as victims of aggression, is an important goal of social research. The present series of studies was designed to examine this issue.

BRIEF HISTORICAL BACKGROUND

What are the effects of erotic or pornographic materials on antisocial behavior? An examination of recent research and reports in the area would suggest that the effects are, if anything, nonharmful. For example:

> It is concluded that pornography is an innocuous stimulus which leads quickly to satiation and that the public concern over it is misplaced.[11]

> If a case is to be made against "pornography" in 1970, it will have to made on the grounds other than demonstrated effects of a damaging personal or social nature. Em-

---

* This paper was written while the author was a visiting professor at the University of Wisconsin. Study III and the writing of this paper was supported by a grant from the National Institute of Mental Health, 1 F32 MH 07788-01.

pirical research designed to clarify the question has found no reliable evidence to date that exposure to explicit sexual materials plays a significant role in the causation of delinquent or criminal sexual behavior among youth or adults.[10]

However, recent criticisms of these findings by a number of investigators[2,3] have led to a reexamination of the issue of erotic exposure and subsequent aggressive behavior. While some individuals, like Cline,[2] have argued that there are major methodological and interpretation problems with the pornography commission report, others[12] believe that the observations might be premature. The major reason for this concern comes, in part, from a recent series of experimental studies that suggests that the relationship between exposure to erotic materials and subsequent aggressive behavior is more complex than first believed. The brief review of this research that follows summarizes the current state of this issue.

Aggression-Enhancing Effects of Erotic Exposure

A number of studies in which subjects have been angered, and later exposed to some form of erotic stimulation, have revealed increased aggressive behavior.[4,13] In fact, there is evidence to suggest that the facilitative effects are greater than those attributed to aggressive films.[4,14] Such findings have been interpreted in terms of a general arousal model, stating that under conditions where aggression is a dominant response any source of emotional arousal will tend to increase aggressive behavior.[15] In accordance with this model, aggressive behavior, in subjects who have previously been angered, has been shown to be increased by exposure to arousing sources such as aggressive or erotic films,[4] physical exercise,[16] and noise.[17] It would seem that because of their arousing properties erotic stimuli can have aggression-facilitating effects under certain conditions. Although there has been research indicating that erotic stimuli might increase aggression without prior anger arousal,[18] the majority of evidence to date would suggest that prior anger arousal is an important condition for a facilitative effect of erotic exposure.

Aggression-Inhibiting Effects of Erotic Exposure

A second group of studies[19,20] have shown that exposure to erotic stimuli can actually reduce subsequent aggression. A number of explanations have been suggested for this effect: erotic stimuli are somehow incompatible, in their emotional state, with aggression;[19,21] the level of anger arousal is inappropriate for an aggressive response;[20] or erotic exposure shifts attention away from previous anger arousal.[6] Whatever the explanation, there is sound evidence to suggest that under certain conditions erotic stimuli can reduce subsequent aggressive behavior.

A Reconciliation of the Research

While at first glance such results seem somewhat contradictory, recent studies by Donnerstein *et al.*[6] and Baron and Bell [7] seem to have resolved this controversy. It is now believed that as erotic stimuli become more arousing, they give rise to increases in aggressive behavior. At a low level of arousal, however, such stimuli act to distract a subject's attention away from previous anger[6] or act as an incompatible response with aggression,[7] thus reducing subsequent aggressive behavior. The evidence for this curvilinear relationship between sexual arousal and aggression seems fairly well established. In fact, Baron[22] has shown that this type of relationship also occurs when females are exposed to mild and highly erotic stimuli.

The Issue of Erotic Stimuli and Aggression against Women

While the current theorizing on the relationship of erotic stimuli and aggression seems fairly conclusive, it is interesting to note that all of the aforementioned studies were concerned with same-sex, primarily male-to-male, aggression. Yet, the social implications of this research would be more applicable by an examination of male aggression toward females. For, as noted by the U. S. Commission on Obscenity and Pornography:

> It is often asserted that a distinguishing characteristic of sexually explicit materials is the degrading and demeaning portrayal of the role and the status of the human female. It has been argued that erotic materials describe the female as a mere sexual object to be exploited and manipulated sexually.[10]

In recent years there has been an increasing concern about the relationship of pornography and violence against women. Writers in both the popular media and the scientific community have addressed this issue. Generally, they have taken for granted that pornography and aggression against women are tightly linked:

> We are somewhat educated now as to the effects of rape on women, but we know less about the effects of pornography . . . we can admit that pornography is sexist propaganda, no more and no less. Pornography is the theory, and rape is the practice.[22]

> Pornography is the undiluted essence of anti-female propaganda . . . does one need scientific methodology in order to conclude that the anti-female propaganda that permeates our nation's cultural output promotes a climate in which acts of sexual hostility directed against women are not only tolerated by ideologically encouraged.[23]

> Even when they do not overtly depict scenes of violence and degradation of women at the hands of men, such as rape, beatings, and subordination, the tone is consistently anti-feminist. . . . The intention would seem to be simply to degrade women, and it is noteworthy that in many cases of rape the men involved either act in the same manner . . .[24]

However, what is the evidence regarding the relationship of pornography and aggression against women?

Some studies have attempted to determine whether or not erotica has a differential effect on aggression against men and against women. The general conclusion has been that no differential effects occur. Thus, in one series of studies, Mosher[25,26] found no increase in "sex-calloused" attitudes, aggressive verbal remarks, or exploitive sexual behavior toward females. More recent research by Jaffe *et al.*[5] and Baron and Bell [27] have also indicated that erotic exposure does not differentially affect men's aggression toward males or females.

There are a number of problems with the research that has examined the link between pornography and male aggression toward females. First, there is strong evidence that prior or subsequent anger instigation is critically important in facilitating aggression following erotic exposure. Given the fact that males are usually hesitant about aggressing against females,[28] and that in the above research subjects were not even instigated by their potential victim, it would seem unlikely that a differential facilitation in aggression would occur. In fact, except for the Jaffe *et al.* study,[5] researchers found that exposing nonangered individuals to erotic films tended to *reduce* aggression or maintain it at a level comparable to that of subjects exposed to a neutral film.[19]

Second, previous researchers have found that only under conditions of high sexual arousal does a facilitative effect in aggression occur. Exposure to mild sexually arousing stimuli seems to reduce aggression, even in previously angered individuals.[19,7,6] Again, except for Jaffe *et al.*,[5] the research that has examined the relationship of erotic stimuli and aggression toward females has employed milder forms of sexually arousing stimuli.

It would seem, therefore, that an appropriate test of the effects of erotic stimuli on aggression toward females would need to employ both some form of anger instigation and high levels of sexual arousal. This particular combination of important factors, which seems to account for the facilitative effects of erotic stimuli on aggression, has not, until recently, been investigated in those studies in which females are the victims of aggression from males.

Experiment I

A recent study by Donnerstein and Barrett[8] was designed to examine these issues using the theory and data of past research in the erotic stimuli-aggression area as a framework. Male subjects were exposed to either a neutral or highly arousing erotic film. The type of erotic stimuli employed was similar to those used in previous studies that have indicated facilitative effects for aggression.[4,13] In addition, prior to stimulus exposure subjects were either angered or treated in a neutral manner by a male or female target of aggression. Both aggressive behavior, in the form of electric shock, and physiological reactions of the subject were observed.

Since the procedures in the studies in this series were all similar, a few words regarding the methodology employed are presented. All subjects were male undergraduates who volunteered for the study as part of receiving extra credit in their course work. They believed that they were interacting with another male or female subject in a study on the effects of stress and performance. Our male subjects were first given an opportunity to write an essay with the understanding that the essay would be evaluated by the "other subject" via the delivery of electric shock. If the subject was in a condition where they were to be angered, they received a large number of shocks plus a negative written evaluation of their essay from the other male or female subject. Nonangered subjects received only one shock and a very positive evaluation. This type of procedure is very common in the literature and produces both physiological responses and self-reports that indicate that subjects have, in fact, been angered. Following this procedure, subjects were then given an opportunity to deliver shock to the "subject" who had evaluated their assay. No shock was actually delivered, but subjects assumed that they were in fact administering various levels of shock to this person. At various times in the studies, physiological responses of the subjects in the form of blood pressure, were measured. It should be noted that in addition to various consent forms that were signed by the subject, a complete debriefing as to the nature of the study was given to the subjects at the end of the session.

With this experimental procedure in mind, the first study in this series made a number of predictions based upon previous research in the area: (1) exposure to erotic films should increase aggressive behavior in angered individuals, while (2) no facilitation in aggressive behavior should occur for nonangered subjects. Of more immediate interest, however, were the following questions: (1) Would exposure to erotic stimuli differentially affect aggression toward males and females in subjects who have previously been instigated to aggress? (2) Might there be an increase in aggression toward females even without prior instigation due to implied sexually aggressive cues in the erotic films? and (3) What are the physiological patterns that emerge during film exposure? This third question was of special interest, in that from a theoretical perspective, the interaction of anger arousal and erotic-film-exposure arousal have been employed in an explanatory manner in this area.[4] To date, however, such results were based upon interactions with only male targets of aggression. There is a suggestion from prior research[29] that although males display less aggression toward females following provocation, physiological arousal is maintained at a high level. It seemed important, in terms of past research in this area, to examine further not only the arousal component of anger instigation from males to females, but also its interaction with highly arousing sexual stimuli. Donnerstein and Barrett[8] also examined the effects of anger, erotic stimuli, and sex on a more prosocial or rewarding response. Since it was expected that less social restraints would be present with this reward response than with the shock response toward females, subjects were given an opportunity in this study to administer rewards (money) to their target. The major results for this first study are presented in TABLES 1 and 2. With regard to aggression, as measured by the intensity and durations of shocks administered to the male or female, two interactions were found. The first, anger × sex of

TABLE 1

MEAN INTENSITY* × DURATION AS A FUNCTION OF EXPERIMENTAL CONDITIONS

	Means	
Condition	Anger	No Anger
Anger × Sex of Target		
Male	1.86$_a$	0.95$_c$
Female	1.55$_b$	1.13$_c$
Anger × Films		
Erotic	1.90$_a$	0.93$_c$
Neutral	1.45$_b$	1.15$_c$

* Means with a different subscript differ from each other at the 0.05 level by Duncan's procedure.

target, indicated that angered subjects were more aggressive than nonangered subjects and that subjects angered by a male were more aggressive than those angered by a female. The second, anger × films, indicated that under nonanger conditions there were no effects for the films shown, but, when subjects were angry the erotic film increased aggression. Thus, when subjects were exposed to highly arousing erotic stimuli there was a possibility for aggression to be facilitated. More important to the discussion is the fact that no differential aggression was observed toward females as a function of film exposure. In fact, as has been the case in past studies,[29] less aggression was administered to the female targets. Does this imply, therefore, that erotic films do not influence aggression towards females as suggested by the pornography commission?[10] The physiological data obtained in this study would suggest that perhaps another process was operating with angered subjects. The blood pressure data indicated that higher levels of arousal were obtained with a female rather than a male target after erotic exposure, and that this arousal was still present after aggressing. It might have been expected, therefore, that aggression would have been higher toward females than males. Results, however, tended to indicate just the opposite. Under anger conditions females were aggressed against less than males. It is interesting to note that Taylor and Epstein[29] also found increased physiological arousal in male subjects who were less aggressive toward a female target under attack conditions. One possible explanation for this type of finding, suggested by Dengerink,[28] is that aggression towards females is generally disapproved of, and that this fear of disapproval could act to inhibit aggression. Further evidence that males were inhibited from acting aggressively toward female targets in this study was suggested by the reward data. Under anger conditions a reduction in reward was found for females. It would seem reasonable to suggest that in the context of this study, changes in rewarding behavior would carry less social restraints than delivery of a noxious stimulus toward a female. If these results were a function of inhibitions toward aggressing against females, then conditions allowing

TABLE 2

MEAN CHANGE* IN BLOOD PRESSURE AS A FUNCTION OF
EXPERIMENTAL CONDITIONS AFTER FILM EXPOSURE

	Film	
Condition	Erotic	Neutral
Mean Blood Pressure		
Anger		
Males	1.8_b	-0.2_b
Females	9.4_a	-3.1_c
No Anger		
Males	8.2_a	-3.9_c
Females	7.2_a	-3.9_c
Systolic Blood Pressure		
Anger		
Males	2.8_b	-1.4_b
Females	11.3_a	-4.8_c
No Anger		
Males	11.2_a	-5.6_c
Females	8.6_a	-6.2_c

* Means with different subscripts differ from each other at the 0.05 level by Duncan's procedure.

for a reduction in inhibitions might reveal differential aggression toward males and females as a function of erotic exposure.

EXPERIMENT II

The purpose of this experiment was to create a condition in which male subjects would be less inhibited or restrained against aggressing toward a female, in order to examine the effects that erotic exposure would have upon such aggression. While there are many potential strategies to reduce aggressive inhibitions (e.g., aggressive models), the present study adopted a situation similar to that employed by Geen, Stonner, and Shope.[30] These investigators found that when subjects were given two opportunities to aggress against an anger instigator, aggression was higher than in a condition in which subjects were not given this initial aggression opportunity. Furthermore, subjects in the double aggression condition reported less restraints against aggressing than individuals in all other conditions. Additional support for this increase in aggression, following an initial opportunity to aggress, has been provided by a number of investigators (e.g., Reference 31). In the context of the present experiment, it was hypothesized that allowing male subjects an initial opportunity to aggress against a female would act to reduce any aggression inhibitions present. If erotic films are capable of facilitating aggression against females, then the present experiment, by incorporating both anger instigation and highly erotic films in ad-

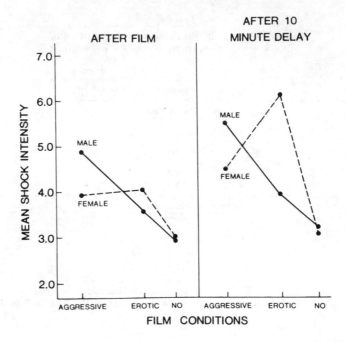

FIGURE 1. Mean shock intensity as a function of film conditions, sex of target, and time of aggression.

dition to a reduction in inhibitions, should allow for a more judicious test of this possibility.

In this study, male subjects were angered by a male or female target prior to being placed into one of three film conditions. Before being given an opportunity to aggress, subjects viewed either a highly erotic film, aggressive film, or no film. After having one opportunity to aggress against the male or female target, subjects waited 10 minutes and were given a second opportunity to aggress.

The results of the present study, as seen in FIGURE 1, would suggest that highly erotic films can act to increase aggressive responses against females under certain conditions. When male subjects were given an opportunity to aggress immediately following film exposure, it was found that highly erotic films did increase aggression beyond that of the no-film controls. This finding corroborates those of other investigators[6, 4] who have found that highly arousing erotica can act as a facilitator of aggression in previously angered individuals. In addition, it was found that during this initial aggression opportunity there was no differential aggression toward males or females. These results are also supportive of previous studies (e.g., References 27, 8, 5) that have indicated no sex-of-target effects following erotic exposure. However, when male subjects were given a second opportunity to aggress against the target, 10 minutes later, aggressive responses were increased against female targets. This finding of an increase in aggression against women in the delayed condition is the first demonstration that this effect can, in fact, occur.

EXPERIMENT III

It has been suggested that a major problem with the conclusion of the pornography commission report[10] was the lack of research on "porno-violence,"or aggressive content in erotic forms of materials.[2] This lack of research was surprising given the results of the National Commission on the Causes and Prevention of Violence,[32] dealing with media aggression and its effect on subsequent aggressive behavior.

Given the nature of most erotic films, in which women are depicted in a submissive, passive role, any subtle aggressive content could act to increase aggression against females because of their association with observed aggression. As noted in the work of Berkowitz,[33] one important determinant of whether an aggressive response is made is the presence of aggressive cues. Not only objects, but individuals can take on aggressive-cue value if they have been associated with observed violence. Thus, in the context of the present research, the viewing of more sexually aggressive films might facilitate aggression towards females because of the aggression-eliciting stimulus properties of the female target from her repeated association with observed violence. This increase in aggression should be especially true for previously angered individuals who are already predisposed to aggress. In the research discussed up to this point the films employed did not contain acts of aggression. If they did, perhaps the results would have differed with respect to female victims.

In order to examine this issue, male subjects in the present study[34] were angered or treated in a neutral manner by a male or female. They were then shown one of three films. Two of the films were highly erotic but differed in aggressive content. While one film was entirely nonaggressive, the other depicted the rape of a women by a man who breaks into her house and forces her at gunpoint into sexual activity. The third film was a neutral (nonerotic and nonaggressive) presentation.

The major results are presented in FIGURE 2. Two interactions occurred which deserve attention. The first, anger × film, indicated that both the erotic and aggressive-erotic film increased aggression, primarily in angered individuals. The largest increase occurred, however, for subjects exposed to the aggressive-erotic film. The second interaction, sex of target × film, indicated that while both types of erotic films increased aggression against a male, only the aggressive-erotic film facilitated aggression against a female, and this level of aggression was higher than that directed against a male. Why would aggression be increased against the female after exposure to the aggressive-erotic film? One potential explanation is that the females' association with the victim in the film made her an aggressive stimulus that could elicit aggressive responses (e.g., Reference 33). The combination of anger and arousal from the film heightened this response and led to the highest

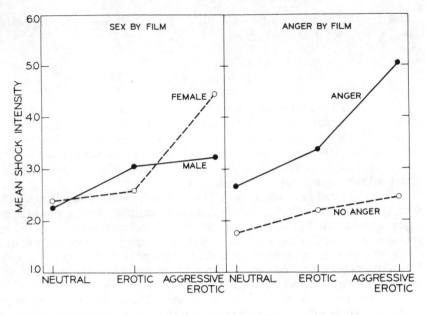

FILM CONDITIONS

FIGURE 2. Mean shock intensity as a function of sex of target by films, and anger by films.

level of aggression against the female. But, even under nonanger conditions aggression was increased. This was not the case for subjects paired with a male. Under nonanger, the aggressive-erotic film did not influence aggression against the male target. It would seem, then, that the female's association with observed violence was an important contributor to the aggressive responses toward her. If this is the case then it would be expected that films that depict violence against women, even without sexual content, could act as a stimulus for aggressive acts toward women. It seems important, therefore, for future research to begin a systematic investigation into the context of women's association with violence in the media.

CONCLUSION AND IMPLICATIONS

It was the intention of the present research to examine the effects that certain media presentations have on aggression against women. Results from these investigation suggest that films of both an erotic *and* aggressive nature can be a mediator of aggression toward women. In addition to the theoretical implications of these results, there is a more applied question that has been the concern of the present paper. When it is found that (1) 50% of university females report some form of sexual aggression,[35] (2) 39% of the sex offenders questioned indicate that pornography had something to do with the crime they committed,[36] and (3) the incidence of rape and other sexual assaults have increased then the question of what conditions precipitate such actions should be examined. The present research suggests that specific types of media account for part of these actions. Given the increase in sexual and other forms of violence against women depicted in the media, a concern over such presentations seems warranted. There is ample evidence that the observation of violent forms of media can facilitate aggressive response (e.g., Reference 37), yet to assume that the depiction of sexual-aggression could not have a similar effect, particularly against females, would be misleading. Given the findings of the present studies, it seems important for future investigations to begin a systematic examination of the role of the media in aggression against women.

ACKNOWLEDGMENTS

The advice and encouragement of Prof. Len Berkowitz in this research is greatly appreciated.

REFERENCES

1. BERKOWITZ, L. 1971. Sex and violence: we can't have it both ways. Psychology Today.
2. CLINE, V. B. 1974. Another view: pornography effects, the state of the art. *In* Where Do You Draw the Line? V.B. Cline, Ed. Brigham Young University Press. Provo, Utah.
3. DIENSTBIER, R. A. 1977. Sex and violence: Can research have it both ways? Comm. 27: 176–188.
4. ZILLMANN, D. 1971. Excitation transfer in communication-mediated aggressive behavior. J. Exp. Soc. Psychol. 7: 419–434.
5. JAFFE, Y., N. MALAMUTH, J. FEINGOLD & S. FESHBACH. 1974. Sexual arousal and behavioral aggression. J. Pers. Soc. Psychol. 30: 759–764.
6. DONNERSTEIN, E., M. DONNERSTEIN & R. EVANS. 1975. Erotic stimuli and aggression: facilitation or inhibition. J. Pers. Soc. Psychol. 32: 237–244.
7. BARON, R. A. & P. A. BELL. 1977. Sexual arousal and aggression by males: effects of type of erotic stimuli and prior provocation. J. Pers. Soc. Psychol. 35: 79–87.
8. DONNERSTEIN, E. & G. BARRETT. 1978. The effects of erotic stimuli on male aggression towards females. J. Pers. Soc. Psychol. 36: 180–188.
9. DONNERSTEIN, E. & J. HALLAM. 1978. The facilitating effects of erotica on aggression toward females. J. Pers. Soc. Psychol. 36: 1270–1277.
10. Presidential Commission on Obscenity and Pornography. 1971. U.S. Government Printing Office. Washington, D.C.
11. HOWARD, J. L., M. B. LIPTZIN & C. B. REIFLER. 1973. Is pornography a problem? J. Soc. Issues 29: 133–145.
12. LIEBERT, R. M. & N. S. SCHWARTZBERG. 1977. Effects of mass media. Annu. Rev. Psychol. 28: 141–173.
13. MEYER, T. P. 1972. The effects of sexually arousing and violent films on aggressive behavior. J. Sex. Res. 8: 324–333.
14. ZILLMANN, D., J. L. HOYT & K. D. DAY. 1974. Strength and duration of the effects of aggressive, violent, and erotic communications on subsequent aggressive behavior. Comm. Res. 1: 286–306.
15. BANDURA, A. 1973. Aggression: A Social Learning Analysis. Prentice-Hall, Inc. Englewood Cliffs, N.J.
16. ZILLMANN, D., A. KATCHER & B. MILAVSKY. 1972. Excitation transfer from physical exercise to subsequent aggressive behavior. J. Exp. Soc. Psychol. 8: 247–259.

17. DONNERSTEIN, E. & D. W. WILSON. 1976. Effects of noise and perceived control on ongoing and subsequent aggressive behavior. J. Pers. Soc. Psychol. **34**: 774–781.
18. MALAMUTH, N. M., S. FESHBACH & Y. JAFFE. 1977. Sexual arousal and aggression: recent experiments and theoretical issues. J. Soc. Issues **33**: 110–133.
19. BARON, R. A. 1974. The aggression-inhibiting influence of heightened sexual arousal. J. Pers. Soc. Psychol. **30**: 318–322.
20. FRODI, A. 1977. Sexual arousal, situational restrictiveness, and aggressive behavior. J. Res. in Pers. **11**: 48–58.
21. ZILLMANN, D. & B. S. SAPOLSKY. 1977. What mediates the effect of mild erotica on annoyance and hostile behavior in males? J. Pers. Soc. Psychol. **35**: 587–596.
22. MORGAN, R. 1978. Going Too Far. Vintage Press, Inc. New York, N.Y.
23. BROWNMILLER, S. 1975. Against Our Will. Bantam Books, Inc. New York, N.Y.
24. EYSENCK, H. J. & H. NIAS. 1978. Sex, Violence, and the Media. Spector. London, England.
25. MOSHER, D. L. 1971. Pornographic films, male verbal aggression against women, and guilt. *In* Technical Report of the Commission on Obscenity and Pornography **8**. U.S. Government Printing Office. Washington, D.C.
26. MOSHER, D. L. 1971. Psychological reactions to pornographic films. *In* Technical Report of the Commission on Obscenity and Pornography **8**. U.S. Government Printing Office. Washington, D.C.
27. BARON, R. A. & P. A. BELL. 1973. Effects of heightened sexual arousal on physical aggression. Proc. 81st Ann. Conv. of the Amer. Psych. Assoc. **8**: 171–172.
28. DENGERINK, H. A. 1976. Personality variables as mediators of attack-instigated aggression. *In* Perspectives on Aggression. R. Geen & E. O'Neal, Eds. Academic Press Inc. New York, N.Y.
29. TAYLOR, S. P. & S. EPSTEIN. 1967. Aggression as a function of the interaction of the sex of the aggressor and the sex of the victim. Pers. **35**: 474–486.
30. GEEN, R. G., D. STONNER & G. L. SHOPE. 1975. The facilitation of aggression by aggression: a study of response inhibition and disinhibition. J. Pers. Soc. Psychol. **31**: 721–726.
31. GEEN, R. G. & M. B. QUANTY. 1977. The facilitation of aggression by aggression: a study of response inhibition and disinhibition. J. Pers. Soc. Psychol. **31**: 721–726.
32. National Commission on the Causes and Prevention of Violence. 1969. U.S. Government Printing Office. Washington, D.C.
33. BERKOWITZ, L. 1974. Some determinants of impulsive aggression: the role of mediated associations with reinforcements for aggression. Psych. Rev. **81**: 165–176.
34. DONNERSTEIN, E. 1979. Pornography commission revisited: aggressive-erotica and violence against women. (Submitted for publication.)
35. KANIN, E. G. & S. R. PARCELL. 1977. Sexual aggression: a second look at the offended female. Arch. Sex. Behav. **6**: 67–76.
36. WALKER, E. C. 1971. Erotic stimuli and the aggressive sexual offender. Technical Report of Commission on Obscenity and Pornography **8**. U.S. Government Printing Office. Washington, D.C.
37. GEEN, R. G. 1978. Some effects of observing violence upon the behavior of the observer. *In* Progress in Experimental Personality Research. B. Maher, Ed. **8**. Academic Press, Inc. New York, N.Y.

TELEVISION VIEWING AND AGGRESSIVE BEHAVIOR IN PRESCHOOL CHILDREN: A FIELD STUDY*

Dorothy G. Singer and Jerome L. Singer

Family Television Research and Consultation Center
Yale University
New Haven, Connecticut 06520

Previous Research

For the past two decades, television, "a member of the family,"[1] has been a major influence on the behavior patterns of children. Extensive research by Bandura[2] has indicated very clearly that children imitate observed acts of aggression whether carried out by live adults or filmed models. Television may also reduce some of the sensitivities to pain in others,[3] and provide a basic moral support for violence since in program after program we witness the good guys physically assaulting or shooting the bad guys.[1] Work by Huston-Stein and Wright[4] and Watt and Krull[5] suggests too that the high rate of activity and the arousal value of television may also predispose children to aggressive action. Laboratory studies under controlled conditions (Friedrich and Stein,[6] Noble[7-9]) indicate that children exposed to aggressive films increase their level of aggression.

In a comprehensive report, supported by the Surgeon General's Committee on Television and Social Behavior,[10] accumulated evidence suggests that children predisposed to be aggressive may increase their level of aggression after exposure to violence on television. The data from field studies[11-13] wherein children have been followed up over longer periods of time than in the laboratory studies show a positive correlation on the order of 0.25 between television viewing and incidence of aggressive behavior. While these correlations are modest, they do suggest some evidence that television contributes to some degree to the many possible causes of aggression in children.

An important longitudinal project involved a ten-year follow-up of boys and girls originally studied in the third grade by Lefkowitz *et al.*[14] Their results indicate that boys who preferred violent television at age nine were the most aggressive both at that time and ten years later. These authors have found that one of the best single predictors at the age of nine of whether a boy will be rated as aggressive by peers or by other criteria ten years later is the amount of *violent* television he watches in childhood. These researchers ruled out possible mediating effects of intelligence, social class, or family background as a means of explaining the correlation for violent television, 0.21 ($P < 0.01$) with concurrent peer-rated aggressiveness

* This study was supported by the Spencer Foundation and by National Science Foundation Grant DAR 6-20772.

and 0.31 ($P < 0.001$) with aggressiveness ten years later. Another study by William Belson[15] in England, following a group of boys between the ages of 12 and 17 over a period of time, indicates that the watching of aggressive material on television, particularly that associated with relatively realistic violent activity such as plays or films in which violence occurs in the context of close personal relations, westerns of a violent kind, programs presenting gratuitous violence, and programs presenting fictional violence of a realistic kind, influences these teenagers to increase their levels of violence. In contrast, he found little or no support for the hypothesis that exposure to sporting programs, science fiction violence, slapstick comedy, or violent cartoons influenced these teenagers to increase their levels of violence.

The Longitudinal Study

One of the objectives of this research was a longitudinal study of the relationship between television viewing within the family setting and possible influences of such viewing on the ongoing patterns of aggression observed during free-play situations in the day-care or preschool setting over a year's time.

Two hundred children from 13 preschool classes in the New Haven, Connecticut area participated in the study. Intelligence, capacity for concept formation, and receptive listening skills were assessed as baseline measures using the Peabody Vocabulary Test, the Do You Know Test (ETS), and Listen to the Story Test (ETS) respectively. In addition, an interview with the child on play activities and television viewing habits was administered.

The children were also observed during their free-play periods for two ten-minute sessions as a baseline for subsequent longitudinal evaluation. Trained observers, working in pairs, simultaneously watched each child and independently recorded all behavior and language. The behavior of the child was then rated independently according to a five-point scale for 20 variables that had been carefully defined in advance. Three such probe periods were conducted during the year's study.

Each family participating in the study kept television log records for a two-week period three times during the year. The log books supplied to the parents consisted of a day-by-day listing of all programs presented by both commercial and educational television stations. Parents were requested to record the degree of intensity and the specific programs watched by the children as well as with whom, if anyone, they viewed each program. Every program recorded in the logbook as having been seen by the child was then coded according to its content.

A detailed informed consent was provided by each family interested in participating in the program. This form follows the guidelines developed by Yale's Faculty of Arts and Sciences Committee. In addition to the consent forms, parents were asked to provide information on the child, some information on family occupational and educational levels (suitable for later use in estimating socioeconomic status), birth order, sex of children, and family size.

Characteristics of the Sample

The eleven participating nursery schools, day care centers, and preschool classes represent institutions that service predominantly lower-middle-class families. Several schools were publicly funded through the state and, in the case of the two public school systems (East Haven and Hamden), through the Federal Title I funds. The structure of each school permitted reasonably unobtrusive observation of the children. The patterns of school activities allowed a sufficient degree of spontaneous free-play behaviors, and the staff were understanding and cooperative.

Pretesting

The following instruments were administered individually to each child involved in the project prior to the observation phase of the first probe: (1) Peabody Picture Vocabulary Test (PPVT) is a nonverbal IQ estimate which requires the child to point to the picture of the item designated by the teacher: e.g., given the word *tackle*, the child points to one of four pictures on the page. (2) Do You Know (Circus, ETS) measures a child's knowledge of facts and concepts necessary for functioning in school and outside. Example: Which of the pictures shows how warm it is outside (thermometer)? (3) Listen to the Story (Circus, ETS) measures the child's ability to listen, understand, and remember information. (4) Interview on imaginative play and television viewing patterns consists of direct questioning of child con-

TABLE 1

SAMPLE CHARACTERISTICS

$N = 199$ Race: White = 144
Male = 89   Oriental = 2
Female = 110   Hispanic = 6
Age 3 = 50   Black = 47
Age 4 = 149   Primary Language: English = 194
    Non-English = 5

	$\bar{X}$	S.D.
SES Index	3.42	0.94
Peabody PVT (I.Q.)	99.29	19.61
Listen to the Story	13.19	3.51
Do You Know	21.64	4.69
Imaginary Playmate, Part A	6.29	2.40
Stuffed Animals, Part B	8.60	2.91
Total Imaginary Playmate Questionnaire	14.84	4.29

cerning imaginative play tendencies, imaginary companions, favorite television shows, characters on television, as well as patterns of viewing.

TABLE 1 presents the basic data on the sample with respect to the pre-dispositional measures. Overall, the IQ scores, concept level, and listening comprehension were within normal range ($\overline{X}$ = 99.29, S.D. = 19.61).

Observational Variables

In each probe period, children were observed on two separate occasions by two observers who independently recorded everything the child did for a ten-minute period (including verbatim speech). These observers subsequently rated the child independently along a series of 20 variables; Imaginativeness of Play, Positive Affect, Persistence, Evidence of Overt Aggressive Behavior, Motor Activity, Interaction with Peers and Adults, Cooperation with Peers and Adults, Leadership, Fear, Anger, Sadness,

TABLE 2

RELIABILITY OF RATERS ON FIRST AND SECOND OCTOBER OBSERVATIONS 1978

Variable	Observation	Kappa	Variable	Observation	Kappa
Imagination	1	0.72*	Leadership	1	0.64*
	2	0.73*		2	0.64*
Positive Affect	1	0.47*	Fearful	1	0.46*
	2	0.51*		2	0.25†
Persistence	1	0.43*	Angry	1	0.42*
	2	0.59*		2	0.56*
Aggression Towards	1	0.74*	Sad	1	0.42*
	2	0.75*		2	0.54*
			Fatigued	1	0.49*
				2	0.44*
Motor Activity	1	0.58*	Sensory Motor	1	0.46*
	2	0.59*		2	0.60*
Interaction Peers	1	0.56*	Mastery	1	0.58*
	2	0.61*		2	0.65*
Interaction Adults	1	0.54*	Make-believe Play	1	0.64*
	2	0.61*		2	0.78*
Cooperation Peers	1	0.51*	Games With Rules	1	0.49*
	2	0.49*		2	0.66*
Cooperation Adults	1	0.48*			
	2	0.59*			

* $P < 0.00001$.
† $P < 0.00003$.
15 pairs of observers
N = 198
Note: Based on D. Cicchetti's interobserver reliability formula

Fatigue, Sensory-Motor Activities, Mastery Play, Make-Believe Play, Games with Rules, Number of Words, and Onomatopoetic Sounds. In effect, these variables represent a priori grouping of behaviors of a general type; e.g., imaginativeness (introduction of make-believe elements into play), positive emotionality (as represented by affects such as interests, curiosity, smiling, laughing, etc.), and persistence at a task for a period of time.

Training of Observers

The observers ($N = 31$), largely Yale undergraduates and graduate students, were selected based on their background in psychology and education.

Observers were provided with 16 typed protocols that were behavioral samples collected in an earlier study and a set of coding instructions. Each variable was discussed in relationship to the instruction booklet. Observers had ample opportunity to discuss reasons for their ratings and a high rate of agreement was attempted on the five-point scale for each variable at each session. During the final sessions, a training tape developed by the Yale Child Study Center was shown that illustrated typical play behaviors in a nursery-school setting. The observers were asked to rate a particular child according to the 20 variables. Observers were given further instructions concerning procedure. Letters of introduction, school etiquette, and actual recording procedures were all discussed in detail.

These sessions were repeated three weeks before the second and third probe for observers who were new to the project. A refresher session was required for those who had participated in previous observations.

Observation Procedures

Observers were told to record in an appropriate place on the record sheet the child's appearance, mannerisms, physical build, time they began and ended each recording, date, sex, and code number of each child. Observations were made only during free-play periods both indoors and out. Observers used a clipboard and stopwatch and tried to be as unobtrusive as possible as they recorded the child's actions and language. Language was recorded verbatim. Observers were instructed not to interrupt behavior, but to accurately record what took place. After the behavior was written down, each observer would then rate the child on the 20 variables, using the five-point scale.

Inter-rater reliability estimates were obtained on the ratings the observers made on the practice protocols and on the actual protocols they collected themselves in the first observational period. Rater reliability was excellent for both training periods, as well as the first probe. Interobserver reliability for all the variables yielded highly significant kappas (TABLE 2).

Development of Logs

The television logs were developed by reviewing the local *TV Guide* and newspaper listing guides for the New Haven area. The daily shows were listed in hour segments of time and recorded on three logging sheets: morning, afternoon, and evening. Space was provided on the sheets for parents to note any programs the child may have watched not listed on the log. A two-week sample of television viewing was obtained for each child; three samples per child throughout the year.

The parents received detailed recording instructions enclosed with the television log packets. They were asked to circle the program watched on the logs. The parents were instructed to note how intensely the child watched a program on a scale of 1 to 5. A rating of "1" meant that the child scarcely watched the program or paid any attention to it, while "5" meant that the child watched with great interest and absorption. In addition, parents were asked to note whether the child watched the program alone, with parents (P), siblings (S), other adults (O), or other children (C) and were instructed to include any combination of people, i.e., other adults and other children.

After each probe period when logs had been returned, the information was transcribed onto a weekly summary sheet. Every show the child watched was noted along with the intensity and with whom it was watched.

Preparation for Statistical Analysis

Time Watched

Each day's viewing was totaled and noted at the bottom of the sheet. A weekly total was achieved by summing all 7 days. The two-week sample was treated as one unit. All statistics are done on a two-week sample. Therefore, when analyzed, if a child watched 5 hours on the first Monday of the logging period and 3 hours on the following Monday, a total of 8 hours was entered for that day. Means and standard deviations were found for the two-week sample, the total sample as well as males and females. Further analysis includes comparisons of a weekday vs. weekend viewing.

Intensity

Finding the mean intensity for each child was based on a half-hour time period. The figure entered would be multiplied by the number of half hours for a show, times the intensity reported on the log. For example, if a child watched an hour and one-half program with an intensity of 4, the intensity would be multiplied by 3. The mean intensity for the sample was achieved by summing all the prorated intensities and dividing by the total number of half hours. As with the viewing time, the mean intensity is based on a two-week period.

Who Watched with Whom

Data on whether the child watched alone or with specific others were based on a half-hour period. Combinations of with whom children watched the shows were entered for analysis. How many hours a child watched television alone, or with parents, and any combination of people were summed for the two-week period and entered for analysis.

Programs Viewed

The programs available for viewing by this group and actually reported on the logs by parents were classified into nine categories and coded:

A. Cartoons, e.g., "Bugs Bunny," "Flintstones."
B. Children's Commercial Shows, e.g., "Captain Kangaroo," "Magic Garden."
C. Educational Shows, e.g., "Sesame Street," "Zoom," "Mr. Rogers."
D. Situation Comedies, e.g., "Happy Days," "I Love Lucy," "Brady Bunch."
E. Game, Variety, Talk, e.g., "Gong Shows," "Mike Douglas," "Jeopardy."
F. Adult Nonviolent, e.g., soap operas, "The Waltons," "Little House On the Prairie."
G. Action-Adventure, e.g., "Wonder Woman," "The Incredible Hulk," "Charlie's Angels."
H. Sports (violent only), e.g., boxing, hockey, auto racing, football.
I. Newscasts and Documentaries.

The categories were divided into the top shows in each category by a quick view of the summary sheets. For example, in Category "A," the shows listed were: "Bugs Bunny," "Scooby-Doo," "Spiderman," etc. If a child watched a show not listed in our program breakdown, it was included under the general category for that type of program, e.g., a special.

The individual programs were combined in categories to determine how many hours children watched a program under the various categories. The programs were also summed individually to determine how many hours a specific show such as "Sesame Street" was watched.

Parametric Characteristics

Our participants' average SES level is in the upper range on the Duncan and Hollingshead-Redlich Scales, clearly a blue-collar to lower-middle socioeconomic status (SES) group. The average Peabody IQ is 99.3; non-whites represent 23–24% of the group; the sample has a somewhat higher number of females than males (110–89), and 4-year-olds predominate over 3-year-olds (149–50).

Predispositional Variables

The children were all administered three types of intelligence tests: the Peabody Picture Vocabulary Test, which yields an IQ based on verbal labeling of pictures; the Listen to the Story and Do You Know scales (newly developed as potentially useful cross-cultural measures of intellectual development by the Educational Testing Service). The scores of our participants on these last two scales were below the currently available normative average although IQs from the PPVT were at the national mean. Subsequent data analyses in this report will be based on the PPVT IQs only, since they have proved to be more reliable with our sample.

In addition to cognitive measures, children were also questioned about imaginary playmates with a scale broken down separately for invisible friends and for stuffed animals.

Results

Patterns of Play and Aggression

As might be expected, certain behavioral variables show significant increases across the probe periods, reflecting particular patterns of growth. Thus, Cooperation and Interaction show steady increases as does Leadership. Aggressive behavior also increased steadily over the year from a mean of 3.01 to a mean of 3.69 [F (2,176), linear trend = 26.6, $P < 0.001$]. This level of aggression is moderately high for such young children.

A factor-analytic examination of the behavioral background and television-viewing variables was carred out. Clearest results emerge from a two-factor principal axis factor analysis with varimax rotation in which the number of hours spent viewing each category of television programming was employed. TABLE 3 presents the results of such a factor analysis across the year with means based on all three probes. The $N = 159$ reflects children from whom full data over the year on all variables were available.

Inspection of TABLE 3 indicates that Factor 1 includes highest loadings for Peer Interaction (0.80), Cooperation with Peers (0.79), Leadership (0.79), Imaginativeness in Play (0.75), and Positive Affect (0.77). This factor corresponds closely with results from our earlier study with middle-class preschoolers[16] and may be labeled *Playfulness*. It essentially indexes a "happy," friendly, and imaginative child. No relationship to television-viewing patterns is in evidence.

The second factor shows its highest loadings for Aggression (0.70) and general Motor Activity (0.68), as well as the affect of Anger (0.52). This factor also reflects sizable loadings for two television variables, the number of hours viewing action-adventure shows (0.44) and game shows (0.36). The

TABLE 3

FACTOR LOADINGS FROM PRINCIPAL AXIS FACTOR ANALYSIS
(VARIMAX ROTATION): TWO FACTOR SOLUTION WITHOUT TOTAL TELEVISION VIEWING

Variable	Factor 1	Factor 2
Sex (1 = M, 2 = F)		−0.45
IQ	0.32	−0.37
Age		
SES		
Ethnic Group (1 = white, 2 = nonwhite)		
Total Imaginary Companion Score		
Imaginativeness in Play	0.75	
Positive Affect	0.77	
Persistence during Play	0.50	
Aggression		0.70
Motor Activity		0.68
Peer Interaction	0.80	
Adult Interaction		
Cooperation with Peers	0.79	
Cooperation with Adults		
Leadership	0.79	
Fear	−0.32	
Angry		0.52
Sad	−0.38	
Fatigue	−0.49	
Sensory Motor Play		
Mastery		
Make-Believe Play	0.65	
Games with Rules		
Number of Words	0.74	
Onomatopoetic Sounds	0.31	0.39
Cartoons		
Commercial Children's Shows		
Educational Television		
Situation Comedies		
Variety/Game Shows		0.36
Adult Drama		
Action Shows		0.44
Sports		
News/Documentaries		
Television Viewing Intensity		

Note: N = 159

factor pattern also reflects Sex and IQ loadings (−0.45 and −0.37, respectively) suggesting that it is somewhat more characteristic of boys and of children with lower IQs. This factor seems to index the linkage of aggressive and high-arousal programming to overt aggressive or unfocused motor activity as reported in our earlier study with middle-class preschoolers.[17] Examples of action-adventure shows viewed by these children are "Six Million Dollar Man," "Battlestar Galactica," "The Incredible Hulk," and "Wonder Woman." The game shows are characterized by much shouting and hysterical motor activity. This factor can tentatively be labeled *aggression-action television-viewing*.

TABLE 4

CANONICAL CORRELATION ANALYSES OF TELEVISION VIEWING WITH
BEHAVIOR AND PREDISPOSITIONAL VARIABLES*

Variable	Loading of First Canonical Variate	Loading on Second Canonical Variate
Television Variables (Set 1)		
Cartoons	0.32	0.45
Children's Commercial Shows	0.05	0.10
Educational Television Children's Shows	0.51	0.26
Situation Comedies	−0.25	−0.08
Variety-Game Shows	−0.57	0.19
Adult/Family	−0.30	0.26
Action/Detective	−0.50	0.60
News/Documentaries	−0.55	0.51
Behavior and Predispositional (Set 2)		
Imaginative Play	0.02	0.04
Positive Affect	−0.09	0.27
Aggression	−0.08	0.42
Motor Activity	−0.16	0.50
Cooperation Peers	0.17	0.14
Angry	0.14	0.62
Sad	−0.29	−0.09
Fatigue	−0.18	−0.10
Socioeconomic Status	−0.34	−0.03
Ethnicity	−0.82	0.23
IQ	0.49	−0.26
Sex	0.04	−0.61
Age	0.19	−0.07

* Based on an average of three probes. First canonical correlation = 0.65, χ^2 = 199, df = 104, P = 0.00001. Second canonical correlation = 0.50, χ^2 = 114, df = 84, P = 0.02.

Although background variables are not strongly implicated in the principal factor solution, a canonical correlation analysis based on the averages of the three probes over the year does add some new information (TABLE 4). This analysis yields two significant canonical variates when television variables are pitted against behavioral and background variables. The first indicates that nonwhites especially and also lower-SES or lower-IQ children are especially likely to be heavier viewers of action, game, and news shows (or adult-oriented fare, more generally) and less likely to be watchers of educational television [Public Broadcasting Station (PBS) children's shows] or cartoons (canonical correlation = 0.65, χ^2 = 199, df = 104, P < 0.00001).

The second canonical variable further confirms the link of action shows to Aggression and high Motor Activity and Anger, indicating also that heavy television viewing of news and cartoons may also relate to action. This relationship again seems especially strong for boys. (Canonical correlation = 0.50, χ^2 = 114, df = 84, P < 0.02).

In effect this analysis suggests that while ethnic background and SES or IQ may be strongly associated with viewing preferences for adult (and less

TABLE 5

RESULTS OF MULTIPLE REGRESSION ANALYSES:
STEPWISE PREDICTION OF AGGRESSION VARIABLES AT TIME 2 FROM INDIVIDUAL SHOWS AT
TIME 1 AFTER ENTERING ETHNICITY, IQ, AND SES

Aggression

Background Variables	Simple R	F-ratio Unique Contribution	Standardized Beta Weight
Ethnicity	0.06	0.5	0.06
IQ	−0.14	2.95	−0.14
SES	0.19*	3.76	0.14
First Five Television Shows			
"Sesame Street"	0.22†	13.5‡	0.27
"Super Heroes"	0.22†	11.3‡	0.25
"Woody Woodpecker"	0.21†	10.4†	0.24
"I Love Lucy"	0.14	7.6†	−0.20
"Talk Shows"	0.14	4.3*	0.15
Multiple R	0.51‡		

* $P < 0.05$
† $P < 0.01$
‡ $P < 0.001$

child-oriented) programming, such a relationship does not account for our finding that aggression is tied to viewing of action-oriented television. We cannot explain the fact that more aggressive children are more likely to be watching the more violent programming by asserting that this reflects only a viewing preference of an ethnic or class group whose behavior is already known to show higher levels of motor activity or fighting in preschool periods. If, on the other hand, the type of television viewed is playing some role in stimulating aggression, it is occurring irrespective of the social class or ethnicity of the children.

Another way of looking at this is through partialling out the effect of background factors on the first-order correlation between aggression and action-television viewing. This correlation for the total sample across the three probes is 0.15 ($P < 0.05$). When IQ, SES, sex, and ethnicity are partialled out individually and then in combination, the correlation drops only a total of 0.04 points suggesting that background factors are not in themselves critical determinants of this linkage, and again confirming our earlier work with middle-class children.[16]

While our data cannot be definitive in suggesting a causal link between viewing television and aggression, we can rule out the fact that the linkage is more a reflection of a viewing preference by already aggressive children through examining cross-lagged correlations. We find for example that the correlation between watching action-adventure television shows at Time 1 (October) is correlated +0.18, $P < 0.05$ with Aggression at Time 3 (April). The correlation of Aggression at Time 1 with action television viewing at Time 3 is only +0.05. This result again conforms to our earlier findings.[16] The effects of total television viewing we had observed before are not evident here, and our data specifically highlight the action-television and aggression link-up with the indications that possible causality goes from viewing towards behavior rather than the reverse. This is not the case for action television and Motor Activity where the correlations from Time 1–Time 3 are significant but equivalent suggesting no clear possible causal direction.

Specific Programming and Overt Behavior

Our data as presented have focused on general categories of programming because these are more consistent across time and less subject to schedule changes. In this study, however, we also examined the links between specific shows and the behavioral variables. This seems an important step because certain cartoons, for example, may be very full of violence while others are not. Hence any modeling or arousal interpretation of television viewing and behavior may be limited if there are contradictory patterns of content subsumed by combining shows under a general rubric. In the next section we will examine correlations and multiple regression predictions of behavior patterns based on the specific programs our children watched.

Examining which specific shows viewed at Time 1 best predicted aggressive behavior at Time 2 yielded a surprise. It turned out that heavy viewing of "Sesame Street" proved to be especially strongly linked to later aggressive behavior. A multiple-regression analysis of the television shows and background variables predicting later overt aggression (criterion) indicates that heavy watching of "Sesame Street" was the best single predictor of aggression three months later. The correlation of "Sesame Street" with Aggression over the year was 0.22, $P < 0.01$, as a matter of fact.

TABLE 5 makes it clear that specific cartoons that have especially violent content, "Superheroes" and "Woody Woodpecker," are also important predictors of aggression. A situation comedy, "I Love Lucy," proves to be negatively linked to later aggression, a result that may chiefly reflect its attraction for girls who prove less aggressive. This result is contrary to our early findings that this type of programming was tied to overt aggression in girls.

The strong influence of violent cartoons or action shows is also supported when one looks across the year—the best predictors from Time 1 to Time 3 for aggression include viewing of "Scooby-Doo" and the "Six Million Dollar Man." The effect of "Sesame Street" drops off by the third probe apparently because viewing of this show also drops sharply, especially by those children who were more aggressive in the second probe.

If we look at Motor Activity at Time 2 after partialling out the effects of IQ, SES, and ethnicity, the role of very active programming is again clear. "Tom and Jerry" cartoons and "Charlie's Angels" (an action show) both yield significant simple rs (0.21, $P < 0.01$ and 0.28, $P < 0.01$, respectively) and highly significant F-ratios for their unique contributions to the prediction equation. The "Muppets," a much-loved but very active "Sesame Street"-like show, also contributes significantly to the Multiple R while "Laverne and Shirley" and the viewing of "Disney World" are negatively linked to later high levels of Motor Activity. Prediction across the year from Time 1 indicates that early viewing of "Spider Man," another active cartoon, and of game shows are positively linked to later Motor Activity while "Disney World" and "Soap" (a humorous but nonviolent or motor-active comedy series) are negative predictors.

In general, our look at the specific programming tied to later aggression or vigorous activity tends to support a combined modeling-arousal model. "Sesame Street," a program characterized by rapid shifts, arousing and sometimes aggressive content,[18] is linked to aggression along with extremely aggressive cartoons or adventure shows. The shifts in viewing and the schedule changes (or the fact that increased afternoon light for outdoor play cuts out viewing of certain shows) weaken the reliability of the specific programs as measures compared with the categories of programming. Still our findings from the individual shows suggest that those shows especially involving considerable physical motion, rapidity of changes, and violence (as in cartoons, action-adventure, or game shows) are linked to aggression as the more general category of action-adventure.

DISCUSSION

The present study is the first to examine the possible relationships between television viewing and spontaneous behavior in day-care settings for a group of preschool children from lower socioeconomic backgrounds. In general our results support the growing body of findings suggesting that heavier viewing of programs characterized by violent action, considerable rapidity of movement, or related arousing activities may be associated with more aggressive and nonfocused motor activity by preschoolers. Two not necessarily contradictory hypotheses have been advanced in the past for the link between television viewing and aggressive behavior, a generalized arousal effect[5] or the imitation of violent actions.[2] Our findings suggest that the specific category of programming most regularly associated with aggressive activity by these children is *action-adventure*. When we look at *specific* shows we find that aggression is also associated with viewing of particularly aggressive cartoons such as "Superheroes" and "Woody Woodpecker" and also certain game shows known for their hyperactivity, screeching, and a hysterical quality. If there is a causal link between programming and the subsequent behavior of preschoolers, our data suggest that heavy exposure to aggressive and also to rapid-cut content (as in "Sesame Street" or the "Muppets"), or to hysterical behavior by adults (game shows), may work together to produce aggression in children.

Of course our data cannot demonstrate causality definitively. We have attempted to rule out alternative explanations for the association between aggressive behavior and television, however. Partialling out the possible effects of class, IQ, or ethnicity does not affect substantially our correlations. It cannot be argued that children who are aggressive are simply reflecting life-style patterns of a subculture which also watches a good deal of more violent or adult-oriented television. It is the case, as the data from our canonical analysis suggests, that nonwhite and lower SES children do watch more adult-oriented shows and less of the "better quality," PBS, child-oriented shows. But that cannot explain the aggression-action show association which emerges in our second canonical variate.

Our cross-lag analyses also seem to rule out the usual argument that aggressive children simply prefer violent programming. What seems more likely is that there is a subtle interaction effect[16] between viewing, arousal and imitation, and then subsequent preference.

These findings must be viewed in perspective. Our participants were small children who, after all, were not violent. Their aggression consisted of pushing, hitting, knocking over others' blocks, or snatching a toy. It remains to be seen whether such early and consistent aggression is predictive of a later history of antisocial behavior. It is clear that by four years of age children are already confirmed television viewers. The accumulating evidence suggests that those children who are regularly exposed, through parental laxity or ignorance,[16] to violent adult programming or to arousing content are also being put "at risk" for the development of later tendencies to uncooperative, antisocial behavior with peers.

ACKNOWLEDGMENTS

We express our thanks to Paul Christoph for his statistical help and to Richard Gerrig for his editorial assistance.

REFERENCES

1. SINGER, J. L. & D. G. SINGER. 1977. Television: a member of the family. National Elementary School Principal 56(3): 50–53.
2. BANDURA, A. 1973. Aggression: A Social Learning Analysis. Prentice-Hall, Inc. Englewood Cliffs, N.J.
3. CLINE, V. B., R. G. CROFT & S. COURRIER. 1973. Desensitization of children to television violence. J. Pers. Soc. Psych. 27: 360–365.
4. HUSTON-STEIN, A. & J. C. WRIGHT. Children and television: effects of the medium, its content, and its form. J. Res. Dev. Ed. (In press.)
5. WATT, J. H. & R. KRULL. 1977. An examination of three models of television viewing and aggression. Human Comm. Res. 3: 99–112.
6. FRIEDRICH, L. K. & A. H. STEIN. 1975. Prosocial television and young children: the effects of verbal labeling and role playing on learning and behavior. Child Dev. 46: 27–38.
7. NOBLE, G. 1970. Film-mediated creative and aggressive play. Brit. J. Soc. Clin. Psych. 9: 1–7.
8. NOBLE, G. 1973. Effects of different forms of filmed aggression on children's constructive and destructive play. J. Pers. Soc. Psych. 26: 54–59.
9. NOBLE, G. 1975. Children in Front of the Small Screen. Constable. London, England.
10. Surgeon General's Scientific Advisory Committee on Television and Social Behavior. 1972. Television and Growing Up: The Impact of Televised Violence. U.S. Government Printing Office. Washington, D.C.
11. BAILYN, L. 1959. Mass media and children: a study of exposure habits and cognitive effects. Psychological Monographs 73(471).

12. CHAFFEE, S. 1972. Television and adolescent aggressiveness. *In* Television and Social Behavior. J. P. Murray, G. A. Comstock & E. A. Rubinstein, Eds. 3. U.S. Government Printing Office. Washington, D.C.
13. SCHRAMM, W., J. LYLE & E. PARKER. 1961. Television in the Lives of Our Children. Stanford University Press. Stanford, Calif.
14. LEFKOWITZ, M. M., L. D. ERON, L. O. WALDER & L. R. HUESMANN. 1977. Growing Up To Be Violent. Pergamon Press, Inc. New York, N.Y.
15. BELSON, W. A. 1978. Television and the Adolescent Boy. Saxon House. Hampshire, England.
16. SINGER, J. L. & D. G. SINGER. 1980. Television, Imagination and Aggression: A Study of Preschoolers. Erlbaum. Hillsdale, N.J.
17. SINGER, J. L. & D. G. SINGER. 1980. Television viewing, family style and aggressive behavior in preschool children. *In* Violence in the Family: Psychiatric, Sociological and Historical Implications. M. Green, Ed. AAAS Symposium Series. Washington, D.C.
18. SINGER, J. L. & D. G. SINGER. 1979. Come back, Mr. Rogers, come back. Psych. Today. **12**(10): 56-60.

CHILDREN AND AGGRESSION AFTER OBSERVED FILM AGGRESSION WITH SANCTIONING ADULTS

Gilbert J. Eisenberg

Union Free School District 13
Valley Stream, New York 11580

INTRODUCTION

This paper is the result of work done on a dissertation at Fordham University. How and why this study came about are, perhaps, just as important as the results of the study itself.

For decades criticism has been leveled against the social scientist, accusing him of carrying out various scientifically controlled studies, performing black magic under the rubric of statistics, and finally making a statement about this or that variable having a significant effect on another variable—all of which was seen as nonsense by the reader. Such an attitude on the part of the reader often merited consideration, since he dismissed the results of the study because the data were collected from a contrived situation and thus had little or no bearing on the real world. It was the attempt to avoid these pitfalls that led me to the "why" of my study. For looking at the "why" points up the need for continued concern on real-life viewing conditions in the area of media violence and points up the powerful impact that media have on our children.

Hopefully, only a few persons will find fault with the conditions under which the following observations were obtained. The observations were taken within the context of the real world; they are descriptive in nature, which implies some degree of objectivity; and they were the *raison d'être* for the study.

I have been employed as a psychologist in an elementary school in a predominantly white, middle-class, suburban community where material needs are fairly satisfied, where lawns are manicured, homes freshly painted—in essence, a community that personifies the American dream. Children come to school well attired and appear cared for. Parents' concern is evidenced by an active PTA and by the willingness of parents to come to school for the numerous meetings that are requested during the school year.

During my 11 years in the district, it became apparent that television was having an effect on the children. When Evel Knievel was the rage and attempted to achieve his jump from a canyon in the Southwest, I watched daily as many of the boys tried to imitate that jump over makeshift contraptions on dirt paths bordering the expressway and noted the resulting injuries. "Kung Fu" had a similar effect—for months the impact of the program was felt in the school as young children interacted with each other using elaborate kung fu techniques.

Not many months later, a television network aired a two-part program

304

on the Manson murders. After the program was aired, I did an informal survey of the intermediate grades in my building. These children were 9 to 11 years of age. I found that of the children I sampled, over 70% had watched the program and, further, most of them had viewed the program alone or with siblings; few had watched with an adult present. I might add that this program was aired at a time other than the "family hour"—at a time when young audiences supposedly do not view television.

Shortly after this survey, I happened to be walking past a third-grade classroom. The coat rack faced the door, and what I saw absolutely astonished me. On the hooks all along the rack I saw a toy arsenal—toy rifles and pistols staring me in the face as I looked in this classroom—a classroom of children who were eight years of age. I spoke with the teacher later that morning in a sincere attempt to get some sort of explanation; she told me that her children were playing "SWAT." That day on the lunch hour, and on subsequent days, I went out to the playground and watched these little children play. What I saw enacted were hostage situations of the type depicted on the television show "SWAT"; children were shooting and yelling at each other. During the times I observed these children at play, I did not once see any attempt by any of them to resolve the conflict through mediation or even surrender—the resolution was always found in the ultimate "shoot-out," with the children play-acting dead all over the grounds. After some days of watching eight-year-old children imitating the violence and killing they had seen on a television program, my dissertation was born.

Human aggression has been present in every era of recorded history. From early times to the present, the history books provide a steady commentary on man's inhumanity toward man. Many explanations have been proposed in an attempt to understand this phenomenon of aggression, which in some of its manifestations is unique to *Homo sapiens*. Hall finds that destructive fighting is practically unknown among baboons,[1] an animal society that most closely resembles human society.

As in former cultures, the present society must look at the nature of human aggression. It is an issue that takes on increasing importance, partly because of mass media exposure and partly because of the nature of modern technology, which enables man to inflict massive destruction on his fellow man. It is an issue from which one cannot hide. Sagan pointed this out when he said:

Human aggression, like Dionysus in Euripides' *Bacchae,* will not go away because we deny its existence. Only if we are willing to look at this destructiveness—undisguised—will we succeed in understanding and conquering it.[2]

While there have been several major theoretical bases that have been proposed as explanations for the origins of aggression—i.e., biological and psychoanalytic instinctual theories and the frustration-aggression theory—the author selected Bandura's theory of aggression.

Bandura proposed a social learning theory arguing that the prevailing theories, those concerned primarily with operant or instrumental conditioning, were much too narrow to encompass the scope of human learning.[3] He maintained that many social responses would not be acquired if social training proceeded solely by the method of successive approximation, and he further felt that in terms of human learning, the operant conditioning model was grossly inefficient. Thus, he proposed a social learning theory in which learning was generally labeled "imitation." He defined this as "the tendency for a person to match the behavior or attitude as exhibited by actual or symbolic models."[3]

According to this theory, prior learning is considered a critical factor in determining the amount of violence later displayed. Bandura maintained that aggressive behavior was learned through the same processes by which other forms of behavior are acquired, that is, by observation and direct experience.[4]

In past years there have been numerous investigations in the area of social learning and the modeling of aggressive behavior.[5-8] These studies have typically employed a research paradigm in which one group of children were exposed to adult models who displayed aggressive behavior, while another group of children were exposed to adult models who displayed nonaggressive behavior. The children were then tested for the amount of new learning in a new setting in which the model was not present. Results from these types of studies provided clear evidence that children who were exposed to the aggressive model learned to imitate more verbal and physical aggression than did the children who were exposed to the nonaggressive model.

It has furthermore been demonstrated that children exposed to filmed aggressive models will display subsequent aggressive behavior.[9-14]

In a classic study, Bandura et al. investigated the effects of exposure to filmed aggressive models on children's subsequent aggressive behavior.[9] The results of the study furnished strong evidence that exposure to filmed aggression heightens aggressive behavior in children. Bandura et al. found that the children who were exposed to the aggressive human and cartoon models on film exhibited almost twice as much aggression as did the children in the control group, who were not exposed to aggressive film content.

With the presence of television in almost every home, the role of symbolic models has taken on great importance. In a random sample taken of grades 3–6 in one school in my district, I found that there was not one home without a television. For the third, fourth, and fifth grades, 61% of the sample had three or more television sets in the home. Bandura and Walters maintain that while children in our culture still learn through real-life models, there is an increasing reliance placed on the use of symbolic models, because of the advent of modern technology and the availability of mass media.[15] These symbolic models are provided in films, television, and other audiovisual sources.

In a subsequent publication, Bandura spoke to the power of television.[4] He stated that television provides a rich source of social learning for children; he maintained that through symbolic modeling, audiences of large magnitude can simultaneously be reached and that, as a consequence, the aggression contagion potential of media presentations is greater than that of direct behavioral modeling.

One must ask how important a role television plays in the lives of American children. Nielsen index figures indicate that by the time a child graduates from high school, he has spent more hours observing television than he has spent in the classroom—15,000 hours of viewing as opposed to 11,000 hours of classroom instruction.[16] Waters found that most children under 5 years of age watch 23.5 hours of television a week.[17] It has been reported that by the time the average American child has reached 18 years of age, he will have seen approximately 350,000 commercials and witnessed some 18,000 murders on television. He will have witnessed numerous additional acts of mayhem and "pretend" death. Of these lesser violent acts, he will have seen an average of about one per minute on cartoons, which, for many children under 10 years old, are standard viewing.[18]

On a recent segment of "Bill Moyer's Journal," young children were asked several questions regarding their preference for television as opposed to other things.[19] The first question asked was, "Would you give up your toys for television?"; all of the children said yes. The second question asked was, "Would you give up your friends for television?"; all the children said yes. The third question was, "Would you give up talking with your father for television?"; most children responded yes.

The television industry—under pressure from social scientists, concerned citizens, and the government—devised a concept called "family viewing hour." This would be an evening hour when children along with their parents would watch what the industry considered appropriate family programs. Children, however, were still being exposed to violent television, and, more frequently than not, they watched these programs without the presence of adults.

Waters found the "family hour" to be a complete fiasco. He reported that, by the time the idea had been dropped, Nielsen figures indicated that 10.5 million children under the age of 12 were still watching television after 9 P.M. when the "family hour" ended.[17]

A study carried out by Dillion, shortly after the assassinations of Robert Kennedy and Martin Luther King, disclosed that television networks continued to show violence as entertainment.[20] The study revealed that in a seven-day period, there were 84 killings and 372 acts of violence on television programs. Violent incidents occurred on an average of once every 16.3 minutes during the early evening hours, a time for which network research estimated an audience of 26.7 million children.

How does violent television programming impact on the lives of American children? Numerous studies investigating the effects of television violence on children have found that children who viewed aggressive television programs and filmed violence were more likely to engage in subsequent imitative aggressive behavior than were children who watched nonaggressive programs.[21-26]

Rothenberg reviewed 25 years of research on the effects of violent television on young children.[27] The studies had involved 10,000 children from every possible background. He found that most studies had shown that exposure to media violence produced aggressive behavior in young children.

The evidence, then, clearly suggests that children can and do learn some forms of aggressive behavior through a process of modeling, or imitation. The literature is replete with studies indicating that children will model aggressive behavior not only from live models, but from filmed models, and even from cartoon characters. There is abundant evidence, as well, showing how aggressive television fare to which children are exposed translates into their daily interactions with their peers and society. There have been, however, few systematic investigations that have looked at the possible effects on subsequent behavior of children who have observed film aggression in the presence of sanctioning adults. The distinction between this study and prior studies—and where I hoped to make a contribution—is that this study faces the possibility that violence is not going to disappear from television in the near future and that, therefore, ways must be found to ameliorate the effects of such programs on children. It occurred to me that if children viewed television in the presence of an adult and the adult reacted to the violent content either positively or negatively, this might have an influence on the degree to which the violence affected the children. Consequently, this investigation studied the effects on children's subsequent behavior of adult presence and sanctions during observed film aggression.

In the experiment reported in this paper, children observed a half-hour segment of a current television show on each of two consecutive days. Both shows fell within the top 10% of those shows ranked as most violent by the National Citizen's Committee for Broadcasting.[28] One group of children observed the television program in the presence of an adult who gave positive sanction to the violent aspects of the program; a second group of children watched the television program in the presence of an adult who voiced disapproval at the violent aspects of the program; a third group watched the television program in the presence of an adult who made no comments at all; while a fourth group watched the television program with no adult present—they were, however, observed unnoticed through a window. Immediately following the experimental procedures, the subjects were tested for posttreatment levels of aggression using the Rosenzweig Picture-Frustration (P-F) Study, Children's Form. The P-F Study allows one to classify responses into "direction of aggression," specifically: extrapunitive (E), which is aggression turned outward on the environment; intropunitive (I), which is aggression turned inward on the subject; and impunitive (M), which is aggression turned off in an attempt to evade the situation.

It was predicted that children in the positive-sanction group, where the adult observer sanctioned the televised violence, would score higher levels of outward aggression (E), as measured by the P-F Study, than would children in the other treatment groups. It was also predicted that girls would show levels of outward aggression (E) as high as those of the boys and, further, that the sex of the adult observer would have an effect on children's levels of aggression. Finally, it was predicted that presence or absence of the adult observer would have an effect on subsequent levels of aggression.

As is often the case, the unpredicted findings—the surprises that are part of the exploratory element in every piece of research—match in interest the predicted results; they also provide the grist for generating future studies. In this study, findings relating to the effects on aggression turned inward and aggression evaded fall into such a category.

METHOD

Subjects

The subjects were 80 white males and females, who were seven years of age and from a New York, suburban, public, elementary school. The pupil population of the school was predominantly white. The socioeconomic levels of the subjects included middle to upper-middle class.

Design and Procedure

Preexperimental Assessment of Levels of Aggression

Forty subjects at a time were brought to a room in the school by an experimenter. The subjects were administered the California Test of Personality, primary form, which measures pretest levels of aggression. The children were ranked according to their scores on aggression and were distributed among the cells* so that levels of aggression among cells were similar. The subjects were then randomly assigned to one of four treatment groups. Ten boys and 10 girls were randomly assigned to positive-sanction, negative-sanction, neutral, and control groups. Half of the male subjects in the treatment groups were assigned to a male adult observer, and half of the male subjects were assigned to a female adult observer. Half of the female subjects in the treatment groups were assigned to a male adult observer, and half of the female subjects were assigned to a female adult observer. There were five subjects in each of the smallest cells in the design (TABLE 1). The major analysis was a $4 \times 2 \times 2$ analysis of variance with main effects of treatment, sex of observer, and sex of subject.

Experimental Treatment

One week after the pretreatment, the subjects were taken, according to their assigned groups, to another room where they were exposed to a series

---

* Cell refers to a grouping resulting from a simultaneous classification of subjects according to their sex, their treatment, and sex of their observer.

TABLE 1

SUMMARY OF EXPERIMENTAL DESIGN*

	Male Adult Observer		Female Adult Observer	
	Male Subjects	Female Subjects	Male Subjects	Female Subjects
Positive	5	5	5	5
Negative	5	5	5	5
Neutral	5	5	5	5
Control	5	5	5	5

* $N = 80$.

of filmed segments on a television monitor for a period of one-half hour on two consecutive days. They were instructed to sit in a semicircle around the television monitor where they also had a full view of the adult observer. The subjects were introduced to the adult observer and were told, "Today we are going to watch a television program. When the program is over we will go back to class."

In the positive-sanction treatment groups, each time aggressive behavior was exhibited, either verbally or physically by the characters on the film, the adult observer would indicate approval with such statements as "he deserved that" and "good."

In the negative-sanction groups, each time aggressive behavior was exhibited, either verbally or physically by the characters on the film, the adult observer would indicate disapproval with such statements as "that was terrible" and "he didn't deserve that."

In the neutral-sanction treatment groups, the adult observer said nothing at all.

In the control group, after the subjects were brought to the room and asked to sit around the television monitor, the adult excused herself from the room and the subjects watched the television program without the presence of an adult.

Posttreatment Assessment of Levels of Aggression

On the third day, five subjects at a time were brought to a room in the school where they were given the P-F Study. After the test, the subjects were returned to their classrooms. The experimenters who administered the posttreatment assessment were unknown to the subjects.

RESULTS

Three separate three-way analyses of variance were performed on the data in this investigation. Each analysis was performed to determine the ef-

TABLE 2

ANALYSIS OF VARIANCE OF AGGRESSION SCORES ON THE E FACTOR

Source	df	MS	F
Treatment	3	808.04	4.10*
Sex of Subject	1	84.0	0.42
Sex of Coobserver	1	96.75	0.49
Treatment × Sex of Subject	3	416.29	2.11
Treatment × Sex of Coobserver	3	59.85	0.30
Sex of Subject × Sex of Coobserver	1	1,394.43	7.09*
Treatment × Sex of Subject × Sex of Coobserver	3	290.87	1.47
Within	64	196.63	

* $P < 0.01$.

fects of treatment (positive, negative, neutral, control), sex of subject, sex of observer, and any interaction between sex of subject, sex of observer, and treatment on amount and direction of aggression.

Analysis of variance of the data for the E factor, overt aggression (TABLE 2), reveals a significant difference at the 0.01 level between treatment groups. A Newman-Keuls a posteriori analysis revealed that the subjects in the positive-sanction group scored at a significantly higher level of overt aggression than did subjects in the negative treatment group and that the differences between the mean scores in the negative, neutral, and control groups were not significant.

Further analysis revealed a significant interaction effect between sex of subject and sex of observer (TABLE 3), with male subjects scoring significantly higher levels of overt aggression with the male adult observer than did male subjects with the female adult observer; and with female subjects scoring significantly higher levels of overt aggression with the female adult observer than did female subjects with the male adult observer.

The presence of the adult observer had no effect on the overt aggression scores. The planned comparison yielded a sum of squares of 0.764, which was not significant. The predictions made earlier were verified with respect to outward aggression. At this point, it is of interest to explore some of the unpredicted findings.

Analysis of variance of the data for the I factor, aggression turned inward (TABLE 4), reveals a significant difference at the 0.01 level, between treatment groups, with the subjects in the negative-sanction group scoring significantly higher levels of aggression turned inward than did subjects in the other treatment groups. A Newman-Keuls a posteriori analysis revealed that the differences between scores in the positive, neutral, and control groups were not significant. No interaction effects were obtained (TABLE 5). It appeared as though children were indeed affected by the violent content of the programs, but because of the disapproval of the adult observer, they turned the aggression inward.

The M factor, aggression avoided or evaded, also produced some surprises. The analysis of variance revealed a significant difference at the 0.05 level between treatment groups (TABLE 6). Subjects in the negative, neutral,

TABLE 3

MEANS OF MAIN EFFECTS AND FIRST-ORDER INTERACTIONS FOR E FACTOR SCORES

	Male Observer		Female Observer		Total
Boys	53.80		47.65		50.72
Girls	47.50		58.05		52.77
	Positive	Negative	Neutral	Control	Total
Male Observer	60.30	43.90	49.90	48.50	50.65
Female Observer	59.90	45.70	50.10	55.70	52.85
	Boys		Girls		Total
Positive	61.90		58.30		60.10
Negative	47.10		42.50		44.80
Neutral	49.40		50.60		55.00
Control	44.50		59.70		52.10

and control groups scored at significantly higher levels of aggression avoided or evaded than did subjects in the positive-sanction group. The positive-sanction groups had a significantly lower mean than did the other treatment groups ($P < 0.05$). Upon further examination, it appeared that the statistical significance resulted from the interaction of the female subjects with the sex of the adult, i.e., female subjects scored significantly higher levels of aggression avoided with the male adult observer than did female subjects with the female observer (TABLE 7).

DISCUSSION

The primary purpose of this study was to determine if the modeling of aggression by seven-year-old children, from filmed aggressive models, was influenced by the presence and sex of sanctioning adults.

The findings suggested that while parent presence did not make a significant difference as to the amount of aggression that was modeled, parent sanction did significantly influence how subsequent aggression was expressed. Subjects in the positive-sanction group, where the adult observer

TABLE 4

ANALYSIS OF VARIANCE OF AGGRESSION SCORES ON THE I FACTOR

Source	df	MS	F
Treatment	3	355.24	7.40*
Sex of Subject	1	59.51	1.24
Sex of Coobserver	1	99.01	2.06
Treatment × Sex of Subject	3	124.74	2.59
Treatment × Sex of Coobserver	3	18.37	0.38
Sex of Subject × Sex of Coobserver	1	59.51	1.24
Treatment × Sex of Subject × Sex of Coobserver	3	104.67	2.18
Within	64	47.98	

* $P < 0.01$.

TABLE 5

MEANS OF MAIN EFFECTS AND FIRST-ORDER INTERACTIONS FOR I FACTOR SCORES

	Male Observer	Female Observer	Total
Boys	14.65	18.60	16.62
Girls	18.10	18.60	18.35

	Positive	Negative	Neutral	Control	Total
Male Observer	14.30	21.80	14.50	14.90	16.37
Female Observer	16.70	25.70	17.60	14.40	18.60

	Boys	Girls	Total
Positive	14.50	16.50	15.50
Negative	20.00	27.50	23.75
Neutral	15.00	17.10	16.05
Control	17.00	12.30	14.65

expressed approval of the filmed aggression, showed a significantly higher level of overt aggression than did subjects in the negative-sanction group. In the negative-sanction group, where the adult observer expressed disapproval of the filmed aggression, subjects turned the aggression inward. The subjects in the positive-sanction group scored significantly lower scores of aggression avoided or evaded than did the subjects in the other treatment groups.

That the treatment effect was so strong and pervasive can perhaps be seen in light of the social-power theory of identification.[29] According to this theory, children will tend more to imitate behavior of an adult who controls positive resources than of an adult who is perceived as powerless. The adult observer voicing approval and disapproval of the filmed aggression might well have been perceived by the subjects as an adult having control and power over their future resources. According to the social-power theory, it seems plausible that the subjects in this study identified with the adult observer—whom they perceived as being powerful—and, in so doing, tended to reproduce behavior consistent with the observer's sanctions, thus producing the significant treatment effect.

Much of the recent research in the area of television and modeling be-

TABLE 6

ANALYSIS OF VARIANCE OF AGGRESSION SCORES ON THE M FACTOR

Source	df	MS	F
Treatment	3	405.14	2.99*
Sex of Subject	1	224.43	1.66
Sex of Coobserver	1	296.43	2.19
Treatment × Sex of Subject	3	153.47	1.13
Treatment × Sex of Coobserver	3	25.08	0.18
Sex of Subject × Sex of Coobserver	1	756.50	5.59*
Treatment × Sex of Subject × Sex of Coobserver	3	145.02	1.07
Within	64	135.16	

* $P < 0.05$.

TABLE 7

MEANS OF MAIN EFFECTS AND FIRST-ORDER INTERACTIONS FOR M FACTOR SCORES

	Male Observer		Female Observer		Total
Boys	31.25		33.55		32.40
Girls	34.05		24.05		29.05

	Positive	Negative	Neutral	Control	Total
Male Observer	24.90	33.80	35.50	36.40	32.65
Female Observer	23.20	30.50	32.10	29.40	28.80

	Boys	Girls	Total
Positive	23.10	25.00	24.05
Negative	32.60	31.70	32.15
Neutral	35.50	32.10	33.80
Control	38.40	27.40	32.90

havior has shown that children will model aggressive behavior after exposure to violent television.[22,25,30] While Waters has made suggestions regarding the effect of parent presence on the impact of television on children,[17] the findings of this investigation have shown that parent presence alone has little effect.

In contrast to previous aggression studies where boys were found to be more imitative than girls,[31, 32] the findings of this investigation showed no significant differences between sex of subject in any of the three aspects of aggression examined. This finding might be explained in terms of the type of programs that girls are exposed to today—such as "Wonder Woman," "Police Woman," and "Charlie's Angels"—where the female model is seen in various roles that were, in the past, traditionally male roles. It may also be seen as a reflection of the changing role of women in society. It is felt that this, coupled with the way women are presented in the media today, accounts for the findings in this study, regarding the lack of any significant differences between the sex of the subjects.

Two significant interaction effects were found between sex of subject and sex of observer for the E factor (overt aggression) and the M factor (aggression avoided or evaded). For the E factor, it was found that male subjects who viewed the filmed aggression with a male adult observer showed higher levels of overt aggression than did male subjects who viewed with a female adult observer. Female subjects who viewed the filmed aggression with a female adult observer showed higher levels of overt aggression than did female subjects who viewed with a male adult observer. These findings can be viewed in terms of both dependency and identification behavior. Bandura and Walters suggest that children in the age group used in this study not only seek to identify with the same-sex adult, but also display a great deal of dependency behavior with the same-sex adult.[15] With respect to the concept of identification, Kagan maintains that the child wants to feel and experience that some of the adult characteristics are his; and, thus, the child will try to identify with the adult, if the child is told or made to feel that he and the adult are similar in appearance or temperament.[33]

For the M factor, there was a significant interaction between sex of subject and sex of observer. An examination of the data revealed that the statistical significance resulted from an interaction of the female subjects with the sex of the adult observer. Female subjects who viewed the filmed aggression with the male adult observer showed higher levels of aggression avoided or evaded than did female subjects who viewed with the female observer.

Johnson maintains that once the Oedipal stage has passed, the relationship between a daughter and her father takes on a new dimension.[34] She senses that his love and caring for her depend on her being feminine and attractive. It is suggested that the female subjects might have perceived the male adult observer as the father figure and thus showed high levels of aggression avoided or evaded, feeling that this was expected of them.

CONCLUSIONS

It was concluded that, within the limits of this study, adult presence while children watch filmed aggression on a television monitor has no significant effect on subsequent aggression. The significant differences, however, on the mean scores between treatments clearly suggest that what the adult observer says, in the way of approval or disapproval of the filmed aggression, does have an effect on how the subsequent aggression will be expressed.

Results from previous studies in the area of television and violence have indicated that children learn aggressive behavior from film-mediated aggressive models.[10,22,23,35-38] Based on past research, then, it is fair to assume that some degree of modeling occurred with the subjects in this investigation during their exposure to filmed aggressive models and, further, based on the findings of this investigation, that adult sanction had a significant effect on how subsequent learned aggression was expressed by the subjects.

The adult observers noted an interesting phenomenon that occurred during the experimental trials: more frequently than not, the subjects appeared to be attending only to the more violent aspects of the program being presented on the television monitor. During the program, the subjects talked, laughed, or played with each other. When the background music became intense and loud—usually the cue for a violent sequence—the subjects would stop what they were doing and focus their attention on the television monitor. When the action sequence ended, the subjects tended to return to their talking and playing. This pattern repeated itself the next time the music became intense and loud. It seems, then, that the subjects were selectively tuning out a good deal of the dialogue and were tuning in all the violence. Further research—looking into the possibility that children are selectively attending to the violent aspects of television—should be considered, as this might offer an explanation as to why television violence has such a powerful impact on children.

Unfortunately, few data have been collected on the relationship between children's viewing of aggressive television and parental sanction. Many more data would have to be generated from different age groups, from different socioeconomic levels, and under different conditions before any definitive conclusions could be drawn. The unforeseen findings of this study indicate that there is a possible conflict situation that develops when an adult just says "bad" to the violent content on television. What appears to result is a residue of learned aggression that is either avoided or internalized by the child. Thus, one might conclude that the issue is much more complicated and that brevity on the part of the parent regarding the violence is simply not enough to vitiate the impact of aggressive television fare. While efforts should be made to teach young children to watch television selectively and critically, efforts should also be put forth in the area of parent education. Perhaps as parents are made more aware of the powerful impact of violent television on their children, they can also be educated as to the importance of having lengthy discussions with their children regarding the programs watched on television. Television industry's latest campaign stresses that families watch television together. Together, while important, is simply not enough. What might be critical are family discussions surrounding the substantive issues in the program and how these issues relate to one's life.

Acknowledgments

With thanks to Dr. Frank Crowley. This paper is based on the author's doctoral dissertation, "Effect on Subsequent Behavior of Seven Year Olds after Observed Film Aggression with Sanctioning Adults," Fordham University, New York, 1978. The author thanks Dr. Belle Wiggens and Carol Eisenberg for their helpful comments; Dr. Thomas Lee, Remo Perini, and the children for making the study possible; and the staff of The Academy their helpful assistance.

References

1. HALL, K. R. L. 1964. Aggression in monkey and ape societies. *In* The Natural History of Aggression. J. D. Carthy & F. J. Ebling, Eds.: 17–26. Academic Press. London, England.
2. SAGAN, E. 1974. Cannibalism: Human Aggression and Cultural Form. Harper & Row, Publishers. New York, N.Y.
3. BANDURA, A. 1962. Social learning through imitation. *In* Nebraska Symposium on Motivation: 211–269. University of Nebraska Press. Lincoln, Nebr.
4. BANDURA, A. 1973. Aggression: A Social Learning Analysis. Prentice-Hall, Inc. Englewood Cliffs, N.J.
5. BANDURA, A., D. ROSS & S. A. ROSS. 1961. Transmission of aggression through imitation of aggressive models. J. Abnorm. Soc. Psychol. 63: 575–582.
6. BANDURA, A. & F. J. MCDONALD. 1963. The influence of social reinforcement and the behavior of models in shaping children's moral judgments. J. Abnorm. Soc. Psychol. 67: 274–281.

7. MAUSNER, B. 1954. The effect of prior reinforcement on the interaction of observer pairs. J. Abnorm. Soc. Psychol. **49:** 65–68.
8. MAUSNER, R. & B. L. BLOCK. 1957. A study of the additivity of variables affecting social interaction. J. Abnorm. Soc. Psychol. **54:** 250–256.
9. BANDURA, A., D. ROSS & S. A. ROSS. 1963. Imitation of film-mediated aggressive models. J. Abnorm. Soc. Psychol. **66:** 3–11.
10. ERON, L. D., M. M. LEFKOWITZ, R. HUESMANN & L. O. WALDER. 1972. Does television violence cause aggression? Am. Psychol. **27:** 253–263.
11. KNIVETON, D. & G. STEPHENSON. 1973. An examination of individual susceptibility to the influence of aggressive film models. Br. J. Psychiatry **122:** 53–56.
12. LIEBERT, R. M. 1972. Television and social learning: some relationships between viewing violence and behaving aggressively (overview). *In* Television and Social Learning. II: 1–42. Surgeon General's Report. Washington, D.C.
13. LIEBERT, R. M. & R. A. BARON. 1972. Short-term effects of televised aggression on children's aggressive behavior. *In* Television and Social Learning. II: 181–201. Surgeon General's Report. Washington, D.C.
14. LOVAAS, O. I. 1961. Effect of exposure to symbolic aggression on aggressive behavior. Child Dev. **32:** 37–44.
15. BANDURA, A. & R. H. WALTERS. 1963. Social Learning and Personality Development. Holt, Rinehart & Winston, Inc. New York, N.Y.
16. KAYE, E. 1974. The Family Guide to Children's Television. Pantheon Books. New York, N.Y.
17. WATERS, H. 1977. What TV does to kids. Newsweek (February 21): 62–70.
18. WILLIAMS, S. & V. CRANE. 1974. Television violence and your child. Paper presented at a lecture series of the College of Marin, California, and the Marin Association for Mental Health.
19. MOYERS, B. 1979. Bill Moyer's Journal. TV program aired July 30. WNET (Public Broadcasting System).
20. DILLION, J. 1968. Violence dominates U.S. summertime TV. Christian Science Monitor (July 25).
21. DOMINICK, J. R. & B. S. GREENBERG. 1972. Attitudes toward violence: the interaction of television exposure, family attitudes, and social class. *In* Television and Adolescent Aggressiveness. III: 314–335. Surgeon General's Report. Washington, D.C.
22. GERBNER, G. 1972. Violence in television drama: trends and symbolic functions. *In* Media Content and Control. I: 28–187. Surgeon General's Report. Washington, D.C.
23. GREENBERG, B. 1974. British children and televised violence. Public Opinion Q. **38:** 531–547.
24. LEFKOWITZ, M. M., L. D. ERON, L. O. WALDER & L. R. HUESMANN. 1972. Television violence and child aggression: a follow-up study. *In* Television and Adolescent Aggressiveness. III: 35–135. Surgeon General's Report. Washington, D.C.
25. LEIFER, A. D. & D. F. ROBERTS. 1972. Children's responses to television violence. *In* Television and Social Learning. II: 43–180. Surgeon General's Report. Washington, D.C.
26. McINTYRE, J. J. & J. J. TEEVAN. 1972. Television and deviant behavior. *In* Television and Adolescent Aggressiveness. III: 383–435. Surgeon General's Report. Washington, D.C.
27. ROTHENBERG, M. B. 1975. Effect of television violence on children and youth. J. Am. Med. Assoc. **234:** 1043–1046.
28. National Citizen's Committee for Broadcasting. 1977. Newsletter. Washington, D.C.
29. MACCOBY, E. E. 1959. Role-taking in childhood and its consequences for social learning. Child Dev. **30:** 239–252.
30. HANRATTY, M. S., R. M. LIEBERT, L. W. MORRIS & L. E. FERNANDEZ. 1969. Imitation of film-mediated aggression against live and inanimate victims. *In* Proceedings of the 77th Annual Convention of the American Psychological Association: 457–458.
31. BANDURA, A. 1965. Influence of models' reinforcement contingencies on the acquisition of imitative responses. J. Pers. Soc. Psychol. **1:** 589–595.
32. BANDURA, A., D. ROSS & S. A. ROSS. 1963. Vicarious reinforcement and imitative learning. J. Abnorm. Soc. Psychol. **67:** 601–607.

33. KAGAN, J. 1958. The concept of identification. Psychol. Rev. **65:** 296–305.
34. JOHNSON, M. 1963. Sex role learning in the nuclear family. Child Dev. **34:** 319–333.
35. LIEBERT, R. M. 1974. Television and children's aggressive behavior: another look. Am. J. Psychoanal. **34:** 99–107.
36. MURRAY, J. 1973. Television and violence: implications of the Surgeon General's research program. Am. Psychol. **28:** 472–478.
37. MUSSEN, P. & E. RUTHERFORD. 1961. Effects of aggressive cartoons on children's aggressive play. J. Abnorm. Soc. Psychol. **62:** 461–464.
38. SAVITSKY, J. C., R. W. ROGERS, C. E. IZARD & R. M. LIEBERT. 1971. The role of frustration and anger in the imitation of filmed aggression against a human victim. Psychol. Rep. **29:** 807–810.

ADOLESCENT AGGRESSION AND TELEVISION

Leonard D. Eron and L. Rowell Huesmann

Department of Psychology
University of Illinois at Chicago Circle
Chicago, Illinois 60680

Most criminal acts in the United States, at least most violent criminal acts, are committed by young males in late adolescence.[1] There could be many reasons why this is so—biological, psychological, sociological, political, and economic. Empirical studies have uncovered relations between aggression and a number of variables from these classes. Some of these relations are causative, some concomitant or perhaps merely coincidental. One particularly striking finding has been that heightened aggression among adolescents is related to the violence of the television programs they watch.[2] However, the extent and the content of a child's television viewing are inevitably correlated with other potential causes of aggression. For example, most violent crimes are committed in lower-class, ghetto areas by individuals of limited IQ, who have dropped out of school, are unemployed, come from disorganized families, and in general have limited resources for coping with problems.[1] These are also the persons who spend much time watching television and who prefer violent programs.[3,4,5] Thus, on the basis of correlational data alone, it is difficult to attribute cause or effect to either of the variables in question.

Causal relations can be best demonstrated by experimental manipulation or inferred from large-scale observational studies done over time using repeated observations on the same subjects. The studies by Berkowitz and his students with college-age subjects exemplify the former approach, and the studies we have done, following youngsters for periods up to 10 years until late adolescence, illustrate the latter approach. Berkowitz, for example, has demonstrated that exposure of university students to violent films increases the likelihood and magnitude of subsequent aggressive behavior, especially if the viewer is angered or frustrated prior to viewing the film.[6]

In our 10-year longitudinal study, we found that the best single predictor of how aggressive a young man would be at age 19 was the violence of television programs he had watched at age 8.[7] By use of a cross-lagged panel design and partial correlation to control for possible third variables, it was demonstrated that the most plausible hypothesis to explain this relation was that continuous viewing of television violence at the earlier age caused the aggressive behavior that was measured at the later age.

FIGURE 1 describes the cross-lag correlational analyses of our 10-year study. These data have already been published, so we will not dwell on them at any length.[7] You see here the significant difference between the two cross correlations over a 10-year lag. The violence of television programs watched by boys at age 8 is more highly related to their aggression 10 years later than is the aggression of boys at age 8 to the violence of television they watched

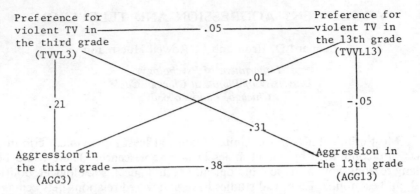

FIGURE 1. Correlations between a preference for violent television and peer-rated aggression for 211 boys over a 10-year lag.

10 years later. This fact, along with other analyses of these data (which are described in Reference 7), reinforces our confidence in the probable causal direction going from violence viewing to aggression. For example, consider those youngsters who at age 8 had been less aggressive but had been watching highly violent television; by the time they were age 19, they were significantly more aggressive than those who initially had been highly aggressive but had been watching less violent programs. This finding contradicts the assertion that it is only highly aggressive individuals or those already predisposed to aggression who are affected by filmed violence.[5]

There can no longer be any doubt that viewing television violence is one important cause of violent behavior among adolescents. The repeated findings of such an effect in rigorously controlled laboratory experiments have been shown to generalize to field investigations in more natural environments.[8] The effect is real. It happens in life, not just in the laboratory. However, not all young people who watch violent television are similarly affected, although a significant number are. The important task for researchers is to isolate and study the relevant mediating variables that determine who the vulnerable ones are, under which conditions, and to devise intervention strategies that will protect those who are susceptible.

One of the mediating variables is gender. Most published studies have shown the television violence effect only for males. For example, in our 10-year study we found there was no relation at all between the violence of programs that girls watched at age 8 and how aggressive they were judged to be by their peers at that age or at age 19.* This obtained difference in results for boys and girls caused us to turn our attention to factors associated with being male or female in our society that might account for the findings. The most obvious factor is the generally higher aggression level in boys. No matter how aggression is measured or what type of aggression is in question,

---

* Actually there was a trend at age 19 for those girls who had been watching violent television to be less aggressive, but this was not statistically significant.

males as a group generally score higher than females as a group. Usually constitutional, hormonal, or other predispositional variables are invoked to explain the differences.[9] However, it cannot be denied that there are some females in our society who are just as aggressive as the most aggressive males and some males who are as nonaggressive as most females. How did these individuals get that way? It is our thesis that they acquired these behaviors, atypical for their gender, at least partially because they were exposed to socialization experiences usually and traditionally reserved for the other sex. In our longitudinal studies of development of aggression in young people, we have continually been confronted by these differences in socialization experiences and by both concomitant and subsequent differences in aggressive behavior.

Another potential mediating variable in the relation between television violence and aggressive behavior might be a child's use of fantasy and the ability to discriminate between fantasy and reality as portrayed on the television screen. Girls may be less affected than boys by television violence because girls may be better able to make this discrimination. In their play and other recreational activities, girls obtain considerable practice in the use of fantasy and have more opportunities to slip back and forth from fantasy to real life than do boys. It is suggested that girls more clearly see television as fantasy and thus are less likely to be influenced by the actions of the characters they observe there.[10] Data we collected in our 10-year study confirm this. In general, girls thought television was significantly less realistic than did boys. Furthermore, the more aggressive a girl was, at both age 8 and age 19, the more realistic she thought television violence was.

Currently we are investigating further these notions about the effect on aggression of differential socialization of boys and girls and how the ability to discriminate between fantasy and reality reduces the effect of television violence on aggressive behavior. We have just completed collection of data in a three-year longitudinal study of approximately 750 children in Oak Park, a suburban Chicago school district, and in two inner-city schools of the Chicago Archdiocese. One-half of these children were in the first grade when we started, and one-half in the third grade. We have not yet completed the three-year longitudinal analyses. However, we do have cross-sectional data obtained from first- and third-grade children in the first wave of the study[11] and some longitudinal analyses from first to second wave. These data are consonant with the interpretation of the previously obtained findings that we have been discussing.

First of all, a positive relation between television violence viewing at home and aggressive behavior was reaffirmed for boys and also emerged clearly for girls. Although the direction of the relation in this study was the same for both sexes, there were interesting differences between the sexes. FIGURE 2 contains cross-lagged correlations obtained across the first year to the second year of our three-year study. The three figures in the top half of FIGURE 2 represent the relation of three measures of television violence to peer-rated aggression in boys over a one-year period, 1977 to 1978. The figure on the left refers to violence of male characters on TV, the middle figure to violence of female characters, and the right-hand figure to sheer frequen-

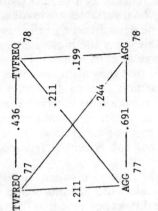

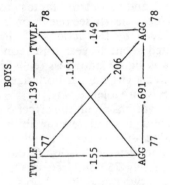

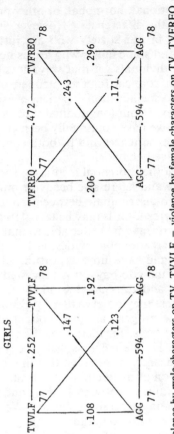

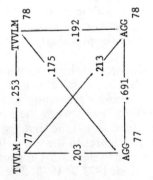

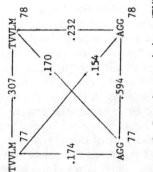

FIGURE 2. Cross-lag correlations. (TVVLM = violence by male characters on TV. TVVLF = violence by female characters on TV. TVFREQ = frequency of TV viewing.)

cy of television viewing. In all cases the correlations are positive, and in all cases the correlation between TV violence in the earlier period and aggression in the later period is greater than the correlation between aggression in the earlier period and TV in the later one. The correlations of course are not great, nor are the differences between the crossed correlations. However, we have always maintained that the effect is cumulative, and it can be predicted that as the years go by, the size of the correlation will increase. Actually, the size of the correlations is of the same order as the contemporaneous correlation in the first wave of our 10-year study.

The cross-lagged correlations for girls are represented in the lower half of FIGURE 2. Here again the correlations are all positive. However, we do not see here the same difference in the cross-lag correlations as is present in the boys' data. Such positive findings for girls were not apparent in our earlier 10-year study and therefore are particularly interesting. Later we will discuss in greater detail the possible reasons for the appearance now of a relation between television violence and aggression for girls when we did not obtain one approximately 20 years ago.

In general, however, this new study of 700 youngsters in a Chicago suburb as well as in the inner city corroborates the findings of our original study done 20 years previously in semirural New York state. We now know that the relation between viewing violence and aggressive behavior has already appeared at age six. Jerome and Dorothy Singer, who observed children's physically aggressive behavior in nursery school over the period of one year, have also recently reported that this behavior was related to the amount of violence that the youngsters, just 3 and 4 years old, viewed on television.[12] By doing a cross-lagged analysis of correlations between aggressive behavior and violence viewing at different times over a year and by partialling out IQ, socioeconomic status, and other background factors—much the same as we did in our 10-year study—the Singers demonstrated that the likely causal direction is from violence viewing to physically aggressive behavior in these three- and four-year-old nursery school children. Their results, based on observed behaviors in nursery school, are even more clear-cut than ours. Interestingly, they also found a positive causal relation for both boys and girls.

TABLE 1 presents the contemporaneous correlations between television violence and aggression in Finland, where our study is being replicated by Kirsti Lagerspetz and where they have now completed the first wave. Our own data are presented again for comparison purposes. Again there are two measures of TV violence and one of frequency of TV viewing. One can see that in both sets of data, the relation of peer-rated aggression to violence by female characters is lower than the relation to male violence. This is true regardless of the subject's sex or age, except for the girls in Finland. The increased effectiveness of the male model is not what we expected. According to modeling theory, female characters should be more salient as models for girls; and it would be predicted that their behaviors would be copied by girls more readily than the behaviors of male characters. In our earlier study conducted 20 years ago, we argued that an important reason for not finding a

TABLE 1

CORRELATION BETWEEN TV VIEWING AND AGGRESSION

	All Subjects	Girls	Boys
Finland 1978			
TVVM*	0.23	0.18	0.14
TVVF†	0.16	0.20	0.07
TVFr‡	0.04	0.09	0.03
USA 1978			
TVVM	0.22	0.23	0.19
TVVF	0.20	0.19	0.15
TVFr	0.22	0.30	0.20
USA 1977			
TVVM	0.22	0.17	0.20
TVVF	0.13	0.11	0.16
TVFr	0.21	0.21	0.21

* TVVM = violence by male characters on TV.
† TVVF = violence by female characters on TV.
‡ TVFr = frequency of television viewing.

TV violence–aggressive behavior relation for girls was that there were far fewer aggressive females on television for a girl to imitate than there were aggressive males for a boy to imitate. This would not seem to be the case, since today we do have aggressive female models on television; and although these models are copied to some extent by girls, the male models seem to be copied more.

It may be that more important than the sex of the model are the behaviors the model is performing and that if masculine activities are intrinsically more appealing to subjects of either sex, then all subjects would be more likely to attend to male characters and imitate their activities. It has been demonstrated that the more powerful the model, the more likely are the model's behaviors to be attended to and copied, regardless of sex.[13] Similarly, it is suggested now that the more appealing are the general activities of the model, the more likely will the observer be to attend to the model and therefore to copy the model's behaviors. Indeed, there is some evidence for this in our data on preference for sex-typed activities among these subjects. Our measure of preference for sex-typed activities comprised a booklet of four pages, each of which contained six pictures of children's activities. Two pictures of each set had been previously rated masculine, two feminine, and two neutral by 67 college students who had designated the activities as popular for boys and girls. The 24 pictures finally used in this procedure were selected with good reliability. The task for the children was to select the two activities they liked best on each page, and the children received a score for the number of masculine, feminine, and neutral pictures they chose. The reason for including a neutral category is that it is much easier for boys to admit to liking neutral activities than to admit to liking feminine ones. Similarly for girls, we anticipated that it would be difficult to admit to liking boys' activities. Here, however, we were surprised. One of our most interesting findings is that *both* boys and girls prefer more traditionally masculine activities as they get older. The mean increase in score is highly significant for both sexes. Therefore, since boys' traditional activities have increasingly more appeal for both boys and girls as they grow older, it is not surprising that male figures stand out as models for both sexes. In Finland, where we have the sole exception to the greater influence of the male model for girls, it is likely that the differentiation between male and female occupational and recreational activities is not as large as it is in this country. Thus for Finnish children, the similarity between model and observer in physical characteristics is more influential in modeling than are the activities in which the male or female model engages.

Furthermore, in this country, the relation between preference for masculine activities and aggression is significant for both boys and girls. Regardless of sex, subjects who score high on preference for masculine activities are likely to be more aggressive. And the relation is stronger from the first to second wave than contemporaneously. The cumulative effect of the socialization experience is obvious. We see the culmination of this socialization experience in FIGURES 3 and 4. These figures describe the results of an experiment by one of our students, Esther Kaplan-Shain,[14] who related scores of men and women college students on scales of masculinity and femininity[15] to performance on an aggression machine. This was an adaption of the Buss-type[16] apparatus, whereby the subject signals a confederate by delivering loud sounds to the confederate's earphones rather than by electric shock—the louder the sound delivered, the more aggressive is the response. Here we see that while masculinity in males has little relation to aggressive responding, femininity in males is significantly negatively related to aggression; similarly, while femininity in females is not predictive of lack of aggression, masculinity in females is positively correlated with the intensity of the aggressive response.[14] Thus it would seem that men—regardless of the masculine attitudes they have—are inhibited from responding aggressively *if* they also have traditionally feminine attitudes and values, while women who subscribe to masculine attitudes and values are facilitated in aggressive

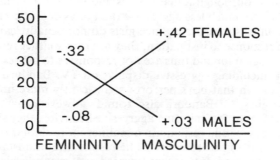

FIGURE 3. Correlations between aggression and masculinity or femininity in male and female college students.

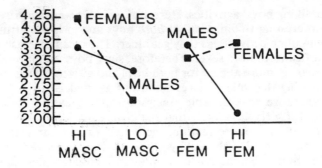

FIGURE 4. Mean aggression scores of high and low masculine and high and low feminine college students (male and female).

responding regardless of their feminine attitudes. FIGURE 4 shows the mean aggression scores according to whether the subjects are high or low masculine or high or low feminine.

There is little difference between aggressive responses of high and low masculine men, but there is a significant difference in the aggressive response of high and low feminine men ($P < 0.02$). Similarly, there is little difference in the responses of high and low feminine women but a large and significant difference between high and low masculine women ($P < 0.01$). The most aggressive responders of all are the high masculine women. Yes, women can learn to be as aggressive as men, despite their low levels of testosterone.

However, within Western societies, women are usually socialized to be nonaggressive, while boys are probably encouraged and reinforced in the direct and overt expression of aggression. Very early in life, girls learn that physical aggression is an undesirable behavior for girls, and so they acquire other behaviors more suitable to expectations for girls. A recent study done with fourth-, sixth-, and eighth-grade youngsters found that while girls endorsed increasingly with age the effectiveness of passive behavior in solving problems, boys increasingly disapproved of such behavior in problem solving.[17] In both of our longitudinal studies and in both the United States and Finland, girls were much less aggressive than boys *at all times*, regardless of how aggression was measured. Since girls do not usually learn physical aggression as a response to instigation, they are rarely either rewarded or punished for such behavior and thus are not responsive to aggressive cues in the environment, including aggressive displays on TV. Bandura's studies have consistently shown that boys perform significantly more imitative aggression than do girls.[18,19] Bandura also found, however, that when girls are positively reinforced for imitating aggressive behavior, they significantly increase such behavior and respond in a manner more similar to boys who are reinforced for the same behavior.[20] The results of Hokanson and Edelman would support this contention that lowered aggression levels in females are a function of lack of reinforcement for aggressive behavior. They found that females did not demonstrate the quickened reduction of physiological arousal after the opportunity to counteraggress against a confederate of the experimenter who had aggressed against them.[21] However, such quickened reduction of heart rate and blood pressure to basal levels was routinely seen in male subjects. Recent studies have shown that the effect of reinforcement on repeated performance of aggressive behavior is relatively independent of the initial modeling of the behavior.[22] What we are suggesting is that different socialization practices have reduced the likelihood that girls will continue to perform aggressive behavior observed on television. In summary, most girls may be trained to be nonaggressive to *such* an extent that aggressive models have little effect on them.

Two related findings are the significant positive relation for girls between aggression and masculine interest patterns as measured by the masculinity-femininity (M-F) scale of the Minnesota multiphasic personality inventory (MMPI) as well as the significant positive relation between aggression scores for girls and the extent to which they watch contact sports on television.[7] Both of these scores related to aggression reflect attitudes and behavior that are normative for boys. For boys, however, there was no relation between viewing contact sports on TV and aggression; nor was there a relation for boys between masculinity on the M-F scale and aggression. It is very probable that the reason for lack of relation with aggression for boys lies in the minimal variability on the other two variables. Most boys, whether low or high aggressive, watch contact sports and also endorse the attitudes and interests comprising the masculinity items on the M-F scale. However, these results indicate that when females are aggressive, some of their interests and activities are deviant from their sex and are similar to the behavior of the male sex group. Parke *et al.* have more recently reported a singular finding in that the level of verbal aggression observed in girls who previously had been exposed to a violent film was higher than that observed in girls who had seen a nonviolent film.[8] However, it should be noted that these girls were incarcerated juvenile delinquents who in the past probably had avoided traditional female values and attitudes and adopted more masculine behaviors.

What about the relation of fantasy behavior to aggression? In our 10-year study, we found that girls who see themselves as masculine at age 19, i.e., those girls who obtain high scores on scale 5 of the MMPI, tend to perceive television as more realistic and also tend to be more aggressive. Thus, the more girls see TV as realistic, the more they are like boys in other respects and the more aggressive they are. We hypothesize that differential ability in using TV as a fantasy experience may account for the difference in the direction of the relation between TV violence and aggression that we found between boys and girls.

In our three-year longitudinal study, we measured each child's fantasy behavior and judgment of TV realism, as well as the variables mentioned previously. The fantasy scales were developed by another of our students, Erica Rosenfeld, from a 45-item questionnaire about daydreams that had been administered to the children.[23] Three major styles of fantasizing were detected in these subjects: "fanciful," in which the youngster daydreams about fairy tales and implausible happenings; "active," in which the youngster daydreams about heroes, achievement, and intellectual pursuits; and "aggressive negative," in which the youngster daydreams about fighting, killing, and being hurt. These styles of fantasy behavior were related to aggression differently for boys and girls.

In the first wave of this three-year study, the major predictors of aggression for boys as indicated by a multiple regression analysis were TV violence viewing, preference for traditional masculine sex-typed activities, and aggressive fantasies. For girls, the best predictors were TV violence viewing, perceptions of TV violence as real, low preference for traditional feminine-type activities, and fantasies about action. In other words, for both sexes TV violence viewing, fantasy behavior, and sex role preference are independently related to aggression, although the nature of the fantasy content that predicts to aggression is different for boys and girls. This is because girls who fantasy about action—heroes and heroines and winning games and achievement—are the most aggressive. For boys, those who fantasy about aggression—beating up other persons—are the ones who are most aggressive. There is no evidence whatsoever in our data that fantasy has a cathartic effect! Especially for boys, those children who *fantasy* about aggressive acts tend to *act* aggressively. Girls, who in general do not score as high as boys on any measure of aggression, also do not daydream much about aggressive themes. However, those girls whose daydreams contain *active* content tend to be aggressive in overt behavior. Active fantasy, it happens, is also generally more characteristic of boys than it is of girls. Thus again we have evidence that girls who are aggressive have interests, values, and attitudes similar to those of boys.

What are the implications of these findings—both from our 10-year longitudinal study and the current studies in Chicago and Finland—for the reduction of aggressive behavior?

Our findings, we believe, point to two areas where efforts can be made that should eventually reduce aggression. The first and most direct is television violence. Significant overall reduction of violence and mayhem on the television screen would, we believe, lower the level of violence in American society. However, we think trying to get any significant change in television programming is like tilting at windmills. Despite the efforts of the American Medical Association, the Parent Teachers Association, and Action for Children's Television, the level of violence on national and local TV has not diminished appreciably. Barring any significant changes in programming, what can be done? For one thing, we can teach parents and children techniques for counteracting the effects of television. Efforts at devising such procedures are going on in at least two places. Dorothy and Jerome Singer of the Yale University Television Research Center are preparing curricula to teach young children and their parents how to be intelligent television consumers; in Chicago we are intervening with groups of children in our longitudinal study to determine the best way to ameliorate the relation between violence viewing and subsequent aggressive behavior in children. It would be nice to report some great breakthrough—the discovery of a vaccine with which we could innoculate children so they would forever be immune to the effects of television violence. However, our first attempts do not appear to have been terribly successful. In the first year of our study, we focused our intervention on teaching children to distinguish between fantasy and reality, e.g., explaining how "Bionic Woman" and "Six Million Dollar Man" simulate the aggressive behaviors and other fantastic actions of these characters and having the children imagine similar feats and how they would simulate them. However, on a criterion test, these children did not distinguish fantasy from reality any better than did a control group of children who had been engaged in different intervening activities. Whether the intervention will have an effect on the relation between violence viewing and subsequent aggressive behavior is still undetermined.

The Singers are having some success in their work with parents—teaching them how to turn off the TV, to monitor the child's watching, to share the viewing experience, to interpret content, to allay fears, and to help the child distinguish real from fantasy figures. Again, the Singers as yet have no data on how these interventions affect the relation between violence viewing and behavior.

However, there is one finding that has obvious implications for the use—or misuse—of fantasy in interventions, and that is the direct positive relation we have found between the extent of aggressive fantasy and the extent of aggressive behavior. It is obviously counterproductive for parents or therapists to encourage their children or clients to engage in fantasy rehearsal of aggressive problem solving in the mistaken assumption that "if you work it out in fantasy, you don't have to work it out in behavior." Such rehearsal often leads to the very acting out one is trying to prevent. We know from simple principles derived from memory studies that the more one rehearses an item, the more apt one is to remember it and therefore to use it in problem solving.

Another finding that suggests a clear direction for intervention is the positive relation between aggression and traditional masculine attitudes and values. The results of our studies to date, as well as those of other researchers, point to differential socialization as crucial in determining the different level of aggression in the two sexes. No matter how aggression is measured or observed, males generally score higher. But not all girls are unaggressive. There are some girls who seem to have been socialized like boys and who are just as aggressive as boys. Thus, although there may be organismically normal conditions, such as sex differences in testosterone level, that are implicated in aggressive behavior, this behavior is not necessarily immutable. Just as some females learn to be aggressive, males could learn *not* to be aggressive. The significant variables are the values and expectations a society holds for the expression of aggressive behavior in one sex rather than another and the rewards it provides or withdraws when that behavior is displayed. We have already discussed the ways in which society discourages aggressive behavior in girls from very early on in their lives and rewards them for engaging in other kinds of activity. We must reexamine what it means to be a man or masculine in our society, since the preponderance of violence in our society is perpetrated by males or by females who are acting like males. It is our contention that if we want to reduce the level of aggression in society, we should also discourage boys from aggression very early on in life and *reward* them for other behaviors. In other words, we should socialize boys more in the manner that we have been socializing girls. Rather than insisting that little girls should be treated like little boys and trained to be aggressive and assertive it should be the other way around. This is where the women's movement has it all wrong. Boys should be socialized the way girls have been traditionally socialized; *boys* should be encouraged to develop socially positive qualities like tenderness, sensitivity to feelings, nurturance, cooperativeness, and aesthetic appreciation. The level of individual aggression in society will be reduced only when male adolescents and young adults, as a result of socialization, subscribe to the same standards of behavior as have been traditionally encouraged for women.

In conclusion, we would like to repeat the old cliché that behavior that is learned can be unlearned; and aggressive behavior is no different—it *can* be unlearned. But how much easier it would be, how much pain and suffering and loss of life and property would be eliminated, if we arranged conditions so that aggression would not be learned in the first place and all youngsters would learn alternative ways of solving problems.

REFERENCES

1. MULVIHILL, D. J. & M. M. TUMIN. 1969. Staff Report to the National Commission on the Causes and Prevention of Violence. **12**. Crimes of Violence. U.S. Government Printing Office. Washington, D.C.
2. CHAFFEE, S. H. 1972. Television and adolescent aggressiveness. *In* Television and Social Behavior. G. A. Comstock & E. A. Rubinstein, Eds.: 31-34. U.S. Government Printing Office. Washington, D.C.
3. COMSTOCK, G., S. CHAFFEE, N. KATZMAN, M. McCOMBS & D. ROBERTS. 1978. Television and Human Behavior. Columbia University Press. New York, N.Y.
4. GREENBERG, B. & J. DOMINICK. 1969. Racial and social class differences in teenagers' use of television. J. Broadcasting **13**: 3331-3334.
5. STEIN, A. H. & L. K. FRIEDRICH. 1975. Impact of television on children and youth. *In* Review of Child Development Research. E. M. Hetherington, Ed. **5**. University of Chicago Press. Chicago, Ill.
6. BERKOWITZ, L. 1973. The control of aggression. *In* Review of Child Development Research. B. Caldwell & H. Ricciuti, Eds. **3**: 95-140. University of Chicago Press. Chicago, Ill.
7. ERON, L. D., L. R. HUESMANN, M. M. LEFKOWITZ & L. O. WALDER. 1972. Does television violence cause aggression? Am. Psychol. **27**: 253-263.
8. PARKE, R. D., L. BERKOWITZ, J. P. LEYENS, S. G. WEST & R. J. SEBASTIAN. 1977. Some effects of violent and non-violent movies on the behavior of juvenile delinquents. Adv. Exp. Soc. Psychol. **5**: 135-172.
9. MACCOBY, E. E. & C. N. JACKLIN. 1974. The Psychology of Sex Differences. Stanford University Press. Stanford, Calif.
10. FESHBACH, S. 1972. Reality and fantasy in filmed violence. *In* Television and Social Behavior. J. P. Murray, E. A. Rubinstein & G. A. Comstock, Eds. **2**: 318-345. U.S. Government Printing Office. Washington, D.C.

11. HUESMANN, L. R., P. FISCHER, L. D. ERON, R. MERMELSTEIN, E. KAPLAN-SHAIN & S. MORIKAWA. 1978. Children's sex-role preference, sex of television model, and imitation of aggressive behaviors. Paper presented at the Third Biennial Meeting of the International Society for Research in Aggression, Washington, D.C., September 22.

12. SINGER, J. L. & D. SINGER. 1978. Television viewing, play and aggression in preschoolers. Paper presented at the Third Biennial Meeting of the International Society for Research in Aggression, Washington, D.C., September 22.

13. BANDURA, A., D. ROSS & S. A. ROSS. 1963. A comparative test of the status envy, social power and secondary reinforcement theories of identification learning. J. Pers. Soc. Psychol. 67: 527–534.

14. KAPLAN-SHAIN, E. 1979. Masculinity, femininity and overt aggression in male and female college students. Department of Psychology. University of Illinois at Chicago Circle. Chicago, Ill. (Unpublished paper.)

15. BEM, S. L. 1974. The measurement of psychological androgyny. J. Consult. Clin. Psychol. 42: 155–162.

16. BUSS, A. H. 1961. The Psychology of Aggression. John Wiley & Sons, Inc. New York, N.Y.

17. CONNOR, J. M., L. A. SERBIN & R. A. ENDER. 1978. Responses of boys and girls to aggressive, assertive and passive behaviors of male and female characters. J. Genet. Psychol. 133: 59–69.

18. BANDURA, A., D. ROSS & S. A. ROSS. 1961. Transmission of aggression through imitation of aggressive models. J. Abnorm. Soc. Psychol. 63: 575–582.

19. BANDURA, A., D. ROSS & S. A. ROSS. 1963. Imitation of film mediated aggressive models. J. Abnorm. Soc. Psychol. 66: 3–11.

20. BANDURA, A., D. ROSS & S. A. ROSS. 1963. Vicarious reinforcement and imitative learning. J. Abnorm. Soc. Psychol. 67: 601–607.

21. HOKANSON, J. E. & R. EDELMAN. 1966. Effect of three social responses on vascular processes. J. Pers. Soc. Psychol. 3: 442–447.

22. HAYES, S. C., A. RINCOVER & D. VOLOSIN. Variables influencing the acquisition and maintenance of aggressive behavior: modeling versus sensory reinforcement. J. Abnorm. Psychol. (In press.)

23. ROSENFELD, E. 1978. The development of an imaginal process inventory for children. Ph.D. Dissertation. Department of Psychology. University of Illinois at Chicago Circle. Chicago, Ill.

THE MEDIA AND CRIME: GENERAL DISCUSSION

Moderator: Flora Rheta Schreiber

Department of Speech and Theater
John Jay College of Criminal Justice
New York, New York 10019

E. DONNERSTEIN (*University of Wisconsin, Madison, Wisc.*): I think we all agreed with each other on the effects of media and violence, that there is an effect on aggressive behavior. I think it's important to note that whether we have correlational, field, or laboratory studies the results are all very similar. I think that's a very important point to make.

L. D. ERON (*University of Illinois, Chicago, Ill.*): Dr. Singer's work is on observations of children in the actual nursery-school situation. Dr. Donnerstein and I have used such things as aggression machines. Dr. Eisenberg used the picture frustration study. Yet they all point to the same kinds of results. I don't think you can quarrel with that anymore.

UNIDENTIFIED SPEAKER: I would like a definition of aggression from Dr. Eron.

L. D. ERON: Aggression has many meanings in society and certainly among lay people, and many of these meanings are positive. For example, for some people aggression connotes achievement, ambition, and pushing ahead, all good middle-class Calvanist ideals.

But this is not the kind of aggression I've been talking about. I define aggressive behavior as behavior that injures another person.

UNIDENTIFIED SPEAKER: How do we teach children the difference?

L. D. ERON: Well, I don't think they have to be inextricably related. There are ways people can get ahead and achieve other than by beating up on other people. Unfortunately, the data that we have show that there's some truth to the lay assumption that these kinds of aggression go together. There's a low-positive correlation between mobility, occupational mobility, aspirations, and physical aggression. But it's certainly not a one-to-one correlation. There is some relationship there. It would seem to me that we ought to be able to devise ways of achieving without beating up on other people.

UNIDENTIFIED SPEAKER: And that should be the job of television, don't you think?

L. D. ERON: I would think so, yes. Television can teach many socially positive, wonderful things, as well as destructive things.

UNIDENTIFIED SPEAKER: If television indeed has such a powerful influence in our society, why don't we have more violence than we do?

L. D. ERON: I have never said that television violence is the only source of aggression in society, and further, there are other factors that tend to ameliorate whatever effect there is. Actually television violence, as far as I can see from the studies I've done, accounts for 10 percent of the variance. Now that's not a great deal, but when you recognize that we have 250

332

million people and I don't know how many thousands of crimes, 10 percent gets to be big number. Further, not every kid watching television is influenced by it for some of the reasons that Dr. Eisenberg mentioned in his paper. Not everybody that smokes gets lung cancer either, but this doesn't mean that smoking is not a cause of lung cancer. Not all adolescents use drugs, but this doesn't mean we shouldn't be concerned about drug use.

R. W. RIEBER (*John Jay College of Criminal Justice, New York, N.Y.*): I would like to respond to the question that Dr. Morse posed to the panel if that's appropriate for the audience to respond to the audience. I think it might be useful to look at the media and its relationship to aggression in two ways. One way would be to say that it is a reflection of the amount of potential aggression in the society. And as such, has the potential both to precipitate and, perhaps in some instances, actually reduce that potential depending upon the viewers. For example, the question that was raised—Why isn't there more aggression given all of the aggressive television and media?— might be answered by saying, well this is not the cause or even the major precipitating factor. It is simply a reflection of the potential amount of aggression that is available at a given moment if there was an easy release for it. Now, if you approach it in that manner, then you might be able to analyze the kinds of aggressive programs on television or in the media and get some insight into what they mean in terms of perhaps social dreams. I prefer to look at these things as social dreams, a reflection of the unresolved problems society happens to have at any given point in time, just as your personal dreams are a reflection of unresolved problems that you have as an individual. I think if one analyzed the aggressive programs, in fact the programs in general, one can get great insight into the psychosocial distress of which violence is only one aspect in the society at this present time.

Further, Dr. Eron responded to values. This all ties in with values. If we examine the Ten Commandments, referred to in Dr. Mednick's paper, as a guide to values in this society I think we fail on just about every one of them. And a lot of them include potential violence. And this must, in some measure, be a reflection of the value system that we have in a contemporary society. It is important for us to take a look at what kinds of values we give lip service to as opposed to what kinds of values we can actually relate to in terms of our human behavior in everyday life. There's a big discrepancy between the values that we say we believe in and the values in our culture that we actually engage in. And the Ten Commandments are a very good example of that.

So I think there is a tie-in and I think there's a fruitful area for research to investigate the relationship between the two.

F. WRIGHT (*John Jay College of Criminal Justice, New York, N.Y.*): This question is directed to Dr. Eron and his point that it might be better for boys to be like girls. How successful have you been, as a college teacher yourself, in presenting this idea to your students? I'd be interested to hear about your experiences.

L. D. ERON: Well it makes some of my more macho colleagues rather nervous if I talk this way, but actually I have no trouble in presenting these findings and making these recommendations to college students. They all seem to agree with them, at least those college students who are in psychology classes. They think it might not be a bad idea. I do have difficulty though when I talk to PTA groups. Parents say: Well what shall I do when my son comes home? I have to teach him to defend himself. He's got to go out and hit the other guy harder. It's very hard to answer that kind of a question. What has to change is the whole society's values. It has to be done on a societal level. I don't think it can be done on an individual level. For example, notice the terrible overemphasis we have on winning in sports. Take the game of basketball, which is not a violent sport like hockey or football: When a player fouls out, for example, because he's done illegal things such as hurting another player, the sympathy does not go to the player who has had the illegal act committed against him but rather to the guy who fouls out. This is the thing that has to change. Further, we are insisting that girls get the same kind of training. This emphasis on winning is now being extended to 100 percent of the population, whereas before we had it for 50 percent.

UNIDENTIFIED SPEAKER: I want to say that it's not a universal finding that a violent program does increase aggressiveness, at least immediately thereafter. I think it's important to note the effect of the context in which the viewing occurs, as Dr. Eisenberg has pointed out. In short, the context effect may overpower the content effects, and too little study of the former has been done.

The findings I'm familiar with show that there are two kinds of children, very aggressive children (who are also very affectionate) and very withdrawn children. Relating that to adults, it seems that the people who commit the most irrationally violent acts tend to be the most withdrawn. Therefore, if we're concerned about preventing later violence, then maybe we should be concerned with learning how to train withdrawn children to come more in contact with peers, even if it is aggressive contact.

L. D. ERON: Actually, there are studies that have done just what you've said. You're talking about the general activity level of the child. Children who are more active than others will engage in more aggressive acts as well as more acts in general, just because they interact with other kids more. In our studies we controlled for activity level. However, I doubt that the bulk of the criminal acts in this country, or in the world, are committed by these loners who, for example, suddenly up and shoot somebody from the Texas tower. These are really isolated incidents. I don't think they're very prevalent, and that's why they come to our attention. But usually criminal behavior or antisocial aggressive behavior is predictive from early life on, at least according to the studies I'm familiar with.

HUMAN NATURE, CRIME, AND SOCIETY: KEYNOTE ADDRESS*

Sarnoff A. Mednick

Social Science Research Institute
University of Southern California
Los Angeles, California 90007

Many months ago, President Carter visited The Bronx in order better to understand the need for urban renewal. His attention was drawn in particular to Charlotte Street, which the *New York Times* had called the worst slum street in New York City. The President duly proclaimed the Charlotte Street Project; it would be a model for national urban renewal programs.

I drove up to The Bronx recently and was rather shocked. The district is almost entirely leveled; buildings that are still half-standing are windowless. The Charlotte Street Project is apparently forgotten.

The experience gave me a sinking, frightened feeling. I spent my childhood and adolescence on Charlotte Street. It was not a rose garden then; but it is still uncomfortable to look for your childhood home and find rubble.

Why did this area disintegrate as so many other areas are disintegrating? Economists and politicians will doubtless propose learned and well-developed reasons. But I can tell you why my family and friends thought they left. A neighborhood boy my age was stabbed to death in front of our apartment house by some cruising youths. Our good friend, the grocer, was held up and shot in the shoulder. Older people hardly dared venture out of their heavily locked doors. It was *danger* that drove them from their homes. And the situation does not seem to be rapidly improving. In 1978, violent crime increased 5%.[15] Most disheartening is the focus of this increase on youngsters; more crimes are now being committed by children under 15 than by adults over 25! In the past 20 years, juvenile crime has increased 1600%.[9] Judging from past experience, these youngsters are not going to be rehabilitated overnight. I don't like to "view with alarm," but many of them are walking time bombs with long criminal careers ahead of them.

I don't know anyone who believes that our methods of dealing with crime have been a blazing success. Perhaps we need to stop and rethink our situation. First, do we want to reduce crime? If so, how? Currently our major efforts to control crime start with individuals *already* delinquent or criminal. We spend fortunes on developing mace, nicer jails, methods of rehabilitation, and faster court systems. Less effort is expended on the primary prevention of crime. I wish to suggest that along with efforts to deal with discovered criminality, we study methods of early intervention to *prevent* the initial onset of criminal behavior.

* The work in genetics is supported by Grant No. MH 31353–02 from the National Institute of Mental Health Center for the Study of Crime and Delinquency.

PRIMARY PREVENTION

I can imagine three avenues in which primary intervention might be explored:

1. Ecological alterations;
2. Systematic societal change;
3. Individual intervention.

Ecological Alteration

By ecological alteration, I refer to environmental manipulation—such as increasing street lighting, improving supermarket and department store security, and developing defensive architectural design. I will not consider this method further in this paper.

Societal Change

In this century, criminology has been dominated by sociological thinking—and for good reason. It seems quite clear that socioeconomic factors provide the reasons for crime for *most criminals.* Sociological thinking has suggested that the etiology of crime lies exclusively in the structure of society. It is expressly assumed that criminals are normal individuals who have been misshapen by an inappropriately arranged social system. If we improve this system, this should prevent criminality.

A critical assumption of this approach to primary prevention is the essential normality of criminals. To the extent that some criminals have deviant psychological or biological characteristics that help predispose them to antisocial behavior, then societal manipulation *alone* will not be sufficient to prevent crime. (I am, in principle, opposed to arguing for societal adjustment for the betterment of the human condition solely on the promise of reducing crime or mental illness. Human conditions should be improved because we are human. Unrealized promises simply promote reactionary backlash.) Thus, in order to better plan the primary prevention of criminal behavior, we must first consider evidence regarding the possibility that some forms of criminal behavior have individual psychological or biological predispositions.

Individual Intervention

This bioindividual approach to understanding the criminal has been less than popular in the social sciences. Let us take a moment and consider the reasons for this. In the beginning, there was no significant conflict. Auguste Comte in 1855 acknowledged that "the whole social evolution of the race must proceed in entire accordance with biological laws. . . ."[7] Perhaps the problems began 23 years later, when Herbert Spencer applied his phrase "survival of the fittest" to social behavior.[24] His prostitution of the theory of evolution for the preservation of class privilege was an outrage to social reformers. Spencer literally urged the "shouldering aside of the weak by the strong. . . ."[24] Social Darwinism inevitably led to racism. Expedient ethics had their day again in the 1920s in the U.S. in the exploitation of spurious intelligence test results to rationalize discriminatory immigration laws. Nazi ideology did not improve the attractiveness of biosocial interactionism. In the 30s, 40s, and 50s, social science academia simply excluded the consideration of biology from the same context as social factors.

Haller has suggested that part of the reason for this was that many of those who had been pointed to as inferior by our immigration laws had struggled to the top of the social-economic status heap (including the academic heap).[10] Politically and emotionally, these individuals turned away from biology. But perhaps even more telling than these emotional factors was a simple intellectual reason: there was very little compelling, empirical, biological evidence that could help us understand social man or (more specifically) criminality. The evidence for genetic influences on criminality consisted mainly of some relatively inadequate and ignored twin studies (some of which were tainted by having originated in Germany or Japan during the Nazi era). In addition, the literature offered some entertaining, well-written, and inventive analogies to observations of animal behavior. Social scientists found biological factors to be not only affectively repulsive, but coincidentally not intellectually compelling.

Within the last 5 to 10 years, however, there have been research developments that are not totally unworthy of the attention of the criminologist. These research developments may have implications for the planning of primary prevention programs. Consequently I will briefly review evidence relating biological factors to crime. I will first focus on three prospective, longitudinal studies.

THREE PROSPECTIVE STUDIES OF ANTISOCIAL BEHAVIOR

The Wadsworth Study

The first study concerns the delinquents in a "sample of 5362 single-born, legitimate, live births in 1946 occurring between March 3 and 9 in England, Wales and Scotland." Wadsworth described the cumulative, officially recorded delinquency when this birth cohort reached 21 years of age.[26] He then went on to examine the relationship of this delinquency to a childhood measure of autonomic nervous system responses to anticipation of stress. The survey members were subjected to a school medical examination when they were 11 years of age. The period of time during which they waited for this examination was designed to be somewhat stressful. Their pulse rates were measured to assess the effects of this stress anticipation. Those who were eventually registered as delinquents at 21 years of age had had a lower pulse rate increase in anticipation of the stress at age 11. Delinquents in this study were defined as those who "either made a court appearance or were formally cautioned by the police between the ages of 8 and 21 years."[27] The delinquent–not-delinquent differences were substantial for those committing indictable and sexual and violent offenses.

The Wadsworth study also makes an important point relating to the interaction of biological and social factors. Within the group of boys who had experienced broken homes early in life, anticipatory pulse rate did not distinguish the delinquents. Within the boys who did *not* experience broken homes, a small anticipatory pulse rate response did predict well to delinquency. This type of interaction of biological (pulse rate) and social (family disruption) data is predicted by Christiansen[5,6] and Sellin,[23] and has been observed repeatedly in our research in Copenhagen. The biological factors predict best in those areas, situations, or among those groups in which social factors (e.g., stable home, middle-class status) do not "explain" antisocial behavior. In those situations, areas, or groups in which social variables (broken home or lower-class status) do predict to antisocial behavior, the biological variables are less effective in prediction.

The Wadsworth study is important because it is based on a large, national birth cohort. The results must be seen as representative. We should also remember that the data on pulse rate were gathered by hundreds of different physicians in different schools, using rather primitive methods. Not all of these measurements were equally accurately taken. About 10 years intervened between the recording of the pulse rate and the ascertainment of delinquency. Despite these conditions, which in most research do not tend to inflate positive findings, the hypothesized results emerged. Those who did not suffer anticipatory pulse rate increase before the examination were those boys who later were more likely to become seriously delinquent. Perhaps this anticipatory response was also lacking before they committed the act (or acts) that gained them access to the delinquent group.

It may be worth underlining one other feature of the Wadsworth study. The low anticipatory pulse rate was observed 10 years before the delinquency was assessed. It is unlikely that the delinquency experience produced the low pulse rate. The prospective nature of the study establishes low pulse rate in anticipation of a stress as a variable worthy of consideration among the potential etiological factors in delinquency.

How salient a predictive factor is pulse rate? Not very. In the Wadsworth study, it predicts to delinquency about as well as the variable "broken home." It is naive to expect that any variable alone (biological or social) will explain large amounts of delinquency variance. Delinquency is likely to be as complex in its causality as it is in its manifestation. Note, however, that when the *interactive* effect of pulse rate and family factors is assessed, prediction improves considerably.

A Second Prospective Study

Janice Loeb and I have reported on a 10-year follow-up of a group of Danish adolescents.[14] In 1962, we examined their skin conductance (a peripheral autonomic measure); in 1972, we ascertained their registered delinquency from the Danish National Police Register. At 10-year follow-up, 7 boys of the 104 adolescents were noted as having been registered for mildly delinquent acts. The predelinquency 1962 skin conductance level, responsiveness, and recovery of the 7 delinquents was below that of the controls. The mean amplitude of response of the delinquents was one-tenth that of the nondelinquents.

Hare's Study

The third prospective study I will cite was conducted by Hare.[11] In 1964, he examined skin conductance in a group of serious, convicted criminals, all in a maximum security prison. Ten years later, he checked to see how seriously recidivistic the prisoners subsequently became. Skin conductance recovery in 1964 predicted to degree of recidivism 10 years later.

I would make several points relating to these prospective studies.

1. In combination with social and familial factors, such biological characteristics that presage the later development of delinquency might be useful in early detection. The development of such early detection techniques would be an important first step in a program of primary prevention.

2. Studies in Philadelphia by Wolfgang, Figlio, and Sellin,[30] research in Stockholm by Gösta Carlsson,[4] research by West and Farrington[28] in the inner city of London, and our own research on a birth cohort of 32,000 men in Copenhagen have rather reliably indicated that only a very small subgroup of the antisocial individuals is responsible for most of the criminal acts and the more serious criminal acts. The biosocial prediction measures seem to be most appropriate to preidentifying this small group of most serious criminals. A program of intervention focused on such a small number of individuals might prove disproportionately effective in crime reduction.

3. All three of the prospective studies are consistent with a description of the predelinquent and prerecidivistic criminal having somewhat underreactive autonomic nervous systems.

GENETIC AND PSYCHOPHYSIOLOGICAL FACTORS AND ANTISOCIAL BEHAVIOR

I will next discuss evidence that such underreactive autonomic nervous systems are characteristic of criminals. I will also consider the possible origins of this state, including genetic factors. Let us examine the evidence that genetic factors are related to the etiology of antisocial behavior. What is the point of examining the genetics literature? Only one of importance from my point of view. If it can be demonstrated that there is some genetic contribution to some forms of criminality, then consideration of a partial biological predisposition for antisocial behavior would be forced upon us. This would have implications for directions of research. There are three genetic research strategies we will briefly describe—family studies, twin research, and adoption investigations.

Family Studies

It has long been observed that antisocial parents raise an excessive number of children who also become antisocial. In the classic study by Lee Robins, one of the best predictors of antisocial behavior in a child was the father's criminality.[21] In terms of genetics, very little can be concluded from such family data inasmuch as it is difficult to disentangle hereditary and environmental influences.

Twin Studies

Twin studies compare criminal outcomes for identical and fraternal twins. The influence of hereditary factors is assumed to be demonstrated to the extent that the identical twins have more similar outcomes than the fraternal twins. From 1929–1977, I have found 10 twin studies in the literature. The early studies report about 60–70% concordance for crime for identical twins and about 15% concordance for fraternal twins.[5]

The most important study of these 10 was conducted by K. O. Christiansen who investigated the fates of all 7,172 twins born in a well-defined area of Denmark.[6] He used a national, complete criminality register about which Marvin Wolfgang has said: "the reliability and validity of the Danish record keeping system are almost beyond criticism. The criminal registry office in Denmark is probably the most thorough, comprehensive and accurate in the Western world."[29] Christiansen notes that "there are several important characteristics of the Danish law enforcement process that relate to its statutory uniformity regarding treatment of the offender and sentencing by the court. Police officers are legally *required* to report cases if they have a suspect. They are not permitted to make judgements in such matters. . . . The social status of a Danish police officer is comparatively high; they are regarded as being incorruptible."[6]

In this, the largest and best designed of the twin studies of criminality, Christiansen reports 35% concordance for monozygotic (MZ) (male-male) pairs and 13% concordance for the dyzygotic (DZ) (male-male) pairs.[6] (Percents given are pair-wise concordance rates.) In this unselected twin population, the MZ concordance rate is lower than in previous studies. In fact, it is important to note that more cases are discordant than concordant. This suggests that genetic factors control a minor but significant portion of the variance. Nevertheless, the MZ rate is 2.7 times the DZ rate. This result suggests the possibility that there is some genetically controlled, biological characteristic (or set of characteristics) that is identical for the MZ twins and that in some unknown way increases their common risk for being registered for criminal behavior.

The results of the twin studies do not contradict the hypothesis that some genetically transmitted, biological characteristic predisposes to antisocial behavior.

Adoption Studies

The problem with twin studies is that the twins are almost always raised together. There is poor separation of genetic and environmental factors. The adoption design does a better job of this separation. Children adopted at birth share no environment with their biological fathers. If criminality in the biological fathers is related to criminality in their adopted-away children, then this suggests that the criminal biological fathers have genetically transmitted some criminogenic biological characteristic to their children.

Crowe studied a small group of adopted children born to women in prison, as well as control adoptees.[8] The adopted children with *criminal* biological mothers were registered for more crimes than were adopted children with *noncriminal* biological mothers. Cadoret reports that among 246 Iowans adopted at birth, criminality in adoptees and their biological parents was significantly related.[3] (He ascertained criminality by telephone interview of the adoptive parents.)

In Copenhagen, Schulsinger finds excessive amounts of psychopathy among the biological relatives of psychopaths who had been adopted at birth.[22] In this study, Schulsinger identified psychopaths from a population of all the 5,483 Copenhagen County adoptions 1924–1947.

From these same 5,483 adoptions, Hutchings and Mednick ascertained the registered criminality of the male adoptees, their biological fathers, and

TABLE 1

REGISTERED CRIMINALITY IN ADOPTEES AND THEIR FATHERS;
"CROSS-FOSTERING" ANALYSIS*

		If Biological Father Is		
		Not Registered	Minor Crime	Criminal
If Adoptive Father Is	Not Registered	10.5	16.5	22.0
	Minor Crime	13.3	10.0	18.6
	Criminal	11.5	41.1	36.2

* Tabled values are percentage of adoptees criminal.

their adoptive fathers.[12] The results are given in TABLE 1. As can be seen in the table, if neither the biological nor the adoptive father is criminal, 10.5% of their sons are criminal. If the biological father is not criminal but the adoptive father is criminal, this figure rises to only 11.5%. Note that 22% of the sons are criminal if the adoptive father is not criminal and the biological father is criminal. Thus, the comparison (analogous to a cross-fostering comparison) seems to favor a partial genetic-etiology assumption. We must caution, however, that the adoption methodology has a number of drawbacks. These have been discussed by Mednick and Hutchings.[18] In an extension of this study, we have now constructed analogous tables for 7,000 adoptees and 28,000 biological and adoptive relatives; the results replicate. We will soon be reporting results for all 14,435 adoptions in our study. These 14,435 adoptions comprise all the adoptions in the Kingdom of Denmark between 1924 and 1947.

It seems that a partial genetic predisposition for antisocial behavior must be considered a serious possibility. I would again emphasize that the expression of the genetic predisposition depends very heavily on social factors. Thus, in middle and upper classes, the genetic effect is more strongly expressed. In the lower classes, the genetic effect is more weakly expressed. As mentioned above, this is in excellent agreement with Sellin's group resistance theory.[23] In social settings that are highly resistant to crime, individuals who become criminal must have strong individual predispositions. Finally, I would say the obvious—this genetic predisposition must be biological.

The three prospective studies have directed our attention to autonomic nervous system "underreactiveness" as possibly being predispositional to antisocial behavior. Twin studies in our Copenhagen laboratories have suggested that important components of the autonomic response system are heritable.[2]

Autonomic Nervous System of Antisocial Individuals

I will now summarize literature that examines the autonomic responsiveness (specifically the skin conductance response) of antisocial individuals. Much of the research began with consideration of psychopaths. Clinical descriptions of the psychopath include such phrases as: lacks emotion, callous, feels no guilt, no shame, no remorse, incapable of love, fails to learn from punishing experiences, cannot emotionally anticipate consequences. Studies of physiological indicators of emotion have noted that these clinical descriptions fit the objective measurements of the physiology of the psychopath. Interestingly enough, the physiological descriptions also fit criminals, delinquents, and (as we have seen) predelinquents. (See Reference 19 for a review of this work.)

For example, in one type of study, physiological measures of autonomic nervous system functioning are continuously monitored. The subject is told that at the count of 9, he will experience a severe electric shock. The more psychopathic, delinquent, or criminal individual does not evidence anticipatory heart rate, skin conductance, or biochemical indicants of fear. This is true even of psychopathic Swedes studied just before they walked into the courtroom for their criminal trials.[13]

The results in this area of research are remarkably consistent and robust across a variety of experimental procedures, definitions of antisocial behavior, and different national settings. The antisocial groups consistently demonstrate hyporeactive autonomic nervous systems. Recall the three prospective studies that find that these same psychophysiological characteristics predict to antisocial behavior ascertained 10 years later. In view of our twin study results,[2] it is tempting to hypothesize that these physiological characteristics may be a part of the biological predisposition passed on from an antisocial parent. Indeed, in our laboratory in Copenhagen, we have found that a group of children with fathers registered for criminality tends to have the very same physiological signs that have been found to be reliably characteristic of the delinquent, psychopath, and criminal.[16]

Biosocial Interactions in the Learning of Morality

Much of this paper has been devoted to reporting literature that finds some biological factors in criminal behavior. Perhaps it would be useful to close with a specific suggestion as to how such biological characteristics might interact with family and social factors to interfere with the learning of moral behavior. It would do no great harm to begin with a discussion of how we define morality. An early publication may be found in TABLE 2. Note that the major thrust of the message is negative—"thou shalt *not* . . ." While subsequent moral authorities have added *some* positive acts to elaborate the definition of moral behavior (e.g., "love thy neighbor"), they

TABLE 2

THE TEN COMMANDMENTS (EXODUS)*

I am the Lord thy God, thou shalt have no other gods before me.

Thou shalt *not* make a graven image nor bow down or serve them.

Thou shalt *not* take the name of the Lord your God in vain.

Remember the sabbath day and keep it holy.

Honour thy father and thy mother.

Thou shalt *not* kill.

Thou shalt *not* commit adultery.

Thou shalt *not* steal.

Thou shalt *not* bear false witness against your neighbor.

Thou shalt *not* covet thy neighbor's home, wife, maidservant, ox, ass.

* Emphasis added.

have also retained the original, basic, inhibitory definitions of moral acts. There are very few who will denounce you if you do not love your neighbor; but if you seduce his wife, steal from him, and/or kill him, you may be certain that your behavior will be classified as immoral. Thus, putting aside philosophical, poetic, or artistic musing on morality, we might admit to ourselves that the statements of moral behavior that are critical for everyday activities are essentially negative and inhibitory in character. The fact that someone took the trouble to enumerate these strictures—and then carve them onto stone tablets—suggests that at some point, there must have been a strong need for insistence on these inhibitions. People must have evidenced—and perhaps still do evidence—a tendency to exhibit aggressive, adulterous, and avaricious behavior. In self-defense, society has set up moral codes and has struggled to teach its children to *inhibit* impulses leading to transgression of those codes.

How are these inhibitions taught to children? As far as I can see, there are three learning mechanisms that could conceivably help parents teach children civilized behavior: modeling, positive reinforcement, and negative reinforcement. I believe that positive acts—such as loving neighbors, helping old ladies across the street, and cleaning the snow and ice from the front walk—can be learned by modeling; but for the more inhibitory moral commands, modeling does not seem to be a natural method. It is possible to imagine arranging circumstances in some artificial way such that modeling *could* teach children not to be adulterous or aggressive. If our civilization had to depend solely on modeling, however, it is conceivable that things might be even more chaotic than they are today. It is also possible to use positive reinforcement to teach inhibition of forbidden behavior; but again, reinforcing a child 24 hours a day while he is *not* stealing seems a rather inefficient method and not very specific.

Following the excellent exposition of Gordon Trasler,[25] we would suggest that childhood learning of the avoidance of transgression (i.e., the practice of law-abiding behavior) demanded by the moral commandments probably is trained, in the main, via contingent punishment applied by society, family, and peers. The critical inhibitory, morality-training forces in childhood very likely are (1) the punishment of antisocial responses by family, society, and friends; and (2) the child's individual capacity to *learn* to inhibit antisocial responses.

Let us attempt to be specific and to relate how children might learn to inhibit an impulse to steal. Frequently when a child steals from his parents, his peers, his siblings, or a five-and-ten, he is punished. After a sufficient quantity or quality of punishment, just the thought of the act of stealing should be enough to produce a bit of anticipatory fear in the child. If this fear response is large enough, the extended fingers will relax and the stealing impulse will be *successfully inhibited*.

Our story suggests that what happens in this child *after* he has successfully inhibited such an antisocial response is critical for his learning of civilized behavior. Let us consider the situation again in more detail.

1. Child contemplates stealing.
2. Because of previous punishment, he suffers fear.
3. Because of fear, he inhibits the stealing impulse.

What happens to his anticipatory fear?

4. Since he no longer entertains the stealing impulse, the fear will begin to dissipate, to be reduced.

We know that fear reduction is the most powerful, naturally occurring reinforcement that psychologists have discovered. So the reduction of fear (which immediately follows the inhibition of the stealing) can act as a reinforcement for this inhibition, and will result in the learning of the inhibition of stealing. The powerful reinforcement associated with fear reduction increases the probability that the inhibition of the stealing will occur in the future. After many such experiences, the normal child will learn to inhibit stealing impulses. Each time such an impulse arises and is successfully inhibited, the inhibition will be strengthened by reinforcement, since the fear elicited by the impulse will be reduced following successful inhibition.

What does a child need in order to learn effectively to be civilized (in the context of this approach)?

1. A social censuring agent (typically family or peers) *and*
2. An adequate physiological fear response *and*
3. The ability to learn the fear response in anticipation of an antisocial act *and*
4. Fast dissipation of physiological fear to quickly reinforce the inhibitory response.

I have indicated earlier that there is consistent evidence that the antisocial individual does not have an adequate fear response and does not learn adequately to emotionally anticipate negative events. The evidence regarding the final point—rate of dissipation of fear—is unequivocal; the antisocial individual tends to evidence very slow fear dissipation.[19] In terms of this theoretical approach, this suggests that under normal rearing conditions, the antisocial individual is not adequately rewarded for inhibiting antisocial responses.

CONCLUDING REMARKS

In these brief remarks, I have attempted to describe recent evidence that biological factors may play some partial role in the origins of antisocial behavior (or perhaps some forms of antisocial behavior). The biological factors can aid in understanding the conditions leading to antisocial behavior in situations or populations where social-familial factors are less successful at prediction. These include, for example, middle- or upper-class background, recidivistic criminality, female criminality, or crime in rural areas. It is in these situations or individuals that the biological variables show stronger relations with antisocial behavior. In circumstances or individuals where social-familal factors would predict elevated crime (such as lower social class rearing), the biological factors are less effective in prediction.

What the implications of these recent findings may be is far from clear at this point. Certainly no social action would be advised without considerable additional research efforts and replication. Perhaps these findings suggest that we reevaluate our ability to predict early who might later become a serious criminal. The complementarity of the social-familial and biological variables suggests that adding the biological variables to the highly effective social-familial factors[20] in a single predictive study might eventually yield acceptably accurate prediction of serious recidivism.

If excellent prediction were possible, what preventive intervention might shield children or adolescents from a crime career? Perhaps the variables that predict to future serious crime will suggest intervention strategies. Acting on the above-reported reliable findings of low autonomic nervous system arousal in antisocial individuals, Allen *et al.* have begun some pilot research attempting to alter this low arousal state by drug administrations to bring delinquents up to normal arousal states. He reports some success with this method, working with an extremely small group of delinquents.[1] An important problem in such drug intervention is that it may result in long-term, unwanted side effects. It was the danger of such side effects that moved us to reject drug intervention in a primary prevention project in the field of serious mental illness (schizophrenia). We chose the conservative step of an excellent, protective nursery school program.[17]

In this Academy meeting, Professor David Bakan has raised the possibility of using severe punishment (his expression was "to terrorize") on individuals who were identified as possible future criminals. This would certainly seem to be an inappropriate model for intervention. While mild punishment is probably the prevailing method that families, peers, and society use to teach small children to inhibit antisocial conduct, it would not seem a likely or promising technique for pragmatic intervention.

I would record one final thought in this paper. As pointed out above, social scientists have had strong negative emotional reactions to attempts to understand the role that biological factors play in the development of social man. These negative emotional reactions have often been responsive to biological scientists' drawing irresponsible or premature conclusions from fallible correlational research. Such scientific carelessness is especially reprehensible in circumstances where political forces may attempt to use such premature conclusions in justifying repressive social action. Responsible criticism of faulty methods or unfortunate, inadequately grounded conclusions is a necessary and important part of a scientist's work. But I would emphasize the word "responsible." Remember that earlier attempts to silence or retard scientific inquiry by public appeals to emotion or public burning of books have not proven as successful as a single intelligent and penetrating methodological analysis.

REFERENCES

1. ALLEN, H., S. DINITZ, T. FOSTER, H. GOLDMAN & L. LINDNER. 1976. Sociopathy: an experiment in internal environmental control. Am. Behav. Scientist **20:** 215–226.
2. BELL, B., S. A. MEDNICK, I. I. GOTTESMAN & J. SERGEANT. 1977. Electrodermal parameters in young, normal male twins. *In* Biosocial Bases of Criminal Behavior. S. A. Mednick & K. O. Christiansen, Eds. Gardner Press. New York, N.Y.
3. CADORET, R. J. 1978. Psychopathy in adopted-away offspring of biological parents with antisocial behavior. Arch. Gen. Psychiatry **35:** 176–184.
4. CARLSSON, G. 1977. Crime and behavioral epidemiology. Concepts and applications to Swedish data. *In* Biosocial Bases of Criminal Behavior. S. A. Mednick & K. O. Christiansen, Eds. Gardner Press. New York, N.Y.
5. CHRISTIANSEN, K. O. 1977. A review of studies of criminality among twins. *In* Biosocial Bases of Criminal Behavior. S. A. Mednick & K. O. Christiansen, Eds. Gardner Press. New York, N.Y.
6. CHRISTIANSEN, K. O. 1977. A preliminary study of criminality among twins. *In* Biosocial Bases of Criminal Behavior. S. A. Mednick & K. O. Christiansen, Eds. Gardner Press. New York, N.Y.
7. COMTE, A. 1855. The Positive Philosophy of Auguste Comte. (Translated by Harriet Martineau.) Blanchord. New York, N.Y.
8. CROWE, R. 1975. An adoptive study of psychopathy: preliminary results from arrest records and psychiatric hospital records. *In* Genetic Research in Psychiatry. R. Fieve, D. Rosenthal & H. Brill, Eds. Johns Hopkins University Press. Baltimore, Md.
9. GODWIN, J. 1978. Murder USA: The Ways We Kill Each Other. Ballantine Books. New York, N.Y.
10. HALLER, M. H. 1968. Social science and genetics: a historical perspective. *In* Genetics. D. Glass, Ed. The Rockefeller University Press. New York, N.Y.
11. HARE, R. D. 1978. Psychopathy and crime. *In* Colloquium on the Correlates of Crime and the Determinants of Criminal Behavior. L. Otten, Ed. Mitre Corp.
12. HUTCHINGS, B. & S. A. MEDNICK. 1977. Criminality in adoptees and their adoptive and biological parents: a pilot study. *In* Biosocial Bases of Criminal Behavior. S. A. Mednick & K. O. Christiansen, Eds. Gardner Press. New York, N.Y.
13. LIDBERG, L., S. LEVANDER, D. SCHALLING & Y. LIDBERG. 1980. Urinary catecholamines, stress and psychopath—a study of arrested men awaiting trial. Psychosom. Med. (In press.)
14. LOEB, J. & S. A. MEDNICK. 1977. A prospective study of predictors of criminality. 3. Electrodermal response patterns. *In* Biosocial Bases of Criminal Behavior. S. A. Mednick & K. O. Christiansen, Eds. Gardner Press. New York, N.Y.
15. Los Angeles Times. 1979. March 28.
16. MEDNICK, S. A. 1977. A bio-social theory of the learning of law-abiding behavior. *In* Biosocial Bases of Criminal Behavior. S. A. Mednick & K. O. Christiansen, Eds. Gardner Press. New York, N.Y.
17. MEDNICK, S. A. 1979. Risk research and primary prevention of mental illness. Int. J. Mental Health **7:** 150–164.
18. MEDNICK, S. A. & B. HUTCHINGS. 1977. Some considerations in the interpretation of the Danish adoption studies. *In* Biosocial Bases of Criminal Behavior. S. A. Mednick & K. O. Christiansen, Eds. Gardner Press. New York, N.Y.
19. MEDNICK, S. A. & J. VOLVAKA. 1980. Biology and crime. *In* Crime and Justice **2.** N. Morris & M. Tonry, Eds. (In press.)
20. ROBINS, L. H. & K. S. RATCLIFF. 1980. Risk factors in the continuation of childhood antisocial behavior into adulthood. Int. J. Mental Health. (In press.)
21. ROBINS, L. N. 1966. Deviant Children Grown Up. Williams & Wilkins. Baltimore, Md.
22. SCHULSINGER, F. 1977. Psychopath: heredity and environment. *In* Biosocial Bases of Criminal Behavior. S. A. Mednick & K. O. Christiansen, Eds. Gardner Press. New York, N.Y.
23. SELLIN, T. 1938. Culture, Conflict and Crime. Subcommittee on Delinquency. Committee on Personality and Culture. New York, N.Y.
24. SPENCER, H. 1878. Social Statistics. Appleton-Century-Crofts, Inc. New York, N.Y.

25. TRASLER, G. 1972. Criminal behavior. *In* Handbook of Abnormal Psychology. H. H. Eysenck, Ed. G. P. Putnam's Sons. London, England.
26. WADSWORTH, M. E. J. 1975. Delinquency in a national sample of children. Br. J. Criminol. **15:** 167–174.
27. WADSWORTH, M. E. J. 1978. Delinquency, pulse-rates and early emotional deprivation. Br. J. Criminol. **16:** 245–256.
28. WEST, D. J. & D. P. FARRINGTON. 1973. Who Becomes Delinquent? Heinemann. London, England.
29. WOLFGANG, M. E. 1977. Foreword. *In* Biosocial Bases of Criminal Behavior. S. A. Mednick & K. O. Christiansen, Eds. Gardner Press. New York, N.Y.
30. WOLFGANG, M. E., R. M. FIGLIO & T. SELLIN. 1972. Delinquency in a Birth Cohort. University of Chicago Press. Chicago, Ill.

A NEUROPSYCHOSOCIAL PERSPECTIVE OF PERSISTENT JUVENILE DELINQUENCY AND CRIMINAL BEHAVIOR: DISCUSSION

Discussant: Lorne T. Yeudall

Department of Neuropsychology
Alberta Hospital
Edmonton, Alberta,
Canada T5J 2J7

Dr. Mednick[1] has presented strong evidence implicating hereditary influences in the genesis of delinquent and criminal behaviors for some individuals. He and his coworkers have shown that biological differences [quantitative electroencephalograph (EEG) abnormalities, low electrodermal responses (EDRs), and slow electrodermal recovery (EDRec)] that have predictive significance characterize individuals at risk for such antisocial behaviors. At least one of these biological markers (EDRec) has an extremely high heritability index. The theoretical model of antisocial behaviors formulated by Dr. Mednick focuses on the inability to inhibit social responses that are not sanctioned by society and is similar in this respect to a number of hypotheses stressing the role of disinhibition of behaviors. It is also a multivariate model, involving the interaction of the social environment with biological factors (adequate fear response, ability to learn a fear response in anticipation of an asocial act, and fast dissipation of fear and/or quick reinforcement of the inhibitory response). The autonomic abnormalities found in some high risk individuals who commit serious and repetitive antisocial behaviors may be significantly related to brain mechanisms underlying the inhibition of behavior, more specifically, those mechanisms that underlie the fast disruption of the fear and/or quick reinforcement of the inhibitory response. The general focus of his theory is a central theme of many researchers currently studying persistent criminal and violent behavior, namely, the failure to develop inhibitory controls.

There can be no doubt that learning plays a crucial role in the development of inhibitory controls. The ability to learn, however, hinges on the integrity of the central nervous system. In my opinion, Dr. Mednick's findings are most relevant to this issue: the integrity of the central nervous system. The demonstration of consistent evidence of psychophysiological abnormalities in high risk populations is indicative of dysfunction or impairment of the central nervous system, particularly in those regions of the brain primarily involved in the control and/or regulation of the autonomic nervous system. Disturbed autonomic functioning has been reported on the basis of a variety of complex psychophysiological response measures. However, Dr. Mednick's findings as well as those of other researchers, including my own research group, are not limited to the investigation of autonomic responses but include such assessment techniques as standard

EEG, quantitative EEG, and neuropsychologic. Such multivariate assessment techniques reveal a broader involvement of other regions of the brain. In this context of more generally altered brain function, many other influences in addition to genetic influences on the pre- and postnatal development of the organism may be fruitfully examined.

It appears that there may be an important relationship between the persistent nature of an individual's criminal history and his being identified as a high risk individual. As Dr. Mednick has pointed out from his own observations and from those of Wolfgang, Figlio, and Sellin,[2] a very small percentage (less than 10%) of the criminal offenders are responsible for over 50% of the serious crimes committed in a given catchment area. It is this unique subpopulation that Dr. Mednick feels may have some specific individual characteristics that increase the probability of persistent criminal behavior. If one focuses on the persistent nature of criminal behavior, then there is emerging evidence that altered brain function may be one of these specific individual characteristics.

The association between disturbed brain function or biogenic influences and persistent criminal behavior, particularly in regard to violent-aggressive and psychopathic criminals, has been supported by research involving EEG studies in prison populations.[3-7] There have been similar findings for noncriminal populations in regard to episodic violent behavior and rage syndromes.[8-10] More recently, neuropsychological studies have also found a high incidence of impairments in violent and nonviolent persistent juvenile delinquent populations.[11-16] Over the last seven years, I and several colleagues have focused our research on the so-called persistent offender with an extensive criminal history. Our investigation of persistent (mean convictions, 10.0) male psychopathic criminals convicted of homicide, rape, and physical assault have consistently found a high incidence (76% to 100%) of neuropsychological impairments.[17] Similarly, our studies on persistent adult sex offenders, violent-aggressive criminals, and adolescents with severe conduct disorders have revealed a high incidence of neuropsychological impairments ($\bar{x} = 90\%$).[18,19] The neuropsychological impairments implicated bilateral dysfunction of the frontal and temporal lobes with a dominant hemisphere emphasis in approximately 72% of the cases. In contrast, persistent male criminals with affective disorders, while showing a similar incidence of dysfunction, were found to have a higher incidence of greater nondominant hemisphere dysfunction.[17] A study just recently completed involved neuropsychological and power spectral EEG analyses of 100 consecutive admissions of persistent juvenile offenders without a violent history and 46 age-matched controls.[16] Of the control group, 12% were found to have abnormal neuropsychological profiles in contrast to 86% of the juvenile offenders. In contrast to the previous persistent psychopathic and violent criminals, these juvenile offenders showed a greater involvement of the nondominant hemisphere in 63% of the cases. Spectral analysis of the alpha frequency band of the EEG, which was recorded during the performance of language and visual spatial tasks, revealed that the juveniles had significantly more power in the frontal and temporal lobe regions with a nondominant hemisphere emphasis. Discriminant function analysis of the alpha band for relative power yielded correct classifications of 94.9% and 97.7% for the juvenile offenders and controls, respectively. Thus our results to date have consistently demonstrated a high incidence of neuropsychological and spectral EEG abnormalities that implicate dysfunction of the frontal and temporal regions of the brain.

The brain-behavior relationships of these anterior regions of the brain may be of particular significance to criminal behavior in that they play an important role in the regulation and inhibition of human behavior.[6,10,20-22] For example, Luria points out that the anterior frontal regions of the brain play a decisive role in the formation of plans and intentions, and in the regulation and verification of complex behaviors.[22] These processes are particularly formulated and elaborated via the speech mechanisms of the dominant hemisphere. Nauta similarly views the frontal regions as playing a special role in monitoring and modulating activity in other neocortical and limbic regions of the brain and suggests that "the reciprocal fronto-limbic relationships could be centrally involved in the phenomena of behavioral anticipation."[21] In contrast to the executive and regulatory functions of the frontal lobes, the temporal lobes appear to be more related to subjective consciousness and to play an integrative role in the individual's personal experience as it relates to the awareness of the relationship between information from his external and internal world. As Williams has pointed out, the functions of the temporal lobes "are much more closely identified with the subject himself; they involve his emotional life, his instinctive feelings and activities and his visceral responses to environmental change . . . that is to say, they include his social as well as his physical milieu."[22] Thus the integrity of the cortical and limbic regions of the frontal and temporal lobes would appear to be very important for the acquisition of moral behaviors and the inhibition of transgressions.

The association between persistent criminal behavior and lower socioeconomic status is well known. Ashley Montagu has elucidated the significance of this correlation and has related it to the effects of impoverished environments on the developing brain.[23] He has concluded that lower socioeconomic status associated with deprived environments increases the probability of brain damage at birth and hypothesized that such social environments could result in altered brain functioning, which then renders the individual more vulnerable to the many challenges in his environment. Stott has also emphasized the interactive role of genetic vulnerabilities and adverse environments (of both the child and mother during fetal development).[24] From his studies of maladjustment and delinquency in children, he has concluded that the association between a number of abnormal physical conditions and behavioral disturbance reflected "congenital insult which in some cases was seen both somatically and in impairment of that part of the nervous system controlling behavior."[24] In addition to the suggested effects of the interaction between genetic factors and/or adverse sociological conditions in regard to the developing brain, there remain many other contributing factors (e.g., birth injury, febrile convulsions, head injuries) that result in altered brain function during the early developmental years of the child. For example, Lewis, Shanok, and Balla, in agreement with other studies, found a significant association between perinatal problems and behavioral disorders in seriously delinquent children.[25] In addition, they found that by the age of two years, these children had sustained significantly more and serious head and face traumas.

Male gender is more frequently found to be associated with behavioral disturbances, which in turn are more prevalent in impoverished environments.[24,26-30] It is well known that there is an excess of males relative to females, approximately 5 to 1, in the incidence of behavioral disorders including juvenile delinquency, persistent violent behavior, infantile autism, learning disabilities, developmental dyslexia and dysgraphia, dysphasia, and stuttering. All of these disorders have now been linked to abnormalities of brain function. Thus a plausible assumption is that the male brain may be more susceptible or vulnerable to adverse events occurring during prenatal or postnatal periods of development. Consistent with this hypothesis is a recent comprehensive 30-year study that found an excess of males (3 : 1) with intracranial abscesses.[31] Several authors have suggested that the excess of males in the previously mentioned behavioral disorders is related to gender differences in brain development.[32,33] Genetic neurohumoral mechanisms are considered responsible for hemispheric differences between the two sexes. Flor-Henry has proposed that these hemispheric differences render the sexes differentially vulnerable to disturbances of cerebral development in regard to the dominant and nondominant hemispheres.[34] Males are viewed as having a relatively superior nondominant hemisphere and a more vulnerable dominant hemisphere, whereas females are thought to have a relatively more superior dominant hemisphere and a more vulnerable nondominant hemisphere during the early developmental years. Thus, as I suggested previously, if the male brain in general is more vulnerable than the female brain to adverse developmental events—and in addition, as others have suggested, is more vulnerable to dominant hemisphere injury—then this would be consistent with the well-known excess of males with language-related disorders. The accumulating evidence for the association of dominant hemisphere dysfunction in the previously mentioned male disorders would also account for the clustering of some of these disorders (e.g., juvenile delinquency and learning disabilities). I have suggested elsewhere that the dominant hemisphere dysfunction of the temporal and frontal regions of the brain may play a critical role in the genesis of persistent criminal behavior.[18] More specifically, I have suggested that dominant hemisphere dysfunction disrupts the role of language in the development of foresight or anticipation of the negative consequences of amoral behavior. In contrast to offenders with dominant hemisphere dysfunction, offenders with nondominant hemisphere dysfunction would be susceptible to behavioral disruption as a possible consequence of mood disorders, which have been linked to nondominant hemisphere dysfunction.[35-37]

The findings of several independent studies have demonstrated a high incidence of neuropsychological impairments in persistent juvenile offender populations. These neuropsychological deficits, particularly in the early developmental years of the child and adolescent, could have significant detrimental effects in regard to the functional, emotional, and cognitive adaptive abilities of the individual with such brain dysfunction. Thus high risk individuals who evolve into persistent criminal offenders may be those who have acquired significant neural impairment or brain damage and have the misfortune to be born into an impoverished environment, which typically lacks adequate attention for medical, educational, psychiatric, and legal problems. In contrast, it would be hypothesized that those individuals born into a similar impoverished environment without significant neural impairment would have a dramatically increased probability of coping with their adverse environment, as well as the biological potential to develop normal inhibitory controls.

The importance of primary prevention in regard to the socioeconomic effects on the developing fetus and child has been made clearly before.[23] However, the consequences of sociogenic brain damage and/or dysfunction will most certainly continue to face mankind. The accumulating evidence of a high incidence of brain dysfunction in persistent juvenile and adult criminal populations has implications not only for the possible identification of high risk individuals, but also for alternative approaches to treatment and rehabilitation.[1,6,11,18,38] In conclusion, the emerging relationships between adverse environments, genetic factors, brain damage, altered brain function or dysfunction, male gender, and behavioral disorders in high risk subpopulations strongly suggest that biological factors interacting with the environment play a significant role in the genesis of persistent juvenile delinquency and criminal behavior. As pointed out emphatically by others, these biosocial influences can no longer be ignored, and a multidisciplinary-multimodal approach is needed to effectively deal with the prevention and treatment of high risk offenders.[23,38,39]

References

1. MEDNICK, S. A. 1980. Human nature, crime, and society: keynote address. Ann. N.Y. Acad. Sci. (This volume.)
2. WOLFGANG, M. E., R. M. FIGLIO & T. SELLIN. 1972. Delinquency in a Birth Cohort. University of Chicago. Chicago, Ill.
3. HILL, D. 1952. EEG in episodic psychotic and psychopathic behavior: a classification of data. EEG J. 4: 419–442.
4. HILL, D. & D. WATTERSON. 1942. Electroencephalographic studies of psychopathic personalities. J. Neurol. Psychiatry 5: 47–65.
5. MONROE, R. R. 1970. Episodic Behavioral Disorders—A Psychodynamic and Neurophysiologic Analysis. Harvard University Press. Cambridge, Mass.
6. MONROE, R. R. 1978. Brain Dysfunction in Aggressive Criminals. D. C. Heath & Co. Lexington, Mass.
7. WILLIAMS, D. 1975. Studies of persons confined for crimes of violence. In Neural Bases of Violence and Aggression. W. S. Fields & W. H. Sweet, Eds. Warren H. Green. St. Louis, Mo.
8. BACH-Y-RITA, G., J. R. LION, C. E. CLIMENT & F. R. ERVIN. 1971. Episodic dyscontrol: a study of 130 violent patients. Am. J. Psychiatry 127(11): 1473–1478.

9. BLUMER, D. & C. MIGEON. 1975. Hormone and hormonal agents in treatment of aggression. J. Nerv. Ment. Dis. 160(2): 127–137.
10. ELLIOTT, F. A. 1978. Neurological aspects of antisocial behavior. In The Psychopath: A Comprehensive Study of Antisocial Disorders and Behaviors. W. H. Reid, Ed. Brunner/ Mazel. New York, N.Y.
11. BERMAN, A. 1978. Neuropsychological aspects of violent behavior. Presented at the Symposium on Adolescent Murderers at the Annual Convention of the American Psychological Association, Toronto, Ontario, Canada.
12. KRYNICKI, V. E. 1978. Cerebral dysfunction in repetitively assaultive adolescents. J. Nerv. Ment Dis. 166(1): 59–67.
13. ROBBINS, D., R. PRIES, D. JACOBS, J. BECK & C. SMITH. 1978. A preliminary report on the neuropsychological development of a group of clinic referred juvenile delinquents. Presented at the Symposium on Adolescent Murderers at the Annual Convention of the American Psychological Association, Toronto, Ontario, Canada.
14. SPELLACY, F. 1977. Neuropsychological differences between violent and nonviolent adolescents. J. Clin. Psychol. 33: 966–969.
15. SPELLACY, F. 1978. Neuropsychological discrimination between violent and nonviolent men. J. Clin. Psychol. 34(1): 49–52.
16. YEUDALL, L. T., D. FROMM-AUCH & P. DAVIES. 1979. Power spectral EEG and neuropsychological findings in persistent juvenile offenders. (In preparation.)
17. YEUDALL, L. T. 1978. Neuropsychological correlates of criminal psychopathy. I. Differential diagnosis. In Human Aggression and Dangerousness. L. Beliveau, G. Canepa & D. Szabo, Eds. Pinel Institute. Montreal, Quebec, Canada.
18. YEUDALL, L. T. 1978. The neuropsychology of aggression. Clarence M. Hincks Memorial Lectures: Psychobiological Approaches to Aggression in Mental illness and Mental Retardation. London, Ontario, Canada.
19. YEUDALL, L. T. & D. FROMM-AUCH. 1979. Neuropsychological impairments in various psychopathological populations. In Hemisphere Asymmetrics of Function and Psychopathology. J. Gruzelier & P. Flor-Henry, Eds. (In press.)
20. LURIA, A. R. 1973. The frontal lobes and the regulation of behavior. In Psychophysiology of the Frontal Lobes. K. H. Pribra & A. K. Luria, Eds. Academic Press, Inc. New York, N.Y.
21. NAUTA, J. W. H. 1971. The problem of the frontal lobes: a reinterpretation. J. Psychiatr. Res. 8: 167–187.
22. WILLIAMS, D. 1969. Temporal lobe syndromes. In Handbook of Clinical Neurology: Localization in Clinical Neurology. P. J. Vinken & G W. Bruyn, Eds. North Holland. Amsterdam, The Netherlands.
23. MONTAGU, A. 1972. Sociogenic brain damage. Am. Anthropol. 74(5): 1045–1061.
24. STOTT, D. H. 1962. Evidence for a congenital factor in maladjustment and delinquency. Am. J. Psychiatry 118(9): 781–794.
25. LEWIS, D. O., S. S. SHANOK & D. A. BALLA. 1979. Perinatal difficulties, head and face trauma, and child abuse in the medical histories of seriously delinquent children. Am. J. Psychiatry 136(4A): 419–423.
26. FERGUSON, T. 1952. The Young Delinquent in His Social Setting. Oxford University Press. London, England.
27. HUTT, C. 1972. Males and Females. Penguin Books. United Kingdom.
28. LEWIS, D. O. & S. S. SHANOK. 1979. Medical histories of psychiatrically referred delinquent children: an epidemiologic study. Am. J. Psychiatry 136(2): 231–233.
29. MONTAGU, A. 1971. Touching: The Human Significance of the Skin. Columbia University Press. New York, N.Y.
30. YEUDALL, L. T. 1977. Neuropsychological assessment of forensic disorders. Can. Ment. Health 25: 7–16.
31. MCCLELLAND, C. J., B. F. CRAIG & H. A. CROCKARD. 1978. Brain abscesses in Northern Ireland: a 30 year community review. J. Neurol. Neurosurg. Psychiatry 41: 1043–1048.
32. OUNSTED, C. & D. C. TAYLOR, Eds. 1972. Gender Differences: Their Ontogeny and Significance. Churchills. London, England.
33. TAYLOR, D. C. & C. OUNSTED. 1971. Biological mechanisms influencing the outcome of seizures in response to fever. Epilepsia 12: 33.

34. FLOR-HENRY, P. 1978. Gender, hemispheric specialization and psychopathology. Soc. Sci. Med. **12B**: 155–162.
35. FLOR-HENRY, P. 1979. On certain aspects of the localization of the cerebral systems regulating and determining emotion. Biol. Psychiatry **14**(4): 677–698.
36. GOLDSTEIN, L. 1977. Characteristics of EEG hemispheric asymmetries on psychopathology. *In* Sixth World Congress of Psychiatry. Honolulu, Hawaii.
37. FOLSTEIN, M. F., R. MAIBERGER & P. R. McHUGH. 1977. Mood disorder as a specific complication of stroke. J. Neurol. Neurosurg. Psychiatry **40**: 1018–1020.
38. JEFFERY, C. R. 1977. Crime Prevention through Environmental Design. Sage Publication, Inc. Beverly Hills, Calif.
39. VAN DEN BERGHE, P. 1974. Bringing beast back in: toward a biosocial theory of aggression. Am. Sociol. Rev.: 77–788.

HUMAN NATURE, CRIME, AND SOCIETY:
PANEL DISCUSSION

Moderator: Robert W. Rieber
Panel Members: David Bakan,
Ashley Montagu, and Lorne T. Yeudall

A. MONTAGU (*Princeton, N.J.*): In the first place, let me say this. When we're dealing with human beings, we're dealing with a very complex series of entities. And to talk about interactionism, namely, the interaction between genes and the environment, has become rather old-hat because by the time we get to the child that is born—whether it is an identical twin, a dizygotic twin, or a singleton—a great many things have happened to the genes, and a great many things have happened to the organism. In the interactionist conception of things, one thinks of the interaction between genes and the environment. This is a rather unsound view to take. What the interaction is, is between the environment and the organism; and the organism is a very different thing from the genotype or the genetic system. An enormous number of things happen. In the first place, in his paper—which I found extremely interesting and well-written and very compellingly so—Dr. Mednick seems to think that monozygotic twins are essentially genetically identical. They are not. No one knows for certain whether they are never so, but the probabilities are very high that they are never genetically identical. They differ in some of their genes at least and sometimes in their chromosomal structure.

Then there are, of course, a vast number of interactions between that growing and developing organism and the environment in the womb. And as you know, in one-egg twins (which should never be called identical twins because they are not identical), often one is larger than the other. When they are born, one may be found to have had its twin's arm around its neck or the amniotic cord twisted around its neck, etc.; the differences between them are very evident.

These differences may be significantly related to the later development of such twins to such an extent that the twins may show considerable differences in their behavior even though they're brought up in the same home. Certainly when they're separated, such twins may show very considerable differences. While we're always citing the remarkable coincidences and concordances in the behavior of twins who have been separated at birth and then subsequently studied, there are differences. Take, for example, Newman and Holzinger's famous case of Phyllis and her sister Gladys, who were separated at birth. One went to college and one did not. As Newman remarked, the benefits that Gladys showed spoke highly in favor of a college education. She showed the advantages of a superior environment. The sister who didn't go to college but was brought up in a lower-class environment showed the lower-class characteristics of such an individual.

356

But what is the point of these remarks to what Dr. Mednick said? Simply this: there is enormous variability in the findings on identical twins and in twin studies. What is often attributed to genes can be very clearly shown to be due in most cases to socioeconomic factors—as for example when Dr. Mednick speaks of low skin conductance level or low pulse level as a good predictor of future delinquency or criminal behavior.

I think it is quite well known that such skin conductance levels and low pulse rates are highly correlated with the emotional condition of the individual at the time of examination. As a child, that individual may have committed no delinquencies whatsoever but still may have been sufficiently emotionally disturbed to show significant changes in his skin conductance and pulse level. Indeed this is what we would expect.

Now to connect this, as Dr. Mednick does, with genetic causes of criminal behavior seems to me an error of scientific methodology. The probabilities indeed are very high that if such children—no matter what their skin conductance levels or pulse rates might be—were removed to an environment that was much more congenial to their healthy development, they would develop as noncriminal, healthy individuals.

This is the long and the short of what I have to say. Let me underscore what I have just said: it is utterly impossible by any method known to me to establish any relationship between genes and criminal behavior.

What we have learned about the interaction of genes in the genetic system is that there is an enormous amount of variability in what happens between genes, that every gene is part of the environment of every other gene, that the interaction between genes and their total environment is very profound indeed, but that no gene ever determines anything. Genes do not make your eyes blue or brown or your skin black or white. What they do is influence the physiological or behavioral expression of a trait. And between the gene and its expression lies a large number of complicating factors.

It is, therefore, my opinion that it is quite impossible with our present knowledge to tease out what part is due to genes and what part is due to environment. It simply can't be done. We just don't have the means of doing this.

So to Dr. Mednick's question as to why it is that people get worried when others begin talking about the genetic determinants of human behavior, the answer is very simple. It is because we have no evidence of any kind that any form of human behavior is genetically determined.

The fact is that everything that human beings come to know and do as human beings they have to learn from other human beings. There isn't a single thing that human beings do—and I don't mean the things they do that they hold in common with other mammals, but the things they do that make them uniquely human—they have to learn from other human beings. And this is not genetically determined. Robert Merton and I wrote a paper about 40 years ago, in the *American Anthropologist,* called "Crime and the Anthropologist" in which we reviewed the first volume of Earnest Hooton's book *The American Criminal,* which was to have appeared in three volumes. As a result of our review, only that one volume was ever published. What Hooton had done was to revive Lombrosianism in a new form. It was not difficult to show how unsound his thesis of inborn criminality was; the crime rates in different societies vary enormously. In New York City last year, there were somewhere in the vicinity of 1800 murders. In England there were somewhere in the vicinity of 300, in Tokyo 50. One can go through a great many examples of such variable statistics. Why the great variation? Is there any genetic difference at work here? The answer surely is that there isn't—that there are socioeconomic, sociocultural factors that are involved here—and that if one really is going to study the origin of criminal behavior, one surely must do this in a wholistic manner.

It is not sufficient to begin with an assumption that genetic determinants are involved in such behavior; I am very well aware that genes are involved in virtually every form of behavior. But the real question we have to ask is: To what extent do genes influence that behavior and especially criminal behavior? I have no doubt that there is some genetic influence responsible in some cases in individuals who have committed criminal behavior. But equally I have no doubt that all of us have genes that under certain conditions would express themselves in the form that Dr. Mednick describes as criminal behavior. We're all capable of criminal behavior. It depends largely on the conditions under which we grow and develop.

D. BAKAN *(York University, Toronto, Ontario, Canada):* May I say something? Dr. Mednick and I have been at it for several times during the day. Perhaps he has changed his position, and that's fine. Maybe for the sake of the *Annals* he's going to rewrite his paper; and maybe for the sake of the *Annals*, when this discussion is published, I'll have rewritten what I have said here. On the other hand, I feel impelled to read at least this, which stimulated part of what I have to say. On page 15 of the manuscript that I received, it goes as follows: "Following the excellent exposition of Gordon Trasler . . . I would suggest that the avoidance of transgression (i.e., lawful behavior) demanded by the moral commandments is probably in the main learned by way of contingent negative reinforcements (punishments) applied by society, family, and peers. I would guess that the critical morality-training forces in childhood are (1) the punishment of antisocial responses by family, society, and friends and (2) the child's individual capacity to learn to inhibit antisocial responses." Okay, so that punishment is certainly the critical factor according to Mednick.

The last thing is in terms of program. Mednick says, I believe, that predelinquents have distinguishing characteristics that could be used to select them for intervention research well before they become serious criminals. Now he says that we're going to intervene, and he says that learning of morality only takes place by punishment. I just put the two things together. If you're going to intervene—and if the critical thing is punishment—it seems to me that there is nothing else that you're going to intervene with except that which you take to be critical. Now I'd like to proceed with my comments.

It is a little-known historical fact that Cleopatra performed some of the earliest experiments on human biological paternity. By controlling the sexual intercourse of women, whom she had imprisoned for the purpose, she was able to explore some of the detailed phenomena of the relationship of sex and childbirth. I mention this because I feel uneasy about the arrogance of the Danish investigators who presume to be knowledgeable about who may be the biological fathers of the children who are put out for adoption. I don't pretend to be an expert on Danish culture or Danish sexual behavior, but I can't believe that the men and women from Denmark are dramatically different from the other Western peoples. Indeed, to this day, we do not have very good data on the gestation period among humans. We have excellent data on thoroughbred dogs, but not on women. So I'm very dubious about the data on the paternity of the children in that study. And I am very concerned that major public policy should be based on such studies.

It is rare for me to find myself in such total and profound disagreement with a paper as I am on this occasion. Indeed, let me say that I even consider the presentation that I have heard to be dangerous.

Let me state what I think are the main points of Mednick's presentation.

The first is that delinquency is to some unspecified extent a function of heredity. The second is that this hereditary defect may be overcome by the use of punishment and the development of anticipatory fear.

Mednick suggests a program of identifying young, predelinquent, hereditarily tainted children and "treating" them. If we take him at his word as to how one learns to be law-abiding, it would seem that the only proper word for his suggested plan is "terrorization."

In response to Mednick, I'd like to make the following three observations.

First, I think that Mednick doesn't understand the proper relationship between statistics, on the one hand, and public policy, on the other.

Second, I think that he is in danger of violating a fundamental principle of legality.

And third, his views are more generally dangerous in connection with public policy.

First, on statistics: Mednick confounds prediction with correlation. They are hardly the same thing. His studies are not predictive. His studies are postdictive, of the past. They describe some presumptive correlations.

Even if it were the case that there were such correlations, there still would be a question as to whether one should use such correlations in connection with public policy in the way that he suggests. The use of presumptive correlation in this way is the essence of unfair discrimination.

Let me give you a very simple example. Suppose we have a test in which more men than women passed. From a statistical point of view, this would constitute a correlation between sex and performance. If one would, on the basis of this correlation, bar women, say, from employment, it would be clearly discriminatory. Similarly, even if most people who display a certain physiological response were later to become criminal, it would be grossly unjust to treat *all* people who display this physiological response as potential criminals.

Consider the basic principle of "innocent until proven guilty." Mednick seems to be recommending a program of large-scale testing to identify potential delinquents, who will then be subjected to some kind of treatment. Mednick would have a needle on an electronic meter not only single people out for suspicion, but subject them to special fear-inducing treatments as well.

I believe that the very notion of such "early detection" of criminality is both heinous—with respect to the individuals that may be so labeled—and mischievous—in connection with public policy. It would be injurious to the individuals, and it would not serve to reduce such delinquency. I would suspect that anyone who might try to implement such a plan would find himself in deep trouble, at least with the parents of children with Mednick's predelinquency signs, those who endowed their children with what Dr. Mednick takes as an unfortunate genetic makeup.

I cannot imagine that the children who are so labeled by Dr. Mednick could develop any respect for the law that might treat them in this manner on the basis of, say, the electrical conductivity of their skins. If such Mednick children were to grow up without any respect for the law, it would be very understandable. The whole thing would constitute an example of the self-fulfilling prophecy.

Let me now speak to the question of the general approach that Mednick seems to be making to public policy. Let me first state what I consider to be a reasonable basic paradigm for apprehending appropriate social behavior. When an individual finds that there's a convergence between the interests of the group of which he is a member and his own interests, then he usually tries to behave well in terms of the norms of that group. On the other hand, when an individual sees his own interests as divergent from those of the group, he may become its enemy. Young people do not become enemies of society of they have hope for a decent life within it. If there is no hope for people, then they can only be controlled by intimidation. However, the limits of the effectiveness of intimidation are set by the limits of the controlling power on the one hand and the amount of courage on the other.

It appears to me that Mednick has not taken either police power or courage into account. Quite the contrary. It appears to me that he has made the assumption that somehow the one that will be carrying out the program he has outlined will have unlimited power and that the target population will be without either power or courage. Mednick has, for example, taken no account of something that is commonplace these days—the power of young people to organize themselves into effective, well-disciplined urban gangs that are capable of returning terror for terror. He has taken no account of justice and fairness as essential ingredients in maintaining the power and credibility of the law-enforcing agencies. I can imagine, for example, the possibility of a pattern of terror loosed on society by some vengeful union of a Mednick-selected group of sluggish-autonomic-nervous-system and low-skin-conductance persons who are outraged against the society that would single them out to be victims of a special fear-inducing program such as Mednick has outlined.

And finally let me mention the following—and this is the deepest paradox associated with the use of punishment at all as a method of social control. Whenever punishment is used as a method of social control, there are always at least two messages involved. The first one is, I am punishing you because you took the cookies out of the cookie jar. That's one thing. But there's always a second lesson. And that second lesson is that it is right and proper to influence another person through the use of force and intimidation; because that is what is modeled when you use punishment. Anytime one uses punishment as a method of control, one is also teaching the person being punished that punishment is a good method of controlling people—at least if one ever gets a chance and if one ever has the power. This means that any kind of use of punishment automatically continues the pattern of terror.

If, then, the Mednick program is ever to be put into effect on the grand scale that he conceives, it would involve the whole society in a massive program of mutual intimidation. There are parts of the world where this has taken place, where everyone is involved in a program of trying to intimidate the others by inducing fear in them.

Indeed, it might well be the tragedy of the world that the program that has been outlined by Dr. Mednick was, in point of fact, put into effect long ago and constitutes the major burden of the modern world. Thank you.

L. T. YEUDALL *(Alberta Hospital, Edmonton, Alberta, Canada):* Thank you. I just have to simmer down a little bit here. It's pretty hard to follow that David; I mean with the adrenalin that is flowing here.

Maybe what I'd like to do is return to a little more sober, scientific attitude. Not that science should be devoid of emotion. But I think one has to pay attention to some of the evidence that's emerging over time.

I find it very interesting that Dr. Montagu is more or less giving the impression that we haven't learned much about genetics and behavior. I don't think that's what he meant really, though possibly he did. But I can't help but think that we've learned something about mental retardation from the genetics of mental retardation. I can't help thinking that we've learned something about the identification of high risk individuals who will become mentally retarded because of genetic structure interacting with developmental fetal environment, which in turn interacts with socioeconomic factors as Dr. Montagu has well pointed out, and as have others before him.

I can't imagine why we have high risk neonatal clinics. Why don't we just scrap them? Because they identify biological markers that will potentially make a life of misery if they're ignored. But now they're not being ignored. Those clinics are increasing the quality of life of individuals both psychologically and physiologically by identifying so-called biological high risk markers.

I find it interesting that when we get into human behavior and start talking about biological markers, everybody gets emotional. But when we talk about physiological factors that don't have psychological behavior associated with them, well that's okay, we can accept that.

I find a similar analogy between neurology and psychiatry. When I'm on a neurosurgery unit or a neurology unit, the doctor goes through the symptoms of temporal lobe lesions and frontal lobe lesions and says, Ah yes, that's an orbital frontal lesion, probably on the left side. If I walk across the hall, I hear the psychiatrist discuss the same symptoms and start talking about dynamics, when the patient is two or three years of age.

Now, there's an interesting parallel here. We have different views of symptoms and behaviors; and what we really have to do, I believe, is examine our own presuppositions, our own belief systems, our own emotional commitments to those belief systems, and then settle down and try to put the picture together in some perspective.

If one looks at human behavior, certainly there are some hints of genetic influences. There are hints of very potent influences during the developmental period, as Dr. Montagu has pointed out in his classic paper entitled "Sociogenic Brain Damage" in the 1972 *American Anthropologist.* There are many factors that interact, not only with the possible genetic structure of the child, as suggested by Stott and others as well as Dr. Montagu, but with the physiological status of the mother and the child, and which covary with a bad environment. We can talk about toxic factors—alcoholism, heavy cigarette smoking, and the list goes on and on—in regard to those things that happen during the prenatal period. Birth injury is another important factor that occurs. The incidence of birth injury, at least in Canada, is phenomenally high. I suspect it's not much lower in the United States. That is, children have their brains injured and become high risk babies for something, whether it's learning disability, juvenile delinquency, stuttering, etc.

The life story doesn't stop. During the child's early development, in those first three years of life, the brain is developing very rapidly. And things happen, such as serious illnesses, convulsions as a consequence of high fevers, battery, and head injuries. As Lewis at Yale has pointed out, the incidence of battering in persistent juvenile delinquents is significantly higher before the age of two, compared to controls.

One other interesting factor is the male gender. The male gender seems to be haunting us in a whole set of disorders. Not only in persistent juvenile delinquency, but in learning disabilities, developmental dyslexia, developmental dysgraphia, developmental dysphasia, stuttering, and hyperactivity, the ratio varies from 5-1 to 10-1, males to females. Ounsted and Taylor at Oxford and Flor-Henry in Edmonton have suggested a male vulnerability hypothesis in regard to dominant brain function. It is a well-known fact that the male is physiologically inferior to the female in a lot of functions and is susceptible to a lot more diseases. I've suggested elsewhere that the male brain in general indeed may be physiologically inferior to the female brain in that it's more vulnerable to adverse developmental effects. Interestingly, a group in Ireland over a 30-year period found that males have brain abscesses at the ratio of 3-1 to females. In addition, there appears to be a greater vulnerability of the left brain—the dominant or language brain—in males that is resulting in disorders pertaining to stuttering, language disorders, learning disabilities, infantile autism (a lack of language), schizophrenia (a thought disorder), juvenile delinquency, and persistent criminality (possibly due to a language disorder, that is, the use of a language to regulate behavior). Thus the evidence indicates that the male-to-female prevalence in pathology involving language disorders is five to one.

There are data to support Dr. Mednick's view about psychophysiological findings of low skin conductance and slow recovery. But there are other data, such as power spectral and quantitative EEG data, from which people are beginning to define characteristics of persistent juvenile offenders and persistent criminal offenders.

There are also neuropsychological data. For example, since around 1972, Dr. Berman from the University of Rhode Island has been consistently demonstrating that persistent offenders have severe neuropsychological impairments—impairments related to cognitive functions involving abstraction and concept formation, as well as anticipation, planning, and organization. Interestingly, all of these functions have been linked to the frontal and temporal lobe system of the brain.

Dr. Pincus and Dr. Lewis at Yale University just recently found that over 94% of violent, persistent juvenile offenders studied had definite neurological disorders. Frank Spellacy in Victoria, Canada, found a similar type of picture with juvenile offenders and violent offenders, that is, a high incidence (over 90%) of neuropsychological impairments. Krynicki and Robbins in the United States have also found similar results. There are lots of data in the literature on persistent chronic offenders, juvenile or adult, that indicate that something is wrong with the offenders' brains.

Now the question is, What percentage of these persistent offenders with brain dysfunction falls into that small group—that 10% that accounts for 60% of the crimes? I don't think we know yet. But my guess is that there may be an interesting relationship between that very small proportion of juveniles who commit a large portion of crimes and brain dysfunction.

Now this links very much to Dr. Montagu's paper, which pointed out that as you go down the socioeconomic ladder, you increase the probability of being born into this world with brain damage, or as I would like to think, altered brain function. It may not be brain damage; it may be altered brain function, which then renders the individual incapable of dealing with the challenges of his environment in the same way as could another child.

Now it's interesting that if you look at the studies of episodic violent people, such as those of Frank Elliott at the Elliott Neurological Institute in Philadelphia, you find that the population of episodic violent adults is very intimately related to damage and dysfunction of the frontal and temporal regions of the brain. And the majority of Elliott's patients came from the middle-class structure—from good homes and good environments. A slight paradox. There is no doubt that the socioeconomic factors are important; however, this could very much depend upon the specific population. For example, it could be that everyone in a given area has primarily a psychosociological reason for their disorder, whereas if you switch to another area, there could be more biological factors operating in regard to the disorder.

Certainly we don't, as you say, know all those influences. But I think we have some parallels in mental retardation where the individual's capacity to learn, to acquire certain things, is diminished. What they can learn, the complexity of what they can learn, and their concept of projecting into the future are impaired. Anybody that's worked with mental retardation knows this. But the retarded are still very amenable to learning and to behavioral techniques. If you focus techniques on what adaptive abilities they have, you can do many, many things indeed. One of the possibilities is that if the persistent offender does have some type of altered brain function, it may indeed be related to the interaction of genetic and developmental influences. But I think it would be unfortunate if we assumed that the persistent offender has the cerebral resources to learn like everybody else. It may not be the case. I don't think we really know yet, but there are some hints that the offenders might be different; and to make that assumption in a sense would be criminal, as it would be to make the assumption that a severely mentally retarded individual could conform in the same way you and I do to the laws of the land or could learn in the same way about the moral laws of the land. I think all we can do is try and find out if indeed that is the case or not. And there are ways of examining those possibilities.

I think the real task is to settle down and try to figure out what are the multivariate possibilities, and then systematically explore those possibilities without getting into the old polemics of the nature versus nurture issue. Let's do the best job we can working together in a multidisciplinary effort, using each other's criticisms and support, and then take the evidence and evaluate it as it comes out. I think those studies have yet to be done; and until we do them, we cannot stand at either end of the polemic pole and say, You're crazy, and I'm right. Thank you.